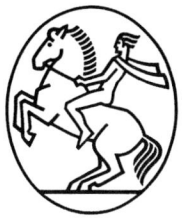

V. V. Frolkis

Aging and Life-Prolonging Processes

Translated from the Russian
by Nicholas Bobrov

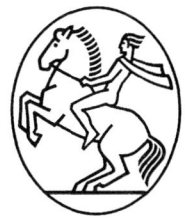

Springer-Verlag Wien NewYork

Prof. Dr. Vladimir Veniaminovich Frolkis
Corresponding Member of the Academy of Sciences of the UkrSSR
Institute of Gerontology of the Academy of Medical Sciences of the USSR
Kiev, USSR

Nicholas Bobrov
Moscow, USSR

© 1982 by Springer-Verlag Wien
Softcover reprint of the hardcover 1st edition 1982

With 91 Figures

Library of Congress Cataloging in Publication Data. Frolkis, V. V. (Vladimir Veniaminovich).
Aging and life-prolonging processes. 1. Aging. 2. Neuroendocrinology. 3. Longevity. I. Title.
QP86.F736. 1982. 612.67. 82-19211

ISBN-13: 978-3-7091-8651-0   e-ISBN-13: 978-3-7091-8649-7
DOI: 10.1007/978-3-7091-8649-7

Preface

There is an Inca incantation which stated said roughly: "Lord, give me spiritual peace so that I can acquiesce to what I cannot change, give me courage so that I can change what I can change, and give me wisdom so that I can distinguish one from the other."

Obviously, this incantation can be regularly repeated by any gerontologist, since it is very difficult to distinguish aging from the processes which enhance the organism's viability, aging from diseases, and the mechanisms of aging in various species of animals.

According to N. Shock, who compiled a valuable bibliography of the works on aging, more than 43,000 works on gerontology have been published in the last decade. Why do we continue to disagree with one another and hold that the most important mechanisms are still largely unknown to us in spite of that flow of information and an enormous number of facts? What is it that we do not know? Could it be that we do not know the sole sacramental fact which can explain everything, such as the hormone of aging, the programmed triggering of a suicide gene, the appearance of a special toxic agent in the axoplasmic flow of substances, and so forth?

Goethe once wrote that a scientist most often holds certain parts, but unfortunately he lacks their sacred link. It could be that what is most important is a one-sided idea of the essence of the processes which occur during individual development and the fact that we still have not established a cause-consequence relationship in the enormous amount of the known changes which occur with age, that we do not know the temporal sequence of their development, that we do not correctly assess them quantitatively, and that we do not always know what is primary and what is secondary. Apparently, all this is important. We still do not know much about the manifestations of aging, and what we do know, we cannot link together.

Therefore, in gerontology, it is important to make a systemic approach, which is not confined to a description of what occurs at various levels of the organism's vital activity, but unites the occurrences into a single system, and to analyze the mechanisms of aging from the standpoint of self-regulation. Regulation, adaptation and aging are three categories. They are three extremely complicated biological processes. The biological essence, principle and direction of the organism's aging can be understood from the standpoint of the relationship between these processes.

Classical gerontology reveals the mechanisms of aging that are connected with the appearance, accumulation and action of the inevitable damaging factors. However, it is important to make a fundamental approach, i.e. to study the processes which make the live systems stable, so as to understand the mechanisms which determine the life span, aging, and the diminution of the organism's adaptive abilities with age.

Making that approach, the author of this book asserts that life-prolonging processes exist. *Vitauct* (from the Latin words "vita", meaning life, and "auctum", meaning to prolong), which stabilizes the organism's viability and increases the life span, occurs together with aging, a destructive process, during individual development. The inseparable link between vitauct and aging determines both development with age and the life span. The next stage of gerontology will largely involve an analysis of the parameters and mechanisms of vitauct that make it possible to maintain vital activity when the damaging factors inevitably act. In this book, the author describes the relationship between aging and vitauct, ascertains the role which the neurohumoral mechanisms play in their development, and then discusses the possible ways of increasing the life span.

Kiev, September 1982   **V. V. Frolkis**

Contents

1. General Biology of Vitauct and Aging 1
Vitauct and Aging 1
General Regularities of Aging 14
Mechanisms of the Life Span of a Species 20
Aging and Evolution 27
Aging and Diseases 30

2. Aging of the Brain 33
General Direction of the Age Changes in the Brain 33
Structural and Metabolic Changes in the Brain During Aging 36
Change in the Brain Functions with Age 52

3. Hypothalamohypophysial Regulation During Aging 70
Regulatory Effects of the Hypothalamus 70
Hypothalamohypophysial Influences 79
Mechanisms of Vasopressin Regulation 83
Feed-backs in the System of Hypothalamohypophysial Regulation in Old Age 87
Adaptive Reactions of the Hypothalamus in Old Age 91

4. Adrenergic Mechanisms of Regulation During Aging 99
Effects of the Adrenergic Influences in Old Age 100
Sympathetic Ganglia During Aging 109
Catecholamine Metabolism 113

5. Cholinergic Mechanisms of Regulation During Aging 124
Acetylcholine Metabolism 124
Effects of Cholinergic Influences 135

6. Insulin Provision of the Organism During Aging 139
Content of Insulin and Carbohydrate Tolerance 140
Structural and Functional Changes in the Insular Apparatus 147
Specifics of the Tissue Reaction to the Action of Insulin in Old Age 150
Regulatory Mechanisms of Insulin Provision 152
Influence of the Change in Insulin Provision on Metabolism 154

7. Thyroid Regulation in Old Age 157
Structural and Functional Changes in the Thyroid Gland 157
Thyroid Hormones in the Blood 163
Hypothalamohypophysial Regulation of the Thyroid Gland Function 166
Specifics of the Influence of Thyroid Hormones on Tissue in Old Age 170
Feed-back Control of the Thyroid System 173
Specifics of the Reactions of the Thyroid Control System 175

8. Neural Regulation of Tissue Trophism in Aging 179

9. Local Mechanisms of Humoral Regulation During Aging 194
Cyclic Nucleotides 194
Adenosine Metabolic System 196
Kallikrein-Kinin System 198
Serotonin 201
Prostaglandins 202

10. Neurohumoral Mechanisms of the Regulation of the Genetic Apparatus ... 205
Genoregulatory Hypothesis of the Processes of Vitauct and Aging 205
Hormonal Regulation of the Genetic Induction of Enzymes 214
Hypothalamohypophysial-Adrenal System of the Regulation of the Genetic Apparatus 225

11. Neurohumoral Regulation of the Energy Processes 230
Oxidative and Glycolytic Phosphorylation During Aging 230
Hormonal Mediatory Influences on the Energy Processes 242

12. Neurohumoral Mechanisms of Cellular Aging 252
Sequence of Cellular Aging 252
Membranogenetic Mechanisms of Cellular Aging 264
Electric Properties of Cells During Aging 274

13. Neurohumoral Regulation of the Cardiovascular System 280
Hemodynamics and Age 280
Hemodynamic Centre in Aging 286
Efferent Neurohumoral Regulation of the Cardiovascular System 288
Reflexes of the Cardiovascular System 298
Regulation of Coronary Blood Circulation in Old Age 303

14. Experimental Life Prolongation 306
Criteria of the Life Span 307
Influence of Physical, Chemical and Biological Factors on the Life Span 314
Influence of Physical Factors on the Life Span 314
    Temperature 314
    Influence of Temperature on the Life Span of Warm-Blooded Animals 320
    Influence of Ionizing Radiation on the Life Span 322
    Influence of the Electric and Magnetic Fields on the Life Span 324
Influence of the Chemical Factors on the Life Span 324
    Influence of Microelements and Chelating Agents on the Life Span 325
    Influence of Antioxidants on the Life Span 326
    Influence of the Stabilizers of the Lysosomal Membranes on the Life Span 326
    Influence of Latirogens on the Life Span 327
    Influence of Other Chemical Agents on the Life Span 328
Influence of the Biological Factors on the Life Span 328
    Influence of the Low-Calorie or Low-Protein Diet on the Life Span 328
    Influence of Physical Activity on the Life Span 332
    Influence of the Hormones on the Life Span 333
    Influence of the Inhibitors of Protein Biosynthesis and Energy Metabolism on the Life Span 335
    Influence of the Genetic Factors on the Life Span 338

In Lieu of a Conclusion 341

References 345

Subject Index 378

1. General Biology of Vitauct and Aging

Vitauct and Aging

Gertsen, a nineteenth century Russian writer, wrote that scientists had come so close to the "shrine of nature" that they sometimes saw only what was before their very eyes. He regarded this as one of the reasons why natural phenomena were interpreted in a one-sided, individual and occasionally erroneous way. The danger of doing this is especially great in gerontology today, because much factual material on the biology of aging has been collected during only the last few decades.

Hence, it is especially important to correctly understand the essence of aging in the general biological sense. Definite mechanisms of aging may be interpreted incorrectly and the significance of aging as well as the development of living matter in a person's life and death may be defined incorrectly if errors are made in this respect. Such errors engender an extreme, likewise erroneous attitude towards controlling the aging process. This attitude may range from the complete rejection of the possibility of controlling the process to an inadequate, light-minded view on the life span, giving rise to promises to greatly prolong a person's life in the immediate future. Today, gerontology is not only a field where disputes are held on the existence of various aging mechanisms, but also a battlefield where views clash. Indeed, vulgar materialistic views on the essence of aging, which almost completely identify the aging and destruction of inanimate objects with the very complicated biological process of aging, and also idealistic views on the existence of "entelechy," "creative energy" and an unknowable beginning, the exhaustion of which causes aging, are being asserted and developed even today. Interestingly many authors of such concepts took a strictly scientific, objective, factual stand in their creative work, but when they go down to biological generalizations, they regarded unexplained facts as something inexplicable. This approach often leads to idealism, which in essence incapacitates a researcher and turns facts which have not been understood into something unknowable.

In gerontology, many facts are now known about a change in various parameters of the organism during individual development and aging. Some parameters progressively decrease when maturity is reached (they include indices of higher nervous activity, the function of analyzers, mental and physical working ability, the secretory activity of the sexual, thyroid and digestive glands, myocardial contractility, and the number of cells). Others do not change substantially by old age (the blood sugar level; some indices of the acid-base balance, the morphological composition of blood, namely, the number of erythrocytes, leukocytes and thrombocytes, the membrane potential of many cells, the activity of some enzymes, etc.), while still others increase (the synthesis of some pituitary hormones, the sensitivity of some tissues to hormones, the activity of some enzymes, arterial pressure, the blood contents of globulin, cholesterol, lecithin and beta-lipoproteins, etc.). Such a non-uniform change in the biological parameters is characteristic of ontogeny as a whole (Fig. 1). Development should be regarded as homeorhesis, which is the course of a change in a system with respect to time. Homeostasis is a stabilized state, while homeorhesis is stabilized flow. What determines the very complicated interaction between the diversely directed, but not chaotic changes and what links them together in age homeorhesis? How do these changes create a live system and maintain its existence, and when do they transcend the bounds of its possible development? Can this seeming diversity be explained by simply stating that an organism at first develops and becomes perfect, and then all the processes occur in the opposite direction, i. e. involution, or regressive development? These questions as well as many others arise when an effort is made to explain the essence of phenomena which occur as the organism ages.

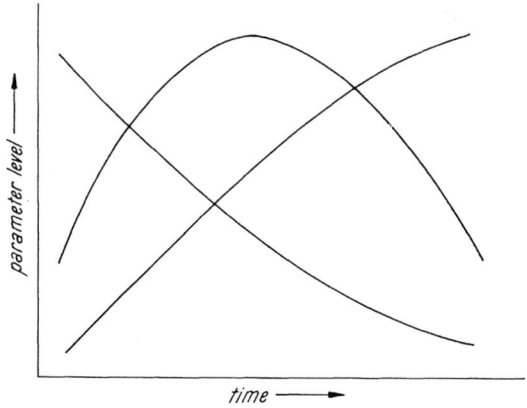

Fig. 1. Dynamics of the age changes of various biological parameters during ontogeny

However, there is a principle which explains how a chance occurrence has become a law, how the initial manifestations of life combined into very intricate biological systems, including man, how all this diversity is incorporated in the viability of the organism, and why there are two opposite tendencies in historical and individual development: vitauct and aging. This is a principle of self-regulation. All the levels of biological organization are self-regulatory ones. However, the organism as a whole is a single self-regulating system, and one of its aspects (neurohumoral mechanisms) controls other levels of biological hierarchy. In this respect, it should be noted that the viability of the organism decreases as it grows old, when the disturbances which occur with time are not compensated by the mechanisms of self-regulation. Owing to these mechanisms, the biological system becomes perfectly adapted to the living conditions at all the levels of biological organization, and an extremely important aspect of life,

i. e. the activation of the processes of restoration, is ensured. If the whole life cycle is nominally divided according to this principle, it can be assumed that restoration with supercompensation occurs in early ontogeny, i. e. during the period of growth, restoration with compensation occurs in maturity, and restoration with decompensation occurs in late ontogeny.

Today, the keen interest taken in the problem of aging, being among the cardinal problems in modern science, is not merely an expression of mankind's aspiration to understand the meaning of aging and to influence its course. This aspiration always existed.

Science is developing in accordance with certain laws, and every stage of its development has its own historical prerequisites. Even the most brilliant predictions are based on the achievements of the previous generations. Biological achievements, i. e. the discovery of the essence of the transmission of hereditary information, protein biosynthesis, successes in cytology, and the discovery of the most important laws of regulating the living, have become the basis of the new, really revolutionary stage in the development of gerontology. Researchers are paying more and more attention to gerontology also because of some socio-economic factors, including an extremely important phenomenon of this century, i. e. the aging of the population of the developed countries and the growth of the share of elderly and old people in the overall population structure. Statisticians predict that the Soviet Union will have 50 million people of pensionable age in the 1980's and 80 million people by the year 2000. In 1970, 15.9 per cent of the population of Hungary, 18.0 per cent of the population of Great Britain and 28.7 per cent of the population of the German Democratic Republic were above the age of 60. Never has the mean life span been so high and the problem of the position of elderly people in society as well as their role in the economy so acute as now. As the number of elderly and old people increases, the state must make greater outlays on social security, and new labor sources must be found. Such an increase affects the entire public health system, because more medical care must be given to these people. Thus, researchers are taking interest in gerontology for not only strictly scientific, academic and cognitive, but also practical reasons.

The history of gerontology is interesting and instructive. Gerontology developed on the basis of definite achievements in the major sciences. As the conception of the endocrine glands rapidly developed at the end of the last century, it was argued that a change in their activity was decisive in the genesis of aging. By thoroughly studying the structure and functions of the cells and elaborating the methods of investigating tissue cultures, it became possible to work out the concepts of a link between the ability of the cells to undergo division and their aging. Molecular genetic hypotheses of aging originated as it became more or less clear how hereditary information was transmitted and how protein underwent biosynthesis.

The formation and development of gerontology are associated with such names as Mechnikov, Bogomolets, Nagorny and Verzar. They all understood the given process and its role in the life of an individual and society after thoroughly studying the essence of phenomena. Their prestige in other fields of natural science has helped to draw some researchers' attention to gerontology.

1*

For decades, this branch of knowledge developed more slowly than the study of the animal kingdom's evolution and the investigation of the early stages of an individual's formation and development. The most important laws governing the mechanisms of heredity, natural selection, evolution, and the link between historical and individual development were formulated and the cytological principles of fertilization and development were described as early as the latter half of the last century. However, the teaching of aging as a science began to be formed only in this century and is associated with the works of Mechnikov (1907, 1908), who is regarded as the "father of gerontology." Such a delay occurred because, among other reasons, it was widely held that evolution and aging were not linked, that aging had no qualitative and biological specifics, and that the existing structures and functions were disturbed and destroyed in one way as the organism aged. In other words, a simple, mechanistic view was held on the essence of aging.

Aging has been defined in many ways during a few decades. However, most researchers emphasized that their definitions were "operational," "transitional," "nominal," and so forth. They were so cautious obviously because the essence of the process must be expressed and something must be artificially cut off from the chain of events, thus often simplifying the significance of the biological process.

Aging is a naturally developing biological process which limits the adaptive possibilities of an organism, increases the likelihood of death, reduces the life span and promotes age pathology.

Gerontologists usually look for mechanisms which limit the life span and increase the likelihood of death. At present, there are a few hundred hypotheses and theories of aging. However, a fundamentally different approach to all these processes can also be made, i. e. it would be quite correct to look for the mechanisms which determine the prolonged (occasionally for tens and even hundreds of years) high level of an organism's vitality, the mechanisms which make it possible not only to maintain, but also perfect an organism's adaptive abilities in spite of the destructive exogenous and endogenous factors, the mechanisms which help to preserve several homeostatic indices even in very old age, and the mechanisms which determine the great differences in the life span of a species and that of an individual. A disadvantage of many aging hypotheses is that they deal with only one aspect of aging.

Twenty years ago, we strongly criticized the assertions that uniform extinction develops, that metabolism, the structure and the function are disturbed in a single direction, i. e. that they are degraded in the aging process. We proposed the concept that important adaptive mechanisms are formed as the organism ages. These mechanisms preserve and perfect an organism's vitality, maintain its homeostasis and increase the life span. They become apparent when aging is considered together with the overall result of development: biological age and the life span. We defined these mechanisms as adaptive regulatory ones, since their biological purpose is to maintain and develop a definite level of the organism's adaptive abilities, while the mechanism of their origin, i. e. their essence, is connected with shifts in the self-regulation processes.

After analyzing the mechanisms of aging, we generalized our conclusions in the adaptive regulatory theory of aging (Frolkis, 1963–1980). A process which preserves the organism's vitality and increases its life span is found at all the stages of the development of living matter together with the aging process, the extinction of metabolism and functions, and the degradation of the organism's structure. We termed this set of adaptive regulatory mechanisms, this process of preserving the organism's vitality and consequently prolonging life, *vitauct* (from the Latin words "vita," meaning life, and "auctum," meaning to prolong). Manifestations of vitauct have been ascertained in our fellow worker's researches at various levels of the organism's vital activity: at the molecular, cellular, organ and systemic levels. This is important theoretically and practically in understanding the essence of aging. Indeed, the life span can be controlled if vitauct is acknowledged and understood. This process should be thoroughly studied. It has its own qualitative specifics and its own biological distinctions, which are manifested at all stages of individual development.

The aging process probably originated in some particular form at the early stages of evolution together with the first manifestations of life. Disturbances in the primary clusters of the protoplasm were the prototype or the specific expression of aging. They were caused by both the damaging action of the factors of the external environment and the biological unreliability of the initial live systems. However, live systems developed and reached a high evolutionary level in spite of the permanency and inevitability of these damaging effects, the invariability and inevitability of individual death. Man was the greatest achievement of evolution. This achievement was made because another process, vitauct, originated and became consolidated together with destruction, degradation, and the development of the aging process. During vitauct, opposite tendencies, i. e. those of maintaining viability, developed. This occurred because adaptation was consolidated on the basis of casual mutations in the form of genetic information. Organisms with clearer manifestations of vitauct had more favourable properties and survived, producing their like. Natural selection occurred in a certain form among live systems at the early stages of development, too. Adaptive shifts took place due to the self-regulation mechanisms, which are the basis of life.

The most important adaptive regulatory mechanisms originated, vitauct was perfected and a viable live system, i. e. the basis of the diversity of the forms of biological organization, developed as evolution continued from coacervates to primary cells with definite organoids.

Opposite processes originate in the course of aging due to the inner contradictory nature of the living, to the mechanisms of its regulation, and to the start (according to the self-regulation principle) of adaptive shifts in response to a change in the state of the system. However, it would be wrong to assume that activation is of adaptive significance, while suppression limits opportunities in this respect. This may be assumed only when one does not understand the inner nature of life, aging, and the dialectics of development. That is metaphysical logic: either good or bad, either prolongation or curtailment, either extinction or activation. In dialectics, good and bad are concomitant, the useful and the harmful are concomitant, and adaptation and its limitation are concomitant. Aging, or age progression, occurs in constant contradiction, in a constant internal struggle.

As biological organization became more complicated, the nature of aging changed qualitatively and the relationship between the extinction, disturbance and adaptation of live systems altered. The self-regulation mechanisms were the essence of these processes. A very important fact is that some random, undirected mutations, which originate during the genetically informative period, can become the basis of adaptation as well as vitauct manifestations before an organism loses its reproductivity, and they can be consolidated in evolution as a result of natural selection. We could substantially change the life span if we knew how to engender directed mutations. If it were not for the adaptive mechanisms which originate on their basis, the aging rate and the extent of the non-compensatory disturbances and damages would be so high that species whose adaptive abilities take decades to be realized could not appear in evolution. The essence of aging, the difference between the aging of live systems and the destruction of the inanimate, will not be understood if account is not taken of that important aspect of aging. The adaptive mechanisms which originate in aging are of relative significance. They do not in any way change the fundamental essence of aging as a process which limits the life span. Moreover, para-adaptation, which causes pathology, may develop in aging. A shift which is of adaptive significance in one process may aggravate age changes in another. For instance, the activation of glycolysis, which is of adaptive significance, can lead to the accumulation of metabolites and, consequently, the disturbance of the rhythmic and contractile functions of the heart. The activation of the beta-cells of the pancreas, while being intended to provide the organism with insulin, may cause exhaustion and diabetes.

Many vitauct mechanisms and the adaptive regulatory shifts associated with age are consolidated in the genome. They are consolidated during natural selection on the basis of casual mutations in the genetic apparatus of the sex cells. At present, it is difficult to thoroughly analyze the cause and nature of these mutations. They are engendered by various endogenous and exogenous factors. Moreover, substantial chemical, physicochemical, biophysical and other shifts occur in aging, and they may cause changes in the genetic apparatus.

Mutations which originate in aging differ in their significance with respect to the aging organism. Some of them cause changes in the genome that promote both aging and the disturbance of the structure and the functions of the organism. Others become the genetic basis of the changes which enhance the organism's viability. Such mutations may occur also in the regulatory part of the genome and thus influence the genoregulatory mechanisms of aging and vitauct.

The vitauct mechanisms, while developing on the basis of the above-mentioned type of mutations, make the organism more viable and have an advantage in natural selection. Therefore, they become hereditary. These genomic changes, which ultimately prolong life, are of adaptive significance also at the early stages of individual development. Thus, the vitauct processes are consolidated not only because they prolong life, but also because they promote the appearance of viable specimens, which are naturally selected in evolution.

We know about the existence of the so-called pleiotropic genes, which influence the formation of various features. According to Medavar (1952), Williams (1957) and Cutler (1979), these genes are of definite importance, since they cause an adaptive shift at one stage of ontogeny and the manifestation of aging and age pathology at another, or they simultaneously determine changes of opposite significance. There are probably pleiotropic genes or genoregulatory mechanisms which determine the origin and formation of the structure and function of the organism at the early stages of ontogeny and the development of the vitauct processes at the later stages. Thus, the evolution of life prolongation is connected with the vitauct mechanisms and the specifics of adaptation at all the stages of ontogeny.

If long-living species had always inhabited the Earth, the evolutionary rate would have been much slower. However, if there were only short-living species, the perfect forms of adaptation to the environment would not have originated, as their formation takes years and decades. Moreover, it should be taken into account that hereditary features are consolidated not only because generations are rapidly replaced. When an animal's life is long, the sex cell is influenced for a longer time (in spite of its protectiveness) by factors which may cause genomic mutation. For instance, the correlation between aging and vitauct determines life span, many features of animal evolution, and the rate at which many adaptive changes are consolidated.

Adaptive mechanisms develop in aging at various levels of the organism's vital activity. They should probably be nominally divided into two groups. One group consists of mechanisms which have been firmly consolidated genetically in evolution and have become part and parcel of the living; they determine the viability of the live systems. The other group constists of current adaptation processes which originate as the organism ages.

The appearance of the cell, which is the main structural element of the vital processes, and membranes, which separate the cell from the external environment and at the same time link it with the environment, was of paramount importance in the origin of life. The plasma membrane with its highly active mechanisms which make it possible for substances to be transported from one cell to another, electric properties which ensure excitability, its participation in both energy production and the receptor mechanisms which ensure interaction between cells, and so forth, have become an extremely important aspect of vitauct that allows the live system to survive despite a great number of damaging factors.

We have shown that the basic properties of the cell membrane and its electrophysiological reactions are formed individually on the basis of protein biosynthesis. According to the data which we obtained together with Martynenko, the stable value of the membrane potential and ionic asymmetry are established in the skeletal muscle fibres between the 19th and 22nd day of life. However, they are established from seven to nine days later when actinomycin D, the transcription blocking agent, or ribonuclease is administered daily from birth (Fig. 2). It has been discovered that the cell membrane is hyperpolarized when the genetic apparatus and protein biosynthesis are activated by various factors (Frolkis, 1969–1979). The hyperpolarization of the membrane is of great adaptive significance, since it creates conditions for protein biosynthesis, enables the necessary substrates to enter the cell, and so forth. These restorative shifts are connected with the formation of a special hyperpolarizing factor in protein biosynthesis. Hence, "finished" structures are created for the cell membrane and a special factor is synthesized during this biosynthesis. The genetic apparatus of the cell controls and regulates the state of the cell membrane with the participation of that factor. The membrane genetic mechanism, its development and formation as well as its change and disturbance play a decisive role in vitauct and aging. Cell division, the development of hypertrophy, multinuclearity, polyploidy in the postmitotic cells, the growth of the nuclear surface, a change in the size of individual organoids, and many other developmental shifts are a manifestation of vitauct at the cellular level.

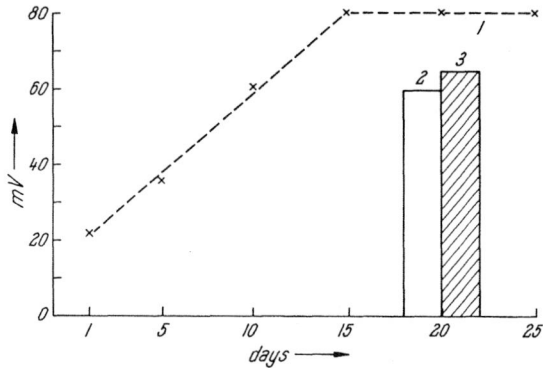

Fig. 2. Formation of the membrane potential of the muscle fibres during the first 15–20 days of the postnatal period *(1)*; slowing down of the formation of the membrane potential when either ribonuclease *(2)* or actinomycin D *(3)* is administered for 20 days

The establishment of the higher forms of neurohumoral regulation during historical and individual development was of decisive importance in the vitauct processes. They managed to influence the organism's viability because they were organized on the basis of the self-regulation principle (direct and feed-back control, which informs about the occurrences in the external and internal environments, including those which are inevitable in aging). This feed-back information about age changes in the organism's internal environment had become the basis for engaging the central neurohumoral mechanisms of adaptation and compensation. Indivisible cells, which are characterized by primary aging, appeared when metazoans were being formed. The organism's longevity depends on the long maintenance of the indivisible cells' viability on a high level. It is determined by the mechanisms of intracellular as well as extracellular neurohumoral regulation. These regulatory effects may stimulate all the aspects of the metabolism of the cell, including the activity of its genetic apparatus and the intensity of protein synthesis, i. e. a set of molecular changes that determines the processes of aging and vitauct. It has been found that the higher the organism is organized evolutionarily, the more clear-cut is that regulatory control. There is enough evidence to show that local and general hormones are important in the formation of the organism in ontogeny. It is well known that the disturbance of the synthesis of transmitters, which act as local hormones (noradrenaline, acetylcholine, serotonin, etc.), upsets cell division at the earliest stages of development.

However, the significance of the neurohumoral mechanisms in maintaining a high level of the organism's viability and a long life span is inadequately assessed. Great structural, metabolic and functional changes occur when neural and hormonal control is weakend. The cessation of neural and many hormonal effects ultimately cause the atrophy, degradation and death of cells. The constant neurohumoral activation of both the metabolism of the cell and the energy and plastic processes in it not only determines its participation in the organism's most important adaptive reactions, but also ensures its viability, makes it possible to maintain optimum activity for a long time, and greatly prolongs the organism's life. It is true that many manifestations of aging resemble shifts which occur when neurohumoral control is impaired. However, it has been found that the primary age changes in the mechanisms of neurohumoral regulation cause secondary shifts in the organs and tissues. Tissues rapidly age when control over the vitauct processes either changes or decreases.

Neurohumoral mechanisms do not merely "engage" or "disengage" the cells and organs in their activity. They regulate trophic process, i. e. the structural and metabolic provision of the function as well as the adaptive effects. Pavlov (1951a–c) and Folbort (1968) have shown that the restorative processes are promoted when activity is carried on and the functional possibilities are exhausted. According to Folbort (1968), exhaustion stimulates restoration. When the organism ages, the relationship between exhaustion and restoration changes and the restorative processes become less intensive. The regulation of trophicity and the neurohumoral "maintenance" of the restorative processes, being an expression of vitauct, are especially important then. However, as we will see in Chapter 8, trophic neural control over tissues is impaired with age. This becomes an extremely important mechanism of age degradation.

The formation of a complex set of neurohormonal shifts, known as the general-adaptation syndrome (Selye, 1952), was an important link in the organism's development. Due to it, the adaptive regulatory processes, which enhance the organism's stability, are formed in a state of tension. A homeostatic disturbance in stress trains the adaptive regulatory mechanisms, which prolong life span. We have shown that rats subjected to moderate stress loads had really lived longer than those protected from all external effects and those subjected to great stress stimuli (Frolkis *et al.*, 1976b). For instance, the average life span of the control rate is 938 ± 19 days, while that of the rats subjected to repeated brief stress influences is $1,120 \pm 34$ days ($p < 0.01$). The half-life of the rat population is 792 ± 12 days and 999 ± 32 days ($p < 0.01$), respectively, while its maximal life span is $1,153 \pm 11$ days and $1,296 \pm 13$ days ($p < 0.01$), respectively. The rats were used in experiments when they were 100 days old. At the same time, the protective action of the general-adaptation syndrome weakens with age and the repeated stress is increasingly detrimental to the aging organism, becoming the cause of the non-compensating homeostatic changes.

The termination of reproductivity is undoubtedly important in adaptation, being connected with a change in neurohormonal control. It has been shown in many works that the frequency of hereditary disturbances progressively grows among the progeny of elderly specimens (Sachs *et al.,* 1977; Frota-Pessoa, 1978). The combination of high sex potency, or reproductivity, and genetic disturbances in the sex cells would be destructive to a species.

The age changes in connective tissue play a definite role in the genesis of aging. Much data show that the aging of connective tissue causes vascular sclerosis, a change in the immune responses and the bone system, and so forth. However, adaptive shifts also occur in the connective tissue cells as the organism ages. Many connective tissue structures are known to perform the trophic function. It has been shown that several substances can pass over from the connective tissue cells to the adjacent cells. The neuroglia is believed to maintain the normal metabolism of the neuron throughout its range and to regulate its excitability. When the nerve cells are stimulated, the number of neuroglias adjoining them grow. It has been observed that when the nerve cells are activated, the number of satellites increases in the cerebral cortex, the geniculate bodies and the spinal cord. Moreover, it is assumed (Galambos, 1965) that the activity of the neuron is programmed in neuroglia. Ionic processes play a great role on the surface in the mechanism of neuroglial contacts. Hence, an increase in the number of glia cells at a definite stage of aging can be of adaptive significance and can promote the trophism of the nerve cells. It should be borne in mind that the connective tissue cells may be of such trophic significance not only in the brain, but also in other organs.

The aging processes are connected with a change in the biochemistry of the live systems. Consequently, the vitauct mechanisms have a molecular basis. Evolutionary shifts in genomic regulation were very important in changing the species life span. The life span of primates increased from eight to a hundred years in a short time from the standpoint of evolution. This was the result of not the quantitative changes in the genome, but the shifts in its regulation. An increase in the number of genic repeats was of great importance in the vitauct processes. It is believed that aging is connected with the disturbance of the state of unique genes.

Biological processes are not absolutely reliable. Therefore, the systems which compensate for the disturbances that occur during vital activity are important to the organism's viability.

Substances which, in a definite amount, can influence the organism's viability, its aging, are always formed during vital activity. Moreover, the organism may become more sensitive to the toxicity of some metabolic products in old age (Frolkis, 1969). For instance, spasmic twitching occurred and the depth and rhythm of respiration, the rhythm of cardiac activity, and the electric activity of the brain changed in rats 24–26 months old when phenol in a dose of 0.2–0.7 mg and guanidine in a dose of 3.0–5.0 mg/100 g of body weight were administered intraperitoneally; that also occurred in mature rats 10–18 months old when 1.0–1.5 mg of phenol and 10–15 mg of guanidine per 100 g of weight were administered intraperitoneally. The system of microsomal oxidation, which ensures many detoxication processes, is an important vitauct mechanism.

It is relatively stable and is therefore important to the viability of the aging organism. Fig. 3 (the data in it were provided by Paramonova) shows that the principal enzymes of the microsomal system of oxidation become less active in rats between 3–4 and 8–10 months old, and that this activity scarcely changes by old age (26–28 months). The data provided by Nedelkina and others (1972) indicate that the system is stable. They showed that the synthesis of individual enzymes of the microsomal oxidation system does not become less intensive even when an inducing agent (phenobarbital) is administered for as long as 140 days. There is a definite relationship between the species life span and the "power" of the microsomal oxidation system.

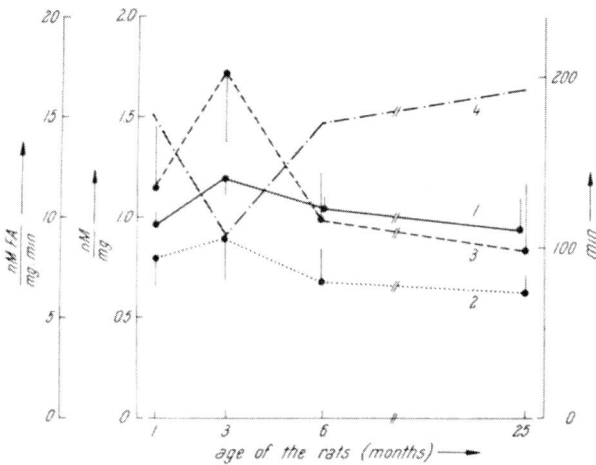

Fig. 3. Content of the cytochromes P-450 and B₅ (1, 2); aminopyridine demethylase activity (3) of the microsomes of the liver and the duration of narcotic sleep (4) in rats of different ages

It was assumed for a long time that DNA is an extremely stable polymer. Indeed, evolution would have been impossible if there was great mobility in the DNA structure and if the genetic code changed during individual development. However, it has been discovered that DNA can be damaged and that its stability depends to a great degree on the mechanisms of its reparation in spite of the special apparatus which stores genetic information (chromatin). It has been shown that there is a direct correlation between the degree of expression of the reparation processes and the species life span. For instance, Hart and Setlow (1976) have demonstrated on seven species (shrew, mouse, rat, hamster, cow, elephant, and man) that reparative DNA synthesis induced by ultraviolet irradiation in fibroblasts is more intensive when the life of a species is longer. There are grounds to assume that the synthesis of some reparative enzymes are under neurohormonal control, whose change may cause shifts in DNA reparation.

However, Kato (1978) did not detect a link between reparation and the species life span when the data obtained were corrected with respect to the dimensions of the genome of diploid cells.

It is now believed that free-radical reactions, the formation of peroxide compounds, the possible damaging action of superoxide radicals, and so forth, play an important role in aging and in damaging macromolecules (Harman, 1962; Emanuel, 1976, 1979). It has been shown in our laboratory that definite changes in cellular reception and the active transport of ions through the membrane are due to the shifts in the free-radical processes in old age. Moreover, it has been found that antioxidants normalize the state of the cell membrane. Powerful systems of antioxidants, including superoxide dismutase, are important in the vitauct processes in this respect. Oxidative processes are known to become less intensive with age. Guskova and others (1979) have shown that the activity of superoxide dismutase and the amount of superoxide radicals uniformly diminish in cell membranes of the old animal liver.

According to the concepts proposed by Orgel (1970), which are supported and opposed by many, "errors" occur during protein biosynthesis at its various stages, causing the synthesis of "erroneous" proteins and the aging of both the cell and the organism. Apparently, the protein biosynthesis system is not absolutely specific and errors inevitably occur. According to Menninger (1977), the number of errors at the stage of ribosomal synthesis ranges from 3×10^{-4} to 3×10^{-5}. Estimates have shown that every tenth or hundredth protein may contain an "erroneous" amino acid. However, aging is not connected with the "catastrophe of errors" because (1) not all the amino acid replacements are fatal to the cell, and (2) there is a powerful vitauct system, a system which eliminates erroneous proteins: their proteolysis, immunological elimination, the hydrolysis of the improperly acetylated tRNA, "ribosomal editing," which consists in the dissociation of peptidyl and tRNA, whose structure does not conform to the mRNA codon, and so forth.

Many adaptive regulatory influences are stimulated by metabolic and functional shifts which develop with age. Our data are presented in Fig. 4. They show that a set of adaptive mechanisms which maintain the energy provision of the heart is formed in response to a diminution of tissue respiration in the myocardium in old age.

There are many examples of the origin of the adaptive regulatory shifts in the aging process. They include the increased sensitivity of some cells to transmitters when the synthesis of these substances decreases in the nerve endings, the higher sensitivity of some hormones when their amount and state change in the blood, the activation of some local systems of humoral regulation when central neural control becomes impaired, and the activation of some links of the anti-coagulation system of blood.

The results of the experiments involving life prolongation show the significance of the vitauct processes. Life can be substantially prolonged when the body temperature is reduced because, generally speaking, aging and vitauct are interconnected. There are grounds to assume that the vitauct processes, which enhance the organism's viability, are connected mainly with enzymic reactions, whose activation energy is 4–12 kcal/mole. Chemical and denaturation reactions (whose activation energy reaches 50–60 kcal/mole), with their Q_{10} being several times higher than that of the enzymic reactions, are especially important in the aging mechanism, which is a destructive process.

Therefore, the vitauct rate can prevail over aging as temperature drops, and this should prolong life.

In analyzing the interaction between vitauct and aging, we can assess the most important factor, i. e. the mechanisms of age-related development, which determine the life span. These mechanisms cannot be understood when only the disturbances of metabolism and the functions are analyzed and the final stage of ontogenesis, old age, is studied. Sacher (1977) emphasized that gerontology is not the science of aging, since such a definition is tantamount to conceding defeat. It is a science of life from the standpoint of its finitude.

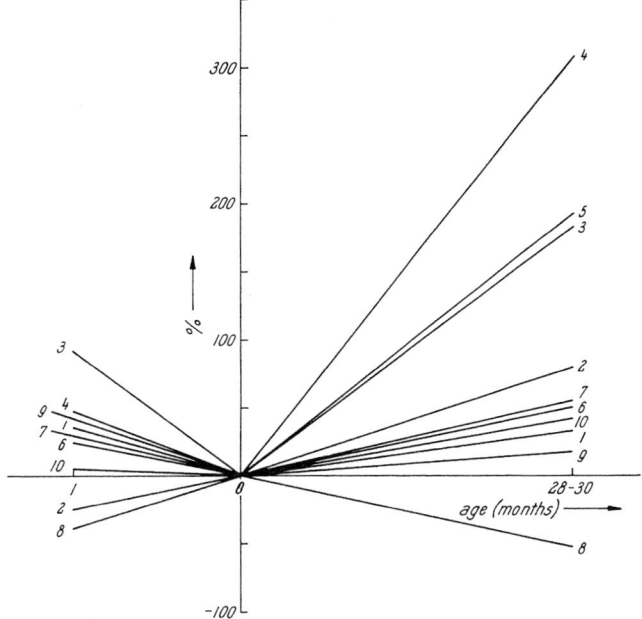

Fig. 4. Comparative characterization of the changes (%) in various links of energy exchange in the heart of rats of different age: *1* oxidation-phosphorylation coupling (P/O) in mitochondria (succinic acid is the substrate); *2* anaerobic glycogenolysis; *3* aerobic glycolysis; *4* aerobic glycogenolysis; *5* influence of the mitochondria of old rats on glycolysis in the cytoplasm; *6* anaerobic glycolysis; *7* activity of the succinoxidase system; *8* glycogen content; *9* summary content of the nicotinamide coenzymes; *10* ADP content. The level in rats 8–10 monts old is taken as 100 per cent

Arshavsky (1976, 1979) supports the concept of the internally contradictory nature of aging. According to him, non-genotrophic processes occur in ontogeny. He believes that they promote progressive development at the early stages of ontogeny. As Arshavsky (1976) put it, individual development is not the continuous unwinding of the organism's biological clock, but (apparently at definite stages) its winding. According to him, active muscular activity, or the function of the skeletal musculature, is very important in the formation of this clock. Similar views are shared by Cutler (1978). He believes that the anti-aging processes, which prolong life, had originated in the course of evolution. According to him, aging is a pleiotropic process, i. e. it is the inevitable outcome, the "by-product" of the most important biological processes that enhance the organism's viability.

General Regularities of Aging

Much factual material is now available on the changes which occur in the organism during aging. They make it possible to establish the most important regularities of development. It has been found that the same level of metabolism and the functions is ensured differently during different age periods. For instance, arterial pressure is the same in mature and old rabbits and rats, but it is maintained due to greater cardiac output in mature animals and to higher total peripheral resistance in old animals. Such hemodynamic relationships may be observed also in two groups of young and elderly persons with approximately the same level of arterial pressure. The membrane potential of many cells (hepatocytes, the neurons of the sensorimotor region of the cortex and the spinal cord, etc.) does not change in old age. However, it is maintained by different correlations of potassium, sodium and chlorine during different age periods. The same blood sugar level is maintained in elderly and old persons by a different change in the glycemia regulation processes. This seeming unchangeability of some homeostatic indices is the outcome of not their stability, but of their dynamics, the constant disturbances of homeostasis, and the mobilization of the adaptive regulatory mechanisms.

The reliability of homeostatic regulation and the possible range of adaptation diminish as the organism ages. This is evident when use is made of various loads which inevitably occur during a lifetime. In this case, their change in old age is observed in spite of the homeostatic level of the functions. Fig. 5 shows that there are different hemodynamic shifts in young and elderly persons with the same initial level of hemodynamics under a physical load. Such differences were demonstrated also by means of the acid-base balance (Sineok, 1975), when the appropriate loads reveal a diminution of the given system's potentialities (Fig. 6A, B).

Aging is characterized by a consecutive change in the functional state of the organism, in its potentialities. This change occurs in four stages: (1) the optimum basal level of the function and its great potentialities, which are revealed during tension; (2) the preservation of the basal and potential level of the function (in spite of age changes) due to the engagement of the adaptive regulatory mechanisms; (3) the preservation of the basal level of the function and the diminution of its potentialities due to an increase in age disturbances and the curtailment of the adaptive regulatory shifts, and (4) a drop in the basal level of the function and its pronounced insufficiency due to the organism's diminishing adaptive possibilities (Fig. 7).

Aging is heterochronic, heterotopic, heterokinetic and heterocateftenitic. It is heterochronic because individual tissues, organs and systems age at different times. In humans, for instance, the thymus begins to atrophy between the ages of 13 and 15, and the sex organs, during the menopause, while some hypophysial functions remain until very old age. Aging is heterotopic because it is expressed differently in various organs as well as structures of the same organ. For instance, the *Zona fasciculata* of the adrenal cortex ages less intensively than *Zona glomerulosa* and *Zona reticulosa*. Different age changes occur in various areas of the cerebral cortex, etc. Aging is heterokinetic because the age changes occur at different rates. They occur rather early and gradually, progressing rather smoothly in some tissues, while they develop later but rather rapidly in others. For instance, change are gradual in the bone-and-joint system, while they are late but rather rapid in definite structures of the brain. Finally, aging is heterocateftenitic because age changes occur in different directions, being connected with the suppression of some vital processes and the activation of others in the aging organism.

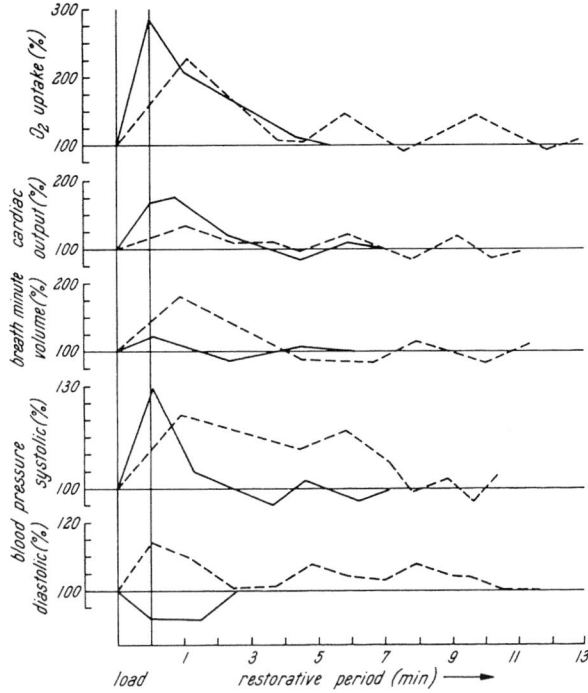

Fig. 5. Changes in some indices of hemodynamics and respiration after brief work in persons of different ages. The continuous line stands for persons who are 25 years old, and the dashed line, for persons who are 75 years old. The initial level of the indices is taken as 100 per cent

An individual's age may be either chronological or biological. Biological age is the objective criterion of the organism's viability at a given moment. It is a very complicated outcome of the interaction between aging and vitauct, and it characterizes the state of the organism as it ages. The biological age of various individuals of the same species as well as species with different life spans obviously changes differently with time. The comparative-gerontological assessment of the dynamics of various age changes in the metabolism, structure and function in animals with a different species life cycle may be of fundamental importance in analyzing the mechanisms of aging. Thus, in using animals with a different species life span, we can see whether the manifestations of aging correlate better with biological or chronological age. The more the changes correlate with biological age, and greater is their significance in the genesis of the aging process.

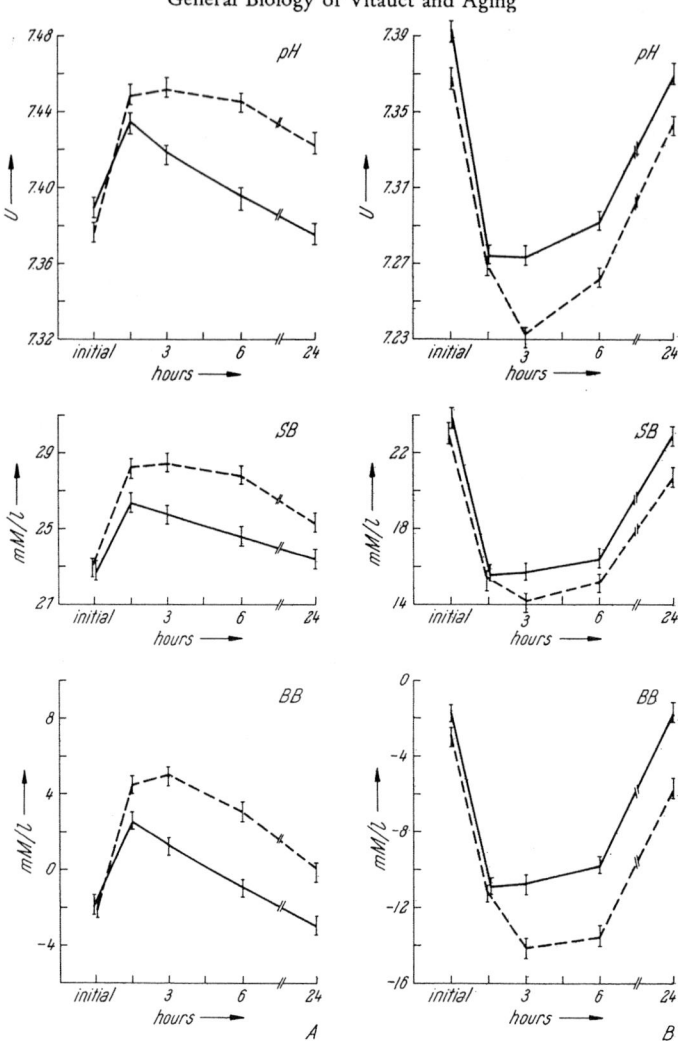

Fig. 6. Dynamics of the changes in the value of the pH of blood, standard bicarbonate (SB) and buffer bases (BB) when sodium hydrocarbonate (A) and ammonium chloride (B) are administered to animals of different age. The continuous line stands for young animals, and the dashed line, for old animals

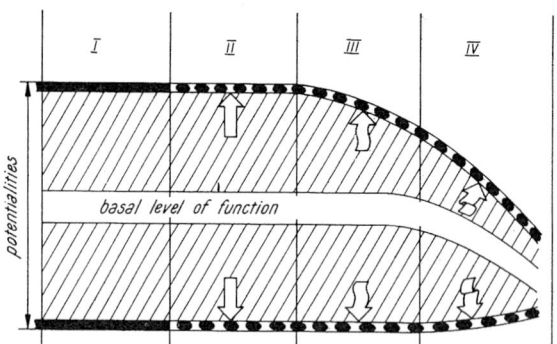

Fig. 7. Change in the basal level and potentialities of the functions in ontogeny. I, II, III, IV – age periods

We compared the hemodynamic shifts in mature and old rats (8–10 and 26–28 months old), rabbits (16–18 and 56–60 months old), dogs (2.0–2.5 and 12–15 years old) and people (20–25 and 70–75 years old). It was found that the level of arterial pressure in rats and rabbits does not change with age, being 78.2 ± 1.6 and 84.2 ± 2.6 mm Hg $(p > 0.05)$ and 93.8 ± 9.2 and 96.5 ± 1.6 mm Hg $(p > 0.1)$, respectively, while it definitely grows in dogs and man, being $123.8 \pm 2,63$ and 139.0 ± 3.13 $(p > 0.01)$ and 116.0 ± 2.6 and 150.0 ± 3.3 mm Hg $(p > 0.01)$, respectively. Cardiac output decreases and total peripheral resistance increases in all cases. However, these shifts are not so substantial in rats and rabbits as to cause changes in arterial pressure. In other words, changes in arterial pressure seem to have no time to develop in animals with a short species life span.

Osteoporosis is one of the main indications that the bone system is aging. The resorption of bone tissue intensifies as the bone-formation processes become less pronounced with age. The morphological indications of osteoporosis include the expansion of the osteon canals, a diminution of the amount of osteons per unit area of bone, a decrease in the amount of cells, and a change in the cellular structure (the wrinkling of nuclei, the deformation of the cytoplasm, etc.).

Osteoporosis is revealed in persons 40–45 by roentgenography. It intensifies as the organism ages further, being fully (by 100 per cent) revealed by the age of 60. It develops earlier and more distinctly in the thoracic area of the spine, the femoral neck, the hands and the ribs.

According to Orlova and Khromyak (1972), the osteon canals expand, their number diminishes and the amount of cells decreases in old rabbits, too. However, these changes are not so great as in human beings and cannot be classified as severe osteoporosis. The resorption of bone tissue in rabbits apparently increases several times as they age, but it does not reach the degree of osteoporosis.

Orlova and Khromyak did not observe severe bone resorption even in the oldest rats. Roentgenography did not reveal any signs of osteoporosis in either rabbits or rats. Thus, osteoporosis correlates not so much with the aging rate as with chronological age. The higher the age, the more clearly defined are the symptoms of osteoporosis.

It has been found that even sclerotic vascular changes correlate with chronological age because, in old age, they are greater in a rabbit than in a rat, while in a dog, they are greater than in a rabbit (Fig. 8 A, B, C).

It follows from these data that vascular sclerosis is not a general biological primary mechanism of aging which limits the life span of various species. However, these changes may be important in the genesis of age changes in long-living animals.

After studying the overall content of water in the organism of various species (mammals, birds, fish, insects and micro-organisms), Calloway (1971) showed that the age changes in this content in animals of different species occurred at the same rate. The mechanical properties of the collagen of the tail of a rat and of a dog as well as the wrist of a person changed at the same rate with age (Rigby et al., 1977). Verzar (1968) as well as Deyl and others (1971) have indicated that

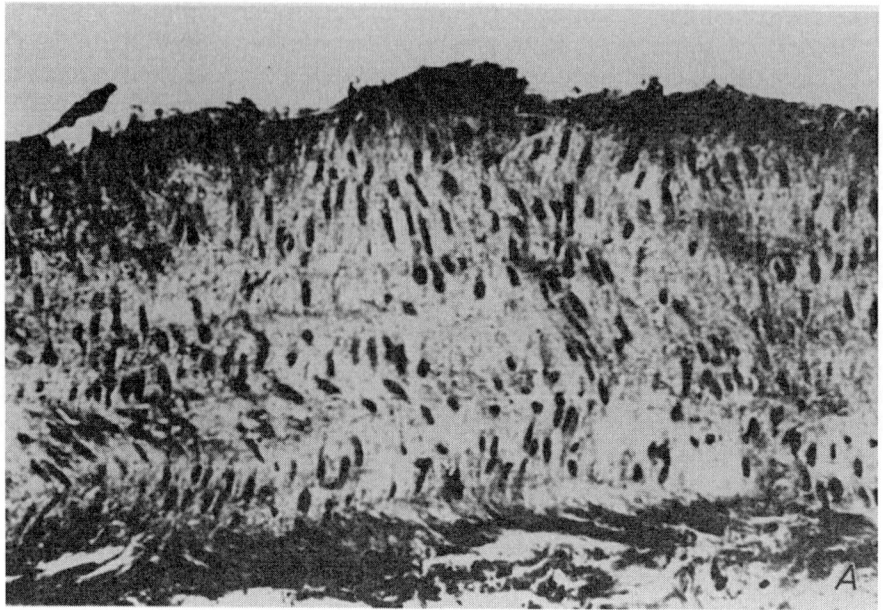

Fig. 8 A

Fig. 8. Specifics of the histological structure of the aorta of old animals: *A* structure of the thoracic part of the aorta of a rat (Van Gieson's stain, 320 ×); *B* sclerosis and separation of the cells in the medium of the thoracic part of the aorta of a rabbit (Van Gieson's stain, 160 ×); *C* desquamation of the endothelial cells of the intima and the focal separation of the medium of the thoracic part of the aorta of a dog (Van Gieson's stain, 90 ×)

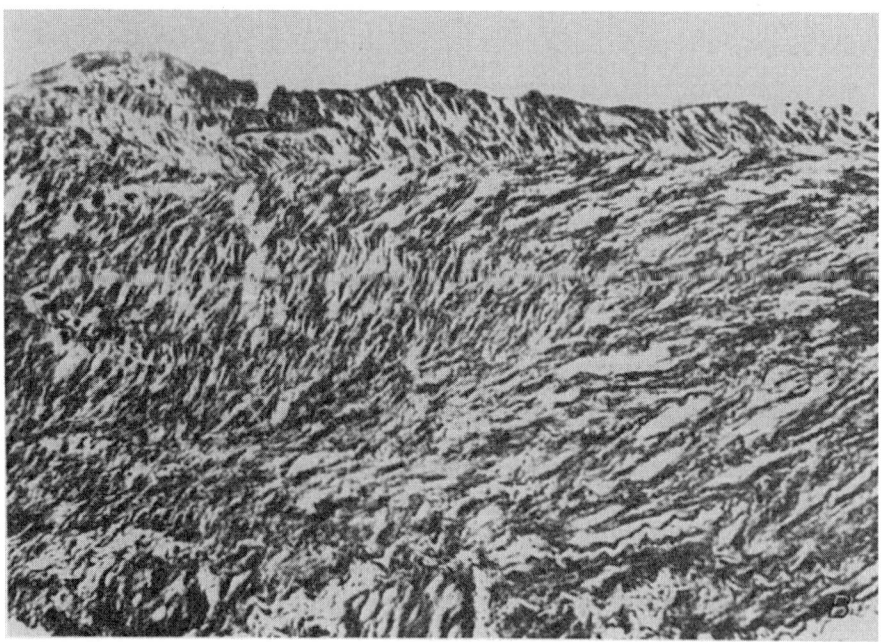

Fig. 8 B

there was no correlative link between the species life span and the formation of the cross linkage of a collagen.

Chronological age, being a temporal factor, apparently influences the development of some types of age pathology. Atherosclerotic lesions occur very frequently in man. However, they are rare in many short-living animals. This is probably because, besides many other factors, the atherosclerotic process has no time to develop.

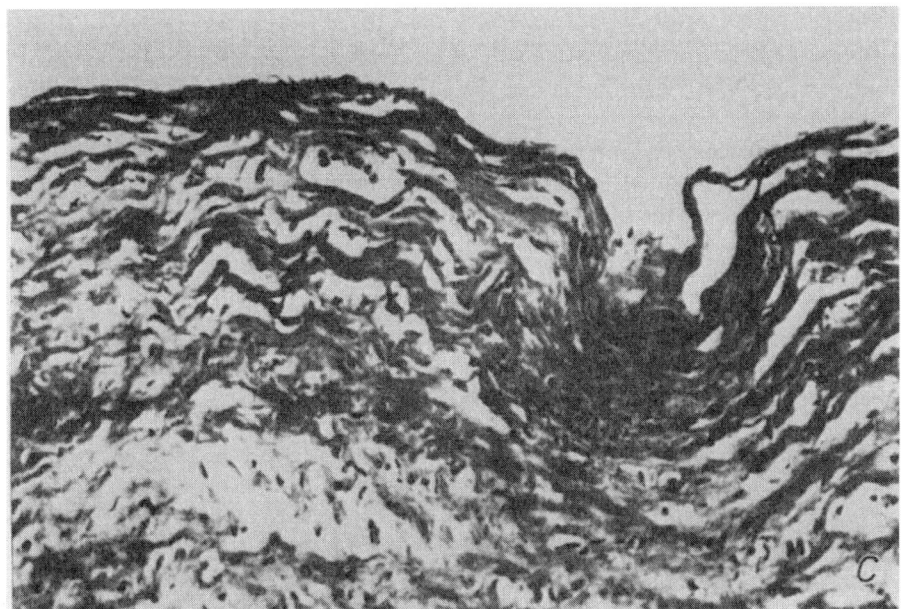

Fig. 8 C

Thus, many manifestations of aging correlate directly with chronological age, while the extent of their changes depends on time. These shifts apparently cannot be regarded as the primary mechanisms of aging. Hence, the aging of short-living organisms mainly differs from the aging of long-living organisms in that, when the process rapidly develops, many age changes which are clearly defined in long-living animals do not occur in short-living ones. Many distinctions of the aging process in various species become clear when the manifestations of aging are divided into two groups. It is undoubtedly important to compare the age changes in the features of animals with a different life span in order to analyze the general biological mechanisms of aging, determine true biological age and understand the specifics of the development of age pathology in a species.

All age-related changes can be subdivided into ontobiological and chronobiological. Ontobiological changes correlate with the species lifespan. The more rapidly they develop, the shorter is species life span. Chronobiological changes correlate with the chronological age. The longer is species life span, the more marked are chronobiological changes, and the greater role they play in an onset of aging.

2*

Earlier, we proposed the "rule of age synchronization" (Frolkis, 1969, 1970). According to one of its principles, the more rapid the aging process, the more pronounced is the non-uniformity of the age changes in the organism, the stronger is the influence of the shifts in one system on the state of the other ones, and the more marked are the primary mechanisms of aging.

The aging of animals of different species has its own essential mechanisms. However, the qualitative and quantitative specifics of their development diversify the manifestations peculiar to a species. According to Strazhesko (1939), there is a syndrome of normal aging. This concept was underpinned by data on the health of persons who lived to a very old age. Modern concepts of the non-uniformity of the aging process suggest that there are several syndromes of old age that differ from one another in the extent and rate of structural, metabolic and functional changes. This explains the development of the mainly hemodynamic syndrome of aging in one case, the neurogenic syndrome of aging in another case, and the relatively harmonious syndrome of aging in yet another case.

There exist intraspecies differences of life span which are especially well studied in man. One should differenciate between accelerated and retarded aging. The accelerated rate of aging promotes an onset of early age pathology. The retarded aging leads to longevity. Acceleration of aging has no common mechanism, and it can be related with essential changes in various links of self-regulation and with deficient vitauct processes. Deficiency of the vitauct processes becomes one of the causes of non-compensatory disturbances in the development of age pathology.

Mechanisms of the Life Span of a Species

The relationship between vitauct and aging determines the species life span.

Francis Bacon wrote that our data are meagre and our observations are careless, while our traditions are fabulous in determining whether some animals will live for either a long or a short time. In any case, longevity is obviously a rare phenomenon in the animal kingdom. Williams (1957) called longevity the "artifact of civilization." Animals must work strenuously with their muscles and respond quickly, their analyzing systems must be very sensitive, the range of the reactions of their cardiovascular system must be wide, and so forth, under natural habitation conditions when they find food to survive, when they run away from predators, when an enemy or a prey approaches, when the seasons change, etc. Aging and even slight changes in the adaptive mechanisms affect the speed of reactions, working ability, and the accuracy with which the surroundings are analyzed. Fatigue then develops more rapidly and to a greater extent, limiting an animal's possibilities in its difficult struggle for survival. It can no longer catch up with a prey, run away from a predator, see or hear danger, and migrate over great distances. Consequently, it is helpless. It starves and eventually dies. The mode of life most animals is such that even the initial manifestations of aging, i. e. the limitation of the adaptive possibilities, become the cause of their death.

Work has changed the relationship between man and the environment, thus affecting man's life span. The age changes and the early manifestations of the limitation of the adaptive possibilities ceased to be fatal owing to man's intellect and the assistance given by the family and society. Moreover, social development as well as science and technology have engendered forms of work in which one may engage even in old age, while the means of preventing and treating several diseases which were a real scourge to mankind have been found in medicine. All this has made it possible for man to live long; it allows him to live even through those changes, in life which animals do not ordinarily reach under natural habitation conditions.

The life span of a person is limited not only by a change on the organism's adaptation to the environment, but also by the great disturbances in regulating the organism's internal environment that cause pathological development.

For almost a century now, attempts have been made to find the most important factor which determines the life span of a species. Even the fact that this life span is genetically determined gives a good reason to assume that a correlation exists between it, on the one hand, and the structure and functions of the genetic apparatus, on the other. The extent of this correlation should apparently be the greater, the more important is the role of the indicator being studied in both aging and the determination of the life span of a species. Unfortunately, comparative gerontological investigations are still at their initial stage. A link is believed to exist between the life span of a species and the number of repetitions of individual genes. However, the relationship between the life span and the size of a genome has not been found (Cutler, 1973). That link is apparently complicated and is exhibited only when large toxonomic groups of animals and plants are compared. As the life span increases, the number of genes of ribosomal RNA (rRNA) grows during phylogeny from one on the plasmid, 5–10 in the bacterial cell, 100–130 in the fruit fly to 250–600 in vertebrates (Cutler, 1979). However, a comparison of the number of repetitions of the rRNA genes in a class or a study of the related classes does not reveal any significant correlative link between them and the life span of a species. This is also more or less the case when the number of genes of the transfer RNA is compared with the life span (Venksuen, 1976). Such a link does not exist either for the frequently repeating loci of DNA or for unique repetitions (Finch, 1976). According to Cutler (1976), the life span of a species is determined by the different extent to which the damaging and anti-aging processes are expressed; the intensity and direction of these processes are also under definite genetic control. To confirm this hypothesis, Cutler presented data on a positive correlative link between the species life span and DNA reparation, the inverse correlation between the rate of accumulation of chromosomal aberrations and the life span of rats, guinea pigs and dogs as species (Curtis, Miller, 1971), the formation of the liver chromosome adducts (Cutler, 1975), and so forth.

The link between DNA reparation and the life span has already been mentioned. A few genetic modifications were made as the life span of a species increased during evolution. For instance, the primary structure of both proteins and structural genes hardly differs in animals with a different species life span. It was suggested that only a few genes with regulatory functions had to be modified in order to substantially increase the life span of a species (Cutler, 1975). For instance, the maximum life span of man increased by 14 years during the last century, but the changes in the genetic apparatus did not exceed 0.5 per cent of 10.000 functioning genes. Thus, the perfection of genomic regulation is apparently the principal molecular factor which determines the evolutionary dynamics of the species life span. The rate and sequence of this regulation had determined the formation and succession of all the stages of ontogeny. Consequently, they influenced the duration of individual development as a whole.

In 1969, we proposed the genoregulatory hypothesis of aging. It shows how the primary mechanisms of aging are formed on the basis of a change in genomic regulation and how the different life span of various species are formed on the basis of the specifics of that regulation, i. e. genomic regulation is a link between aging and the life span.

Many attempts have been made to link the species life span with the organism's constitutional properties. Such a link may be regarded as a well documented fact of the inverse correlation between the life span and the animal mass. Korchagin and others (1973) used literary data relating to 177 species of mammals to calculate the coefficient of this correlation, which turned out to be very high: 0.82. Other researchers (Rockstein *et al.*, 1977; Kohn, 1978) have also observed that this coefficient was high. Of course, there are many exceptions to this rule. Bourlière (1957) was quite right in emphasizing that it was enough to compare the masses of a person, a horse and a cow in order to see that this rule had its limits.

Rather high correlation coefficients were observed when a comparison was made of the life span of mammals with the duration of pregnancy (0.75), maturation (0.78) and especially maturity (0.98) (Korchagin *et al.*, 1973). However, in comparing the average and maximal life spans of a species with the duration of the estrous cycle, pregnancy, puberty and growth in 21 mammalian species which were studied best of all, Rockstein (1977) did not deny that a correlative link existed between these indices, but he stressed that there were difficulties in making an unequivocal estimate of the link between the parameters under consideration.

It has been shown that there is a definite link between the species life span and the length of various parts of the intestine, the relative body mass (Storer, 1967) and the heart rate (Arinchin, 1966). It is widely believed that cephalization is an extremely important factor which determines the life span of a species (Friedenthal, 1910; Sacher, 1977, etc.).

According to Sacher (1978), the mechanisms of homeostatic regulation are more perfect in animals with a large brain, and this determines their longevity. But according to Storer (1967), a natural link between the life span and the mass of both the body and the brain as well as the intensity of metabolism is still not revealed within the framework of a species. In his experiments involving 18 different strains of mice, he found that metabolism is more intense in the long-living strains.

Aging is ultimately a metabolic process and all the structural and functional changes develop on its basis. Hence, the attempts to find a link between the life span and the level of metabolism. Rubner (1908) proposed the "surface rule," which substantiated the existence of a direct link between energy consumption and the life span. He believed (this is mainly where he was wrong) that a species had an energy reserve whose consumption determined the life span. However, much data which are now available show that an inverse relationship does not always exist between metabolic expenditures and the life span. In studying mammalian species, Sacher (1977) showed that the life span of a species is inversely proportional not to the level of metabolism, but to its square root. According to Arshavsky (1976, 1979), the species life span is determined by the energy rule of the skeletal muscles. Eurybionic animals, whose motor activity is great and oxygen consumption is low (e. g. hare, squirrel, horse), live much longer than their related stenobiontic animals, whose motor activity is inconsiderable and oxygen consumption is high (rabbit, rat, cow).

The more intense the metabolic processes, the greater is the likelihood of the formation of free radicals. Indeed, a comparison of the intensity of the signals of the electron paramagnetic resonance (EPR) of the quick-frozen sections of the brain of 11 mammalian species with that of 11 avian species has revealed an inverse correlation between the species life span and the intensity of the EPR signals. The nature of this link is of a single type in mammals and birds, although the intensity of the signals is about 40 per cent higher in birds than in mammals. However, this index of a short-living species (mouse) differs little from that of a long-living species (human). Hence, this link was not detected in the same mammalian species (Rahman, 1976).

A clearer correlative link between the species life span and the possible damaging effect of free radicals has been detected when the activities of the microsomal oxidases of mixed functions were compared with one another. The damaging effect of most mutagens and cancerogens, which act in accordance with the free-radical mechanism, is known to be exhibited only after their transformation under the influence of the given oxidases. Using the fibroblast cultures of animals which greatly differed from one another in their species life span, Schwartz and Moore (1978) showed that there was a clear inverse relationship between the life span and the activity of the microsomal oxidases of mixed functions as regards the mutagens of the anthracene and benzpyrene series. The peroxide radicals, being natural oxidation products, are destroyed by superoxide dismutase in the cell. It has been shown that there is a positive correlation between the life span of a species and the activity of that enzyme in the brain of the short-living (A/J) and long-living (LP/J) mice (Kellogg, Fridovich, 1976). In other organs which were studied, the activity of dismutase differs little in the mice of the given strains.

The nature of the energetic processes is almost always used in the attempts to find a link between the intensity of metabolism and the species life span. Using the concept of the essence of aging, it is important to ascertain the link between the intensity of the processes of protein biosynthesis, the activity of the genetic apparatus and the life span. In our laboratory, Muradian and Timchenko are now regularly doing research work in this respect (Fig. 9). According to their data, the longer the life span of a fruit fly, the less is the "load" of the genetic apparatus of the cell.

It can be seen that the life span of a fruit fly, the intensity of the synthesis of total RNA and protein, and temperature are directly correlated with one another in a definite temperature range. A change in the activation energy of the processes under consideration is interesting. This energy increases as the habitation temperature is elevated and the life span is shortened. The mechanisms which limit the life span are apparently replaced, and the degradative denaturation processes become most important when temperatures are high and the life span is short.

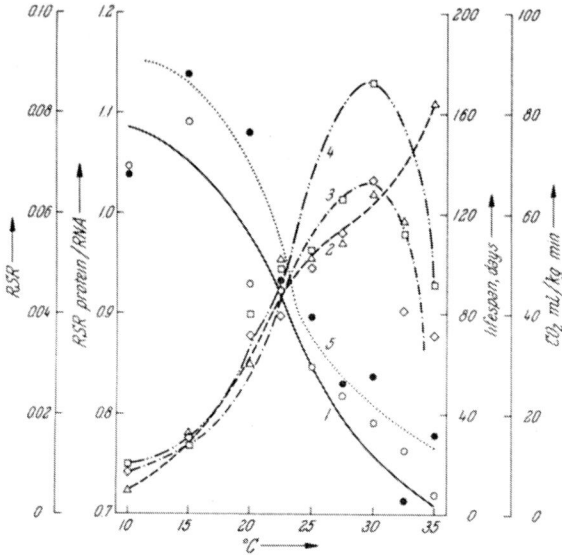

Fig. 9. Influence of incubation temperature (°C) on the duration of life *(1)*, the amount of carbon dioxide which is exhaled *(2)*, the relative specific radioactivity of protein *(3)*, RNA *(4)* and the relationship between the relative specific radioactivity of protein and RNA *(5)* in the imago of the fruit flies of the wild type of the D-18 strain

However, there is another technique which is scarcely used when the correlation between certain aging mechanisms and the life span is analyzed. If the life span can be substantially changed by altering the rate of a certain biological process, the process is apparently important in aging. We studied the effect of olivomycin, an agent which blocks transcription, on the life span of white rats and fruit flies (Frolkis *et al.*, 1976b, 1979b). The maximal life span of both species increased by 25–30 per cent. For instance, it was 1,153 ±11 days in the group of control rats and 1,481 ± 9 days in the group of test rats. Olivomycin precluded age changes in several important metabolic cycles. Hence, the life span can be increased by delaying the rate of the age changes in protein biosynthesis. When the life span is short, the turnover of RNA and protein is especially great. It should be noted that the term "intensity," which is used in this text, applies likewise to the changing relationships between opposite biological tendencies, i. e. processes in which metabolic potentials are not only spent, but also restored; consequently, complicated links are created between them and the life span. Whatever the case, there is a natural link between the duration of the stages of ontogeny, the intensity of metabolism and the species life span.

Thus, the species life span is a function of ontogeny as an intricate interaction between vitauct and aging, and not simply the rate of aging, which is erroneously believed to begin with the loss of reproductivity. This loss is not the beginning, but rather the result of aging.

Researchers seem to be divided in their evaluation of the aging mechanisms. Some researchers believe that aging is a genetically programmed process, i. e. the outcome of the natural sequence of the repression and depression of genes that causes the succession of various stages of aging. Other researchers, however, regard aging as a stochastic process, i. e. the outcome of the natural action of casual damaging factors, including thermal and radiation microeffects, free radicals, active metabolites, and the inert analogues of many other factors which inevitably originate during vital activity. They also include the inevitable "inaccuracies," "blunders" and "errors" of the biological processes which occur during the microintervals of time in microspace and which require very accurate interaction. The objective laws governing the vital processes as well as those governing the origin of these damaging factors engender the objective laws of the aging of a certain species. There is apparently no need to compare closely those two approaches.

Muradian's data on the age changes in the turnover of total RNA in various organs are given in Fig. 10A, B. An interesting fact is that the intensity of RNA synthesis diminishes to the greatest extent during a rather short age span, i. e.

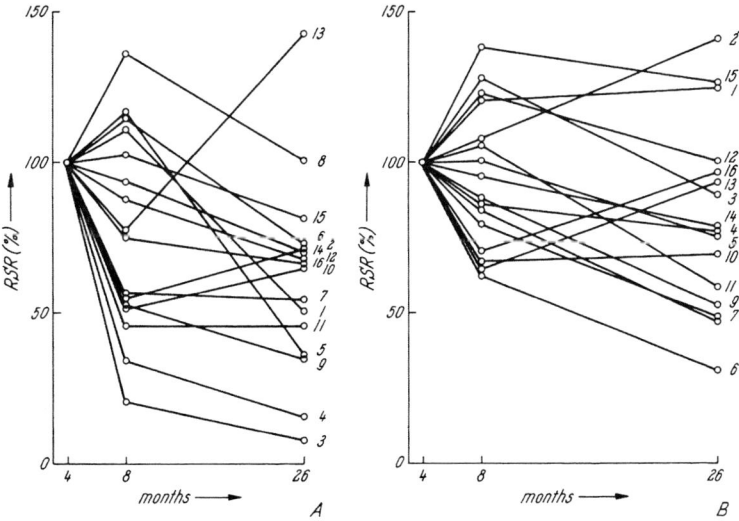

Fig. 10. Age changes in the relative specific radioactivity of RNA (A) and protein (B) in the following organs of young rats (4 months), adult rats (8 months) and old rats (26 months) (relative specific radioactivity in young rats is taken as 100 per cent): 1 frontal cortex; 2 motor cortex; 3 caudatum; 4 hippocampus; 5 brain stem; 6 hypothalamus; 7 pituitary; 8 spinal cord; 9 skeletal muscle; 10 myocardium; 11 adrenal gland; 12 testes; 13 intestinal epithelium; 14 bone marrow; 15 liver, 16 kidney

when the rats are between four and eight months old. The intensity of transcription does not substantially change during the remaining period of the rat's life, i. e. when it is from 8 to 26 months old. Such dynamics of the age changes is characteristic of many other extremely important metabolic cycles, too. The diminution of the intensity of metabolic processes is of great adaptive significance. It protects an animal from excessive plastic and energy expenditures, which can rapidly cause death, and from inadequate growth. Thus, it helps the organism to become adapted to the environment and prolongs the life span. However, the mechanisms of programmed aging, i. e. the mechanisms of the growing extinction of metabolism and regulation, are formed in this programmed "restraint" of metabolism, in the switch-over from the regulation of the genome to its repression.

Stochastic changes become increasingly important as the organism ages, because they not only occur more frequently with age, but also progressively accumulate, doing more and more damage to the structure and the metabolism of the cell. Damages grow because the means of defence become less effective, while the vitauct processes, less intensive.

According to the adaptive regulatory theory of aging (Frolkis, 1970–1980), the primary mechanisms of aging are connected with a change in genomic regulation. This may have three effects: (1) the activation of the genes which were repressed earlier and the appearance of proteins which were not synthesized earlier (the genes of aging?); (2) the complete repression of the genes which were active earlier and, if a gene is unique, the dropout of the synthesis of a definite protein, and (3) a change in the correlation between the activities of individual genes and in the correlation between the syntheses of various proteins. Of course, these possibilities can occur simultaneously. It could be that the first one plays the greatest role in actively engaging the mechanisms which cause the death of the cell and the animal's organism. The death of annual plants and the Mexican agave, which lives for decades until it flowers, is also considered from this standpoint. The May fly lives only several hours. During this time, it flies, pairs in the air, lays eggs and dies. Comfort (1964) gives data on the substantial difference in the life span of the fecundated and non-fecundated specimens of the butterfly *Fumea crassiorella*. The Pacific salmon is known to die after spawning, which entails great stress. However, its life span was prolonged by ovariectomy and adrenalectomy, which prevent that stress from developing. Consequently, Kogan (1972) believes that aging and death are the active destructive functions of the organism, i. e. the manifestation of self-regulation which is biologically expedient for a species but is "unfavourable" for an individual.

In their review, Rockstein and others (1977) have shown that all these examples are an exceptional phenomenon. Most species of animals continue to live after their progeny are born, after they lay eggs, and so forth. They age not because reproductivity diminishes; their reproductivity diminishes because they age. As the age changes grow, the organism is eliminated from the population. There is another possibility, which is quite real and which has been proved on the basis of much factual material. It presupposes a change in the correlation between the activities of various genes in aging. These shifts in genomic regulation may cause a change in the state of the cell membrane: a diminution of the number of receptors and ionic canals, the weakening of the mechanism of the active transport of substances, and the abatement of the synthesis of a special hyperpolarizing factor. All these membranogenetic shifts disturb the cellular function and the intercellular relationships. Their occurrence in the nerve cells limits the organism's adaptation to the external environment, reduces the reliability of homeostatic regulation, promotes secondary age changes in the organs and tissues, and causes the organism to age.

Aging and Evolution

There are a few dogmas in gerontology. According to the most widely accepted one, aging is involution, i. e. the organism's regressive development. Consequently, a peculiar relationship exists between ontogeny and phylogeny: at the early stages of ontogeny, the organism develops from the simple to the complex, passing the stages of the ancient forms of the manifestation of life to the more perfect ones (recapitulation), while at the late stages of ontogeny, the opposite occurs as the organism ages, i. e. the organism develops from the complex to the simple, from the new, the perfect to the phylogenetically more ancient, to a more rudimentary form. Ontogeny is divided into two parts: development and its reflected image, i. e. regressive development, involution, aging. Spenser's philosophical views and Jackson's neurological conception played a certain part in the formation of these concepts.

Indeed, many perfect, phylogenetically late mechanisms suffer in the aging process. It is enough to recall the substantial shifts in mentality, i. e. in higher nervous activity, or the fact that the more perfect form of energy generation, namely, oxidative phosphorylation, suffers earlier in the aging process, while the more ancient form, namely, glycolysis, is even activated in some tissues. But this does not mean that changes always occur in this direction as the organism ages. In many cases, the evolutionary more ancient mechanisms age sooner than the mechanisms which originated later and are more perfect. It is enough to trace the changes in the number of neurons, the number of cell receptors, and the shifts in the turnover of transmitters at various levels of the central nervous system. For instance, the greatest number of neurons which are lost in the human brain is in *Locus ceruleus* (Brody, Vijayashankar, 1975). In the zones 4 and 8 of the cortex of the major hemispheres, deterioration in the aging process is expressed more distinctly in the phylogenetically more ancient formations (projection neurons of the fifth layer) than in the phylogenetically late associative neurons. In some structures of *Truncus cerebri,* substantial shifts occur in the intensity of tissue respiration and glycolysis (Potapenko, 1974). The turnover of dopamine and its uptake by the striatum synaptosomes are especially retarded in the striapallidal system (Finch, 1973; Ponzio *et al.,* 1978). The metabolism of acetylcholine substantially changes in the cerebellum (McGeer *et al.,* 1971). The shifts which occur in aging do not fall into the given pattern even whithin the limits of a single structure, such as the hypothalamus. In old age, for instance, the density of the neurons falls by 30 per cent in the arcuate nucleus and 37 per cent in the ventromedial nucleus (Hsu, Peng, 1978), while it virtually does not change in the lateral mamillary and the perifornicate nuclei (Mezhiborskaya, 1970).

Thus, aging as pure involution, as a simple return from the evolutionarily new to the ancient form has actually not been confirmed and theoretically substantiated. We have shown that the manifestations which occur in old age and which are similar to the early stages of ontogeny have a different mechanism of development (Frolkis, 1975). Aging is regressive development only from the preformative standpoint. It is quite wrong to believe that the evolutionarily new form is always more vulnerable. Aging is not the mechanical suppression of the new levels of biological organization; it is a process of a qualitative change at all the levels of the organism's vital activity.

The interconnection between aging and evolution is still greatly debated. Weisman (1889) was among the first to discuss this problem. He believed that life span limitation and death were of adaptive significance, since they reduced the duration of life to the limits which ensure the most favourable conditions for the simultaneous existence of a maximal number of viable individuals. In this respect, we can refer to present-day evolutionists (Astafev, 1972), who emphasize that populations with a poor survival of individuals and a short life span are populations with a poor organization. These populations are very productive, thus compensating for their high mortality rate, and are not economical. According to other researchers, evolution does not influence aging. They believe that this is connected with the fact that aging is neither adaptively significant nor genetically consolidated.

The advocates of the concepts concerning the adaptive significance of aging believe that aging, while reducing the life span, promotes the succession of generations and the consolidation of the acquired features, thus furthering the evolution of the animal kingdom. However, this is a one-sided approach in trying to understand the aging of all species of animals. This is evident from the conception proposed by Shmalgausen (1968) with respect to the mobile and stabilizing form of selection, a form which is designed to transform the structure and the functions of the organism and bring about new adaptation, a form of selection which is designed to maintain the optimally stable state and "eliminate" unsuccessful features. According to Shmalgausen (1968), at every moment stabilizing selection consolidates the results which were produced, links them into an integral system and makes their reproduction most reliable.

The species life span varies greatly due to that combination of opposite tendencies, i. e. mobility and stability. Much time is needed for the adaptive mechanisms which were engendered during evolution to fully develop in some species of animals. For instance, decades are needed for the most important mechanisms of the higher nervous activity of man, a perfect mobile mechanism of adaptation, to develop. In the organism with good survival, the systems which are responsible for its viability are highly economical and reliable. Evolution, which is governed by the laws of self-regulation, causes the progressive accumulation of information. However, much time is needed for coding, transforming and realizing this information.

Species were perfected during evolution due to the shortening of the life span and the more rapid consolidation of features as well as to an increase in both life stability and the life span of individuals and, consequently, to the greater opportunities for substantial shifts to occur within a lifetime, shifts which then become hereditary. Thus, an important way of adapting to the environment is not only the succession of generations, but also the prolongation of the life span of each individual. The more highly is an animal organized, the more stable is its system of homeostatic regulation and the more perfect are the mechanisms of the reparation of the genetic apparatus. Under these conditions, definite changes occur at great intervals in the hereditary apparatus and are important in the evolutionary process. Therefore, an increase in the life span is of positive significance in evolution.

There is now much data which show that the life span of many species grew during evolution. For instance, Cutler (1979) took 59 species of hoofed animals and 32 species of carnivores to show that their evolution entailed life prolongation, especially since the Paleogenic era. For instance, the maximal potential life span of carnivores was 9 years in the Archean era, 14 years in Paleogene, 17 years in Neogene, and 21 years in the New Era. The figures for hoofed animals are 10, 15, 21 and 30 years, respectively. The life span of primates also grew approximately to that extent. An exception are hominids, whose life span increased much more rapidly. For instance, the maximal potential life span of man increased by 14 years during the last 100,000 years; that was accompanied by the modification of only 0.5 per cent of the genome (Cutler, 1978). The dominant and superdominant inheritance of longevity apparently plays an important role in the evolutionary increase in the life span. This has been shown by many researchers on the basis of various species of insects and mammals, including man (Vanyushin, Berdyshev, 1977).

The link between evolution and longevity can be correctly understood when the relationship between vitauct and aging is considered. The whole life cycle of the organism can be nominally divided according to its reproductivity into genetically informative and genetically uninformative periods. The adaptive regulatory shifts, which originate during the genetically informative period on the basis of casual mutation, can be genetically consolidated and can influence the formation of the life span in evolution. Therefore, genetically programmed vitauct processes are formed and consolidated in the course of evolution. It is their program together with the age disturbances (which accumulate in conformity with the specifics of metabolism) that determines the life span. This consolidation of vitauct explains the steady increase in the mammalian life span. This increase is especially great among primates. The occurrences in the post-reproductive period cannot be genetically consolidated. They are thus irreversible in evolution.

The forms of regulation and adaptation were perfected as the biological organization became complicated in the course of evolution. At the same time, definite aging mechanisms changed and were transformed. The mechanisms of vitauct and aging qualitatively changed as they came under central, neurohumoral control. The general regulatory shifts were superimposed on the main, basal, purely cellular aging mechanisms, modifying them, since the organism ages as a complex system and not as a simple totality of cells. The higher the evolutionary level of the organism, the more important are these neurohumoral mechanisms in the genesis of vitauct and aging. Their significance may serve as a basis for correct understanding the mechanisms of the whole organism's aging.

Aging and Diseases

There is a close connection between aging and some diseases from which man suffers. This is evident from both the sharp growth of the occurrences of diseases (atherosclerosis, myocardial and cerebral ischemia, arterial hypertension, malignant tumours, diabetes, etc.) in elderly and old persons and their higher mortality.

Mortality is higher among men than among women. However, this sex difference is levelled out with age. For instance, the death rate is 3.3 times higher among men aged 20–29, 3.1 times higher among men aged 30–39, and 1.4 time higher among men above 60 than among women of the same age. Mortality due to cardiovascular diseases and malignant tumours increases with age. For instance, mortality due to cardiovascular diseases is 195.7 times higher and that due to cancer is 80.9 times higher among men above 60 than among those aged 20–29 (*Vestnik statistiki*, 1973, No. 12, p. 81).

Mortality due to ischemic heart disease sharply increases among men as early as the age of 35–44. This shows that the pathology of the cardiovascular system originates and rapidly develops not only among elderly and old persons, but also among younger persons. In this respect, it should be noted that the given pathology, i. e. ischemic heart disease, myocardial infarction and arterial hypertension, occurs more and more frequently among young persons, although it is true that the average life span is increasing.

The age dynamics of mortality due to various pathologies of the cardiovascular system differs at different stages. In Japan, mortality due to stroke sharply increases with age, while mortality due to myocardial infarction is rather low in comparison with other countries. It is interesting to compare the dynamics of mortality caused by the disease of the cardiovascular system in such European countries as Finland, France, Italy and Poland. The dynamics of the rise of mortality due to cardiovascular diseases differs from one country to another, although the average life span in them is about the same.

Many elderly and old people fall ill because many diseases occur more frequently at their age, and also because the diseases which began at other age periods accumulate by the time they reach their elderly or old age.

Age pathology is a group of pathological processes and diseases which develop mainly during a certain age span; it is a group of pathological processes for whose development the age changes in the organism create the main prerequisites. The relationship between aging and diseases is among the most disputed problems. It is an important problem not only in gerontology, but also in medicine as a whole.

Enough facts are now known to maintain that the organism's adaptive possibilities are curtailed in the aging process. Consequently, vulnerable spots are engendered in its self-regulation system and the prerequisites are created for some diseases. Diseases cannot be regarded as aging processes proper, just as aging cannot be identified with diseases.

The organism's biological properties sharply change during ontogeny, starting from the zygote to very old age. Every stage of ontogeny has its own level of adaptation and its own age characteristics of the organism's metabolism, structure and function. All this qualitatively, or fundamentally, distinguishes every stage of the organism's development in its reactions to an environmental change. These qualitative features of development largely determine the specifics of age pathology, i. e. the disappearance or growth of definite diseases with age and a change in the specifics of the occurrence of the same pathology during different age periods. From this standpoint, it is quite correct to single out pathology which is characteristic of mainly the antenatal and postnatal periods, children's diseases, the pathology of puberty, and the diseases from which elderly and old people suffer. For instance, there is antenatal pathology, which includes gametopathy, embryopathy and fetopathy. Intrauterine asphyxia is among the most frequently occurring types of antenatal pathology. Pathology associated with labour is clearly defined. All that age pathology is obviously timed for definite conditions of the organism's formation.

The prevalence of a disease among people of a given age is most frequently regarded as evidence of aging. According to sectional data, fibrous patches are found in 95–99 per cent of the cases after the age of 50. However, such prevalence of some diseases is observed also in childhood, although they are justifiably not regarded as a property of a child's physiological development. The specifics of the development of a child's organism create prerequisites for their occurrence. For instance, 96 per cent of the children in Russia suffered from rickets at the beginning of this century. In the 1950's, between 66.3 per cent and 92.8 per cent of all children in the Federal Republic of Germany suffered from rickets. In childhood, rickets is caused by some specifics of the metabolism of vitamins, especially vitamin D. Transient dyspepsias and gastroenterites are observed in most children as both the function of the digestive glands and the motility of the gastroenteric tract originate. However, they should not be regarded as a manifestation of a child's physiological development.

Age changes in the organism also promote the development of a definite group of diseases. For instance, the organism is provided with less insulin and becomes less tolerable with respect to carbohydrates as it ages. This fact is due to a change in the structure and function of the beta cells of the pancreas as well as to a decrease in both the physiological activity of insulin and the reactivity of tissues to insulin. Such a set of shifts as well as less tolerance to carbohydrates promote the development of diabetes in elderly persons. However, certain conditions are needed for a predisposition to be realized in a definite disease. Indeed, according to various authors, less tolerance to carbohydrates is observed in 50–85 per cent of elderly persons, while diabetes develops only in 7–9 per cent of them. Incidentally, a definite set of conditions involving age also promotes diabetes in children.

The occurrences of parkinsonism sharply increase among elderly persons. Cases of parkinsonism are much more common among persons above 60 than among young persons. In young persons, this disease is the outcome of either the primary degenerative changes in the subcortical structures or postencephalitic disturbances, while in elderly persons, the vascular factor is mainly responsible for it. The neurophysiological mechanisms of parkinsonism are connected with a disturbance in the motor regulation centres, the striapallidal system, and *Substantia nigra*. In this respect, the metabolism of catecholamines is disturbed and the dopamine content is sharply reduced. Definite shifts in this system occur in many elderly persons, i. e. the electric activity of the muscles is higher at rest, light tremor is frequent, and so forth. Clearly expressed parkinsonism develops when the brain vessels are greatly affected by atherosclerosis against that background in some of these persons.

The relationship between aging and atherosclerosis is an especially acute problem. Atherosclerosis and its manifestations are among the main causes of death of elderly and old persons. Some researchers believe that this disease is connected with the specifics of the living conditions in modern society, because it frequently occurs today. Atherosclerosis and its manifestations are becoming more frequent as the average human life span grows and the number of elderly and old persons increases. It could be that the long human life span is a factor which promotes the development and revelation atherosclerosis, whose formation takes a definite length of time. The same investigations in the United States and some European countries have shown that lipids are deposited in the aortic intima in all persons of both sexes, beginning with the age of ten. Fibrous patches in the abdominal aorta have been discovered in 16 per cent of persons aged 10–19. Lipid spots take up 9.9 per cent of the inner membrane of the aorta in men and 17.1 per cent of that in women aged 10–19. The overall area of the atherosclerotic changes in the coronary arteries increases from 2–3 per cent of the inner membrane surface in men aged 10–19 to 60–62 per cent in men aged 80–89. All this shows that Vichert (1977) was quite right in saying that the investigations of human atherosclerosis today should be concentrated on children and youths, because when atherosclerosis is already developed, i. e. at the age of 40–50 or even 30–40, it is difficult to determine what played the most important role at the stage of its origination, which occurs during the early periods of human life.

Thus, the prerequisites for the development of certain age pathology are created at every stage of ontogeny due to the specifics of the organism's adaptive possibilities. Diseases accumulate and many of them occur anew by old age, acquiring qualitative and quantitative features. They cause the organism's death because its adaptive possibilities diminish. Old age only brings a person to the edge of the precipice from where diseases push him over.

2. Aging of the Brain

General Direction of the Age Changes in the Brain

Kozma Prutkov, an image created by a group of Russian authors in the last century, once said: "If you are asked what is more useful, the sun or the moon, answer the moon, because the sun shines during the day, when it is light, but the moon shines at night." In some ways this aphorism applied for a long time to the investigation of the central nervous system's aging. In most cases, the researchers concentrated on the role which the change in the brain function plays in the aging of the whole organism without taking account of the fact that both the processes which increase the organism's viability and the vitauct processes are connected with the activity of the nervous centres.

It can now be maintained that the most important manifestations of the organism's aging are the result of the age changes in the brain. The aging of the central nervous system causes changes in mentality, higher nervous activity and in the ability to analyze the external environment, shifts in behavioural and emotional reactions, some loss of memory, a decrease in mental and physical working ability, motor activity, reproductive ability, changes in the regulation of the organism's internal environment, and so forth. These disturbances are so significant that they cause the death of animals, which cannot survive because they are less able to adapt themselves to the constantly changing conditions of the external environment. Man, however, survives these disturbances because of the high level of mental activity, the society's care for an individual, and the new, perfect level of the organism's adaptive regulatory processes. The main causes of his death are the disturbances of the autonomic ensurance of the organism's activity as well as specific age pathology. The significance of the age changes in the nervous system during the organism's aging has been shown even with respect to invertebrates. For instance, if a flatworm (*Stenostomum incaudatum*) is repeatedly cut in two, the head part dies, but the tail part continues to divide infinitely.

All this seems to suggest that the age changes in the brain are the main mechanism of the whole organism's aging. However, there is another direction of the relationships between the brain's activity and the life span.

The activity of the central nervous system, or the brain's function, determines the most important manifestations of the vitauct process, which is intended to increase the organism's viability and life span. It should be taken into account that the adaptive regulatory mechanisms, such as those connected with man's higher nervous activity, take decades to develop.

Many researchers (Friedenthal, 1910; Hansche, 1975; Sacher, 1975; Shvarts, 1976) acknowledge that the life span of a species and the brain's regulatory abilities are interconnected. Friedenthal (1910) was the first to correlate the life span of a species and cephalization. He regarded cephalization as the ratio of the brain mass to the body mass or, to be more exact, to the protoplasm mass. Definite parallelism proved to exist between the value of the cephalization ratio and the life span of a species. Hence, he assumed that a wiser person lived longer. However, the mass of the brain does not reflect the possible realiability and perfection of its regulation, which is very important to the organism's viability. Indeed, the life span of many species does not adequately correlate with cephalization (Sacher, 1975, 1977). Sacher proposed the following formula which, besides the brain mass, includes some metabolic indices:

$$L = 8 \times E^{0.6} \times S^{-0.4} \times M^{-0.5} \times 10^{0.025T}$$

where L = life span, months;
       E = brain mass, g;
       S = body mass, g;
       M = level of metabolism at rest, cal/g/h;
       T = body temperature, °C.

This ratio correlated well with the value of the life span of 85 mammalian species ranging from mice to the elephant (Sacher, 1975). Shvarts (1976) believes that the lagging of the brain mass behind the body mass is the main mechanism of aging of a large group of mammals with definitive body dimensions. Although the calculations are limited and conditional, a definite regularity has been observed, i. e. the brain development level and the viability enhancement mechanisms which are apparently connected with it determine the life span of a species to a certain extent. This correlation would even be greater if the objective criteria of reliability, or durability, of the mechanisms of neurohumoral self-regulation were found. Economos (1980a, b) has shown from the calculations made for 63 species of mammals that the coefficient of the correlation between the logarithms of the life span and the brain mass is 0.88, while that between the life span and the body mass is 0.77. The coefficient of the correlation between the life span and the brain mass is greater than that between the life span and the mass of the liver or the adrenal glands. The coefficient of the correlation between the life span and the brain mass is greater in primates than in rodents, carnivores and ungulates.

There is another approach which proves that the functions of the central nervous system play a definite role in vitauct and life prolongation. Some aspects of the function of the long-living person's brain have their own specifics. The prolonged preservation of several extremely important functions of the long-living person's brain is an interesting fact (Mankovsky, 1973). According to Malinovsky (1962), longevity is closely connected with man's higher nervous activity. Belonog and Kuznetsova (1973) indicate that there are no great differences in the intensity of slow rhythms (delta and theta rhythms) as well as in alpha-activity and fast rhythms (beta and gamma rhythms) in long-living persons and in the control group of young persons. However, such differences exist in elderly and old persons of the average population. The assimilation of imposed rhythms, an important indicator of the great lability of the brain structures, remains on a high level in long-living persons. These shifts in the bioelectric activity of their brain corroborate the views held by Mankovsky (1973), who developed the principle proposed by Bekhtereva (1974). The bioelectric phenomena which are recorded on the EEG not only reflect the occurrences in the brain, but also maintain a definite state of the brain structures, a definite level of their activity. This assumption is underpinned by modern concepts of the membrane mechanisms of the bioelectric phenomena in the neuron, the role which ionic shifts play in this respect, and the participation of active ionic transport in restorative processes. It should be taken into account that when the neuron's electric activity changes, ionic shifts influence the most diverse aspects of cellular metabolism, including the activity of the genetic apparatus.

An interesting fact is that mental and muscular working ability of long-living persons can be optimized to a definite extent by training (Litovchenko, 1973; Sichinava, 1973). In long-living persons, the changes in mental activity are greater than rheoencephalographic changes (Mints, 1973), which do not reveal any clear-cut signs of the development of atherosclerosis. Hence, the former changes are not caused by the disturbance of vascularization, but are connected with the primary shifts in the nervous tissue.

All those specifics of the nervous system of long-living persons are largely genetically determined, since they are observed also in their relatives. According to Mankovsky and others (1975, 1976), the long-living person's relatives have a higher frequency of alpha-activity during all the age periods. Their alpha index is also relatively stable.

The frequency spectrum of the alpha rhythm, its extent of expression, regularity and zonal topography reflect the level of the functional adjustment of the complex cortical and subcortical mechanisms which ensure the harmonious activity of various brain systems. Therefore, the higher frequency of the alpha rhythm in the relatives of long-living persons is probably a peculiar reflection of the high functional activity of the central nervous system.

The duration of the latent period of a reaction to light and the nature of the distribution of the ranges of assimilation of imposed rhythms during light stimulation also indicate the constitutional specifics of the formation of the bioelectric reactions of the brain of the long-living person's relatives. Reactive bioelectric shifts develop more rapidly in these relatives during all the age ranges. Hence, adaptive regulatory mechanisms can be genetically consolidated and can influence both the life span and the aging rate.

Such distinctions of the reliability of brain activity are characteristic of not only individuals with a different life span, but also species with a different life span. The great, prolonged reliability of the brain makes it possible to optimally regulate the trophism of various tissues for a long time and reduces the rate of development of the age changes, which are the basis of pathology.

There is another way of proving the existence of a link between the functional state of the brain and the organism's viability and life span. Many manifestations of the organism's aging can be simulated by disturbing the functions of the central nervous system for a long time. Such experiments have been carried out long ago by Petrova (1946), who showed that the systematic disturbances of higher nervous activity cause the development of signs of premature aging in experimental dogs and reduce their life span. This is evident also from the fact that frequent great stresses reduce the life span of rats (Frolkis, 1975).

Thus, the adaptive regulatory theory of aging suggests that the adaptive mechanisms which increase the life span and preserve adaptation to the environment are formed and that the most important vitauct processes occur due to brain activity during aging. However, adaptive abilities are curtailed and the whole organism ages when age disturbances naturally and inevitably occur in the central mechanisms of regulation.

Structural and Metabolic Changes in the Brain During Aging

Metabolic disturbances during aging ultimately cause the destruction of neurons and their replacement by glia cells. The destruction of neurons is not only a certain objective measure of various brain structures' aging, but also an important mechanism of a change in their functions. The functions of a nerve centre are inevitably affected when the number of neurons decreases by 30 or 40 per cent in it. The structure of the neuron chains and the plurality and duplication of the interneuronal links are an extremely important mechanism of vitauct, which helps to preserve the functions when a part of the nerve cells dies.

Table 1, taken from the monograph by Frolkis and Bezrukov (1979), gives some data on the loss of neurons in various parts of the brain. These data show that different brain structures age non-uniformly. In mice and rats, the neuronal loss may be as much as 25–75 per cent in some regions of the cerebral cortex (Peng, Lee, 1975; Brizee, Ordy, 1979), but in others, the number of neurons hardly changes. This number decreases especially in the frontal region. It

Table 1. *Age changes in the brain neuronal population*

Brain structures	Changes %	Species	Age	Sex	Reference
Whole brain	−70	Swiss albino mouse	1 vs. 29 months	M, F	Johnson, J. E.; Miquel, J. (1974)
Cerebral cortex	−20	human	19–28 vs. 77 years	M, F	Shefer, V. F. (1972)
Area 6	−22	human	19–28 vs. 77 years	M, F	Shefer, V. F. (1972)
Subiculum	−29	human	19–28 vs. 77 years	M, F	Shefer, V. F. (1972)
Frontal polar region (area 10)	−28	human	19–28 vs. 77 years	M, F	Shefer, V. F. (1972)
Middle temporal gyrus (area 21)	−23	human	19–28 vs. 77 years	M, F	Shefer, V. F. (1972)

Table 1 *(continued)*

Brain structures	Changes %	Species	Age	Sex	Reference
Cerebral cortex (frontal pole, area striata, cingulate gyrus, precentral gyrus)	−44	human	to 90 years		Colon, E. J. (1972)
Visual cortex (area 17)	−24	Fischer 344 rat	11 vs. 29 months	M	Ordy, J. M.; Brizzee, K. R.; Kaack, B.; Hansche, J. (1978)
	−18	Fischer 344 rat	17 vs. 29 months	M	Ordy, J. M.; Brizzee, K. R.; Kaack, B.; Hansche, J. (1978)
Indusium griseum	no (+8)	ASH/TO mouse	5 vs. 18 months	M	Sturrock, R. R. (1977)
Cerebellar cortex	no	guinea pig	to 7, 6 years	M, F	Wilcox, H. H. (1959)
	−25	human	1 vs. 100 + years	M, F	Hall, T. C.; Miller, A. K. H.; Corsellis, J. A. N. (1975)
Lateral mammillary nucleus	− 8	rat	1 vs. 28 months	M	Mezhiborskaya, N. A. (1971)
	− 8	rat	6 vs. 28 months	M	Mezhiborskaya, N. A. (1971)
	− 7	rat	10–12 vs. 28 months	M	Mezhiborskaya, N. A. (1971)
Perifornicate nucleus	− 7	rat	1 vs. 28 months	M	Mezhiborskaya, N. A. (1971)
	− 5	rat	6 vs. 28 months	M	Mezhiborskaya, N. A. (1971)
	no (− 2)	rat	10–12 vs. 28 months	M	Mezhiborskaya, N. A. (1971)
Posterior hypothalamic nucleus	−18	rat	1 vs. 28 months	M	Mezhiborskaya, N. A. (1971)
	no (−12)	rat	6 vs. 28 months	M	Mezhiborskaya, N. A. (1971)
	no (− 4)	rat	10–12 vs. 28 months	M	Mezhiborskaya, N. A. (1971)
Brain stem Ventral cochlear nucleus	no	human	0–90 years	M, F	Konigsmark, B. W.; Murphy, E. A. (1970)
Inferior olive nucleus	no	human			Monagle, R. D.; Brody, H. (1974)
Locus ceruleus	−42	human	14 vs. 87 years		Brody, H.; Vijayashankar, (1975)

decreases somewhat less in the basal ganglia, the thalamus, the subthalamic region, the cerebellum, and the brain stem. An interesting fact is that the number of neurons decreases less in the hypothalamus (except some regions, namely, *Nucleus arcuatus* and the preoptic region) than in other brain structures.

Rafalowska (1980) studied the segments of the spinal cord at the C_8-Th_1 level in persons of different age (fetuses, children one to three years old, persons 15 to 58 years old without any pathology of the spinal cord, and persons 72 to 93 years old who died of strokes) and found that different changes occur in the dimensions and number of neurons in the retroposterolateral nucleus of the spinal cord. The linear dimensions of the motor cell of *Cornu anterius* are minimum in fetuses (32.41 μm); they increase in children of an early age (45.80 μm) and in persons 16 to 58 years old (52.23 μm), but decrease in old age (49.39 μm). The number of cells in that nucleus decreases on the right-hand side as well as the left-hand side with age (on the right-hand side, there are 3.78 cells in a section in children, 2.75 cells in persons 15 to 58 years old, and 1.74 cells in persons 72 to 93 years old; on the left-hand side, the figures are 3.75, 2.88 and 1.61, respectively).

There is a definite correlation between the extent of the neuronal loss and a change in the appropriate brain functions (regulation of the motor sphere, the reproductive function, the perception of afferent impulses, etc.).

Besides the destruction of neurons, gliosis develops and the ratio between the glia cells and the nerve cells grows (Brizzee, Ordy, 1979; Peng, Lee, 1975). Morphometric as well as biochemical and histochemical methods have been used to show that the number of neurons decreases and gliosis develops. For instance, it has been shown that the content of neuronine and the proteins S_4 and S_5 (which are characteristic of neurons) decreases, while the content of the protein S-100 (which is localized mainly in glia) increases with age (Perez, Moor, 1970). According to Vernadakis (1975), the activity of acetyl-cholinesterase (which is specific for neurons) decreases, while that of butyryl-cholinesterase localized in the glia cells increases in old age. The number of glia cells in various brain structures changes differently in old age. For instance, the number of these cells in the grey matter of the brain increases, but it decreases in its white matter (Sturrock, 1977).

When the number of glia cells increases, the blood supply of the neurons may worsen, their position with respect to the capillaries may alter, and the interneuronal relationships may change substantially. However, neuronal trophism may be preserved at a definite stage of the growth of the number of glia cells. It could be that the trophic function of glia is stimulated, intercellular transport occurs and plastic substances are transferred from the glia to the neuron. It has been shown that the content of protein, several enzymes and RNA decreases in the glia cells and increases in the neurons when certain nerve structures of the brain are stimulated. Gliacytes may secrete amino acids and proteins into intercellular clefts, from where they penetrate into neurons (Globus *et al.*, 1973). Data show that the number of neuroglia cells increases around the actively functioning neurons. An extremely important function of the glia, i. e. the recapture of the brain mediators, greatly influences the realization of the regulatory effects. According to Aprikyan and others (1978), the capture of amino acids by the neurons of the cerebral cortex of old rats is affected more than their capture by the glia cells. It is believed that the glia cells participate in the formation and consolidation of temporary links (Roitbak, 1969). The changes which occur in the state of the glia with age probably influence that process in old age.

The destruction of neurons is preceded by many morphological changes in the cells. Machado-Salas and Scheibel (1979) studied morphologically more than 200 C57BL/6J mice of both sexes and found great changes in several limbic formations. In the hippocampus, the outlines of the bodies of neurons and dendrites are upset, spinae are lost, axons are fragmented, terminals swell, and astrocytes proliferate. Some of these changes are found also in the olfactory bulb. The membrane nuclei change far less. Freddari and Giuli (1980 studied morphologically the glomeruli of the cerebellum of the Wistar female rats 3, 18 and 28 months old. The surface density of the synaptic contact zones decreased by 20 per cent, the overall length of these zones, by 19 per cent, the numerical density of synapses, by 42 per cent, while the average length of the synaptic contact zone increased by 19 per cent in old rats as compared with mature ones. Hence, the brain functions decrease with age because of the great reduction of synaptic contacts.

According to all the researchers, intact cells and, what is more, cells with clear signs of hyperfunction are found together with atrophied, or destroyed, cells in old age (Mezhiborskaya, 1970; Stupina, 1978; Brizzee, Ordy, 1979; Artyukhina, 1979). Electron microscopy has revealed three types of neurons: (1) neurons which have hardly changed; (2) neurons with hypertrophied cellular organelles in the cytoplasm with vacuoles, i. e. the nucleus has many outgrowths, the cavities of the cytoplasmic reticulum and the reticulate apparatus are enlarged, the number of ribosomes is reduced, and swollen mitochondria occur, and (3) neurons with signs of dystrophy, i. e. the nucleus is dense, perinuclear space has cisternae and pores, mitochondria are without cristae, the lysosome membranes are damaged, and so forth (Artyukhina, 1979). The deposition of lipofuscin, or the "pigment of aging," is universal. According to many researchers, this fact is so typical of aging that it can be used as an objective criterion of the extent of the changes which occur with age. However, not all the researchers uphold this view. The topographies of the maximum deposition of lipofuscin and the maximum destruction of neurons do not coincide. According to Brizzee and Ordy (1979), lipofuscin in monkeys accumulates most rapidly in the structures of *Medulla oblongata* and *Mesencephalon*, but most slowly in the cerebellum and the neocortex. Much more lipofuscin is deposited in monkeys 4 to 9.5 years old than in those 9.5 to 19.5 years old. A comparison of the life span of various strains of fruit flies with the rate of accumulation of lipofuscin in the nerve cells has revealed no correlation between them (Biscardi, Webster, 1977). Karnaukhov (1973) has presented interesting data on the adaptive role of the accumulation of lipofuscin, which contains elements of the respiratory chain, in old age. Morphological changes in neurons have been thoroughly described (Dalakishvili, 1967; Andrew, 1971; Stupina, 1978; Artyukhina, 1979). They are reflected in all the cellular structures: mitochondria, the endoplasmic reticulum, the nucleus, the lysosome, etc. Certain disturbances have been observed also in the cell membrane. It is believed that they are less significant than those in several other ultrastructures of the cell. However, it is not taken into account that the nerve cell cannot exist when its membrane is greatly damaged. The cell continues to function when a part of the mitochondria is destroyed, a part of the endoplasmic reticulum is disturbed, and so forth, but it ceases to exist as an independent structure when its membrane is irreparably ruptured. The restoration of the cell membrane is an extremely important mechanism of vitauct.

The definite direction of the structural changes which occur in neurons with age is a general biological regularity. It is characteristic of animals which belong to species of different life spans and can be seen in mammals as well as invertebrates. Stupina (1978) has shown that the changes which occur with age in the neurons of molluscs (*Lymnaea stagnalis*) are the same as those which occur in the neurons of mammals. The hyperplasia of the lysosomal apparatus and the accumulation of secondary lysosomes are observed in the neurons of ganglia together with the changes in the protein-synthesizing system. At the same time, some compensatory rearrangements occur, i. e. the area of the nuclear membranes increases and individual organoids become hypertrophied (Fig. 11 A, B).

According to the adaptive regulatory theory of aging, important adaptive shifts occur together with atrophy and destructive changes as the organism grows old. This principle has been confirmed by an analysis of the structural changes in the brain. Those manifestations are expressed to a different extent in various parts of the brain. They include the hypertrophy of many neurons, the appearance of polyploid nerve cells, the growth of the surface of the cell and its nucleus, an increase in the number of nucleoli, the intensified coloration of nuclear chromatin that is not connected with pyknosis, an increase in the volume of mitochondria as their number decreases, the growth of dendrodendritic and axosomal contacts in some structures, a change in the spina apparatus, the hypertrophy of microtubules as a part of them is destroyed, etc. (Andrew, 1971; Artyukhina, 1979; Mezhiborskaya, 1980; and others). These adaptive changes allow definite central nervous structures to function in spite of the great morphological changes. Hence, the functions of some nerve centres are preserved even when many neurons are lost (Fig. 12 A, B, C, D).

The extent and sequence of the structural changes in various parts of the brain do not fit into the involutional scheme, according to which age disturbances occur first of all in the phylogenetically late formations of the brain. An important fact is that great structural changes in neurons are observed in higher and lower animals with different life spans. This confirms their direct link with the chief mechanisms of aging.

Metabolic shifts are the basis of the change in the structure and functions of the brain during aging. Blood circulation in the brain strongly influences its metabolism. Blood supply changes more in the frontal and temporal regions of the cerebral cortex and less in the parietal and occipital regions (Mankovsky, Lizogub, 1976; Naritomi *et al.*, 1979). Fujishima and Omae (1980) have shown that the average time which is needed for blood to pass through the brain greatly

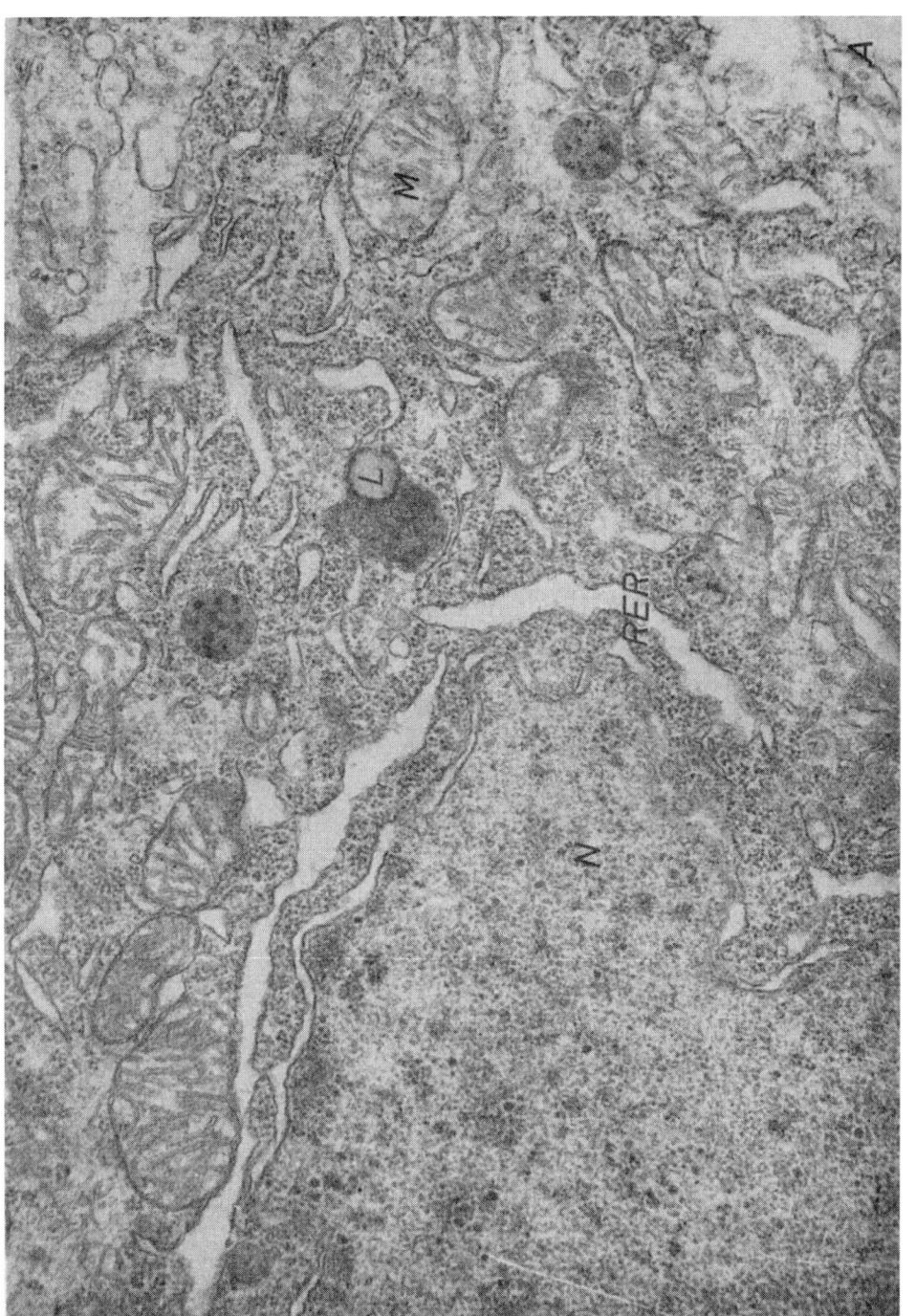

Fig. 11A

Fig. 11. A portion of a spinal cord neuron of an old rat (A) and a ganglion neuron of an old snail (Lymnaea stagnalis) (B). Lipid granules (L), residual body enlargement of rough endoplasmic reticulum profiles (RER) with a small amount of ribosomes in the cytoplasm. N nucleus; M mitochondria. 20,000×

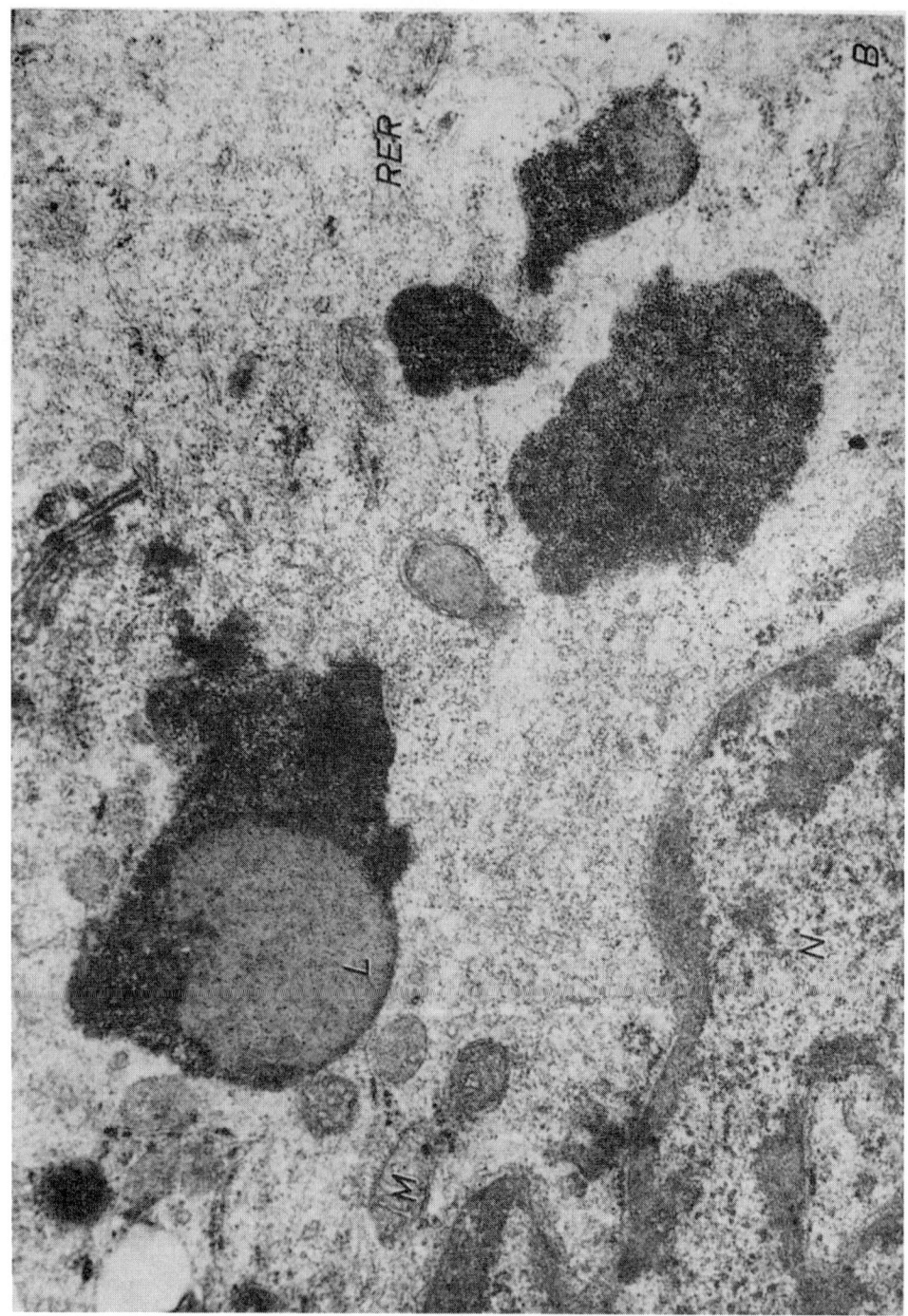

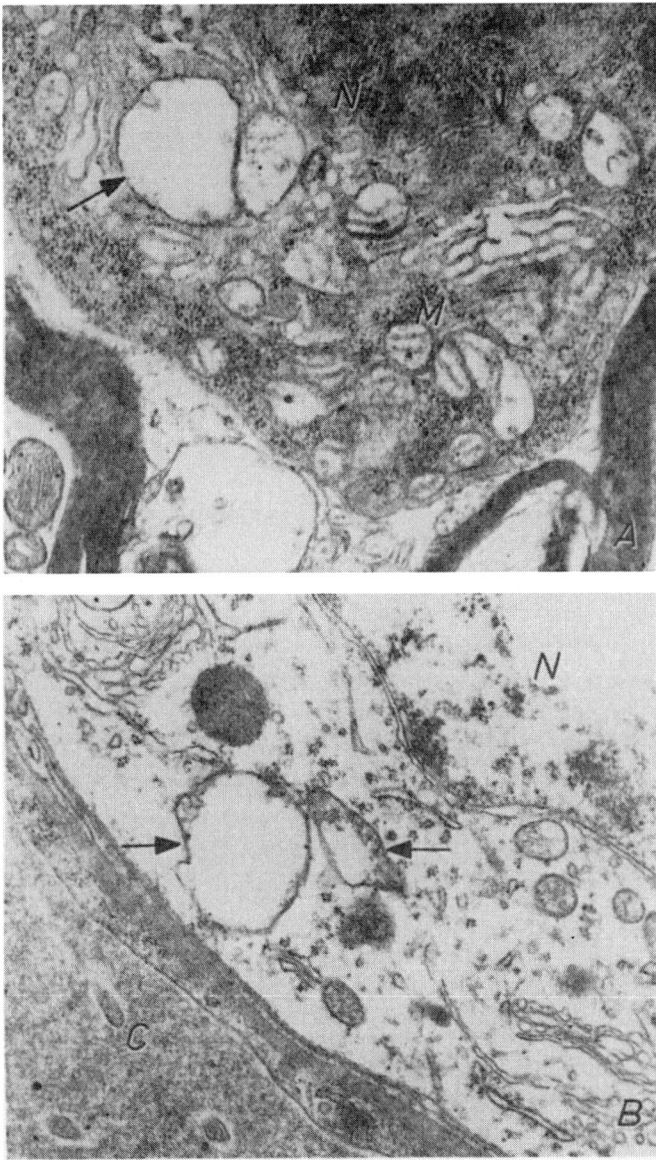

Fig. 12 A, B

Fig. 12. Neurons of the mammillary lateral nucleus of an old rat. *A, B* reduction of cristae and the sharp swelling of mitochondria (arrows), 30,000 ×. *C* expansion of the cisternae of the endoplasmic reticulum (arrows), 20,000 ×. *D* signs of intensive protein synthesis: the granular endoplasmic reticulum is well developed; mitochondria (arrows) are near the membranes of the reticulum; a large nucleolus is near the nuclear membrane, 20,000 ×. *ER* endoplasmic reticulum; *C* capillary; *M* mitochondria; *N* nucleus; *Nu* nucleolus; *Nb* Nissl body

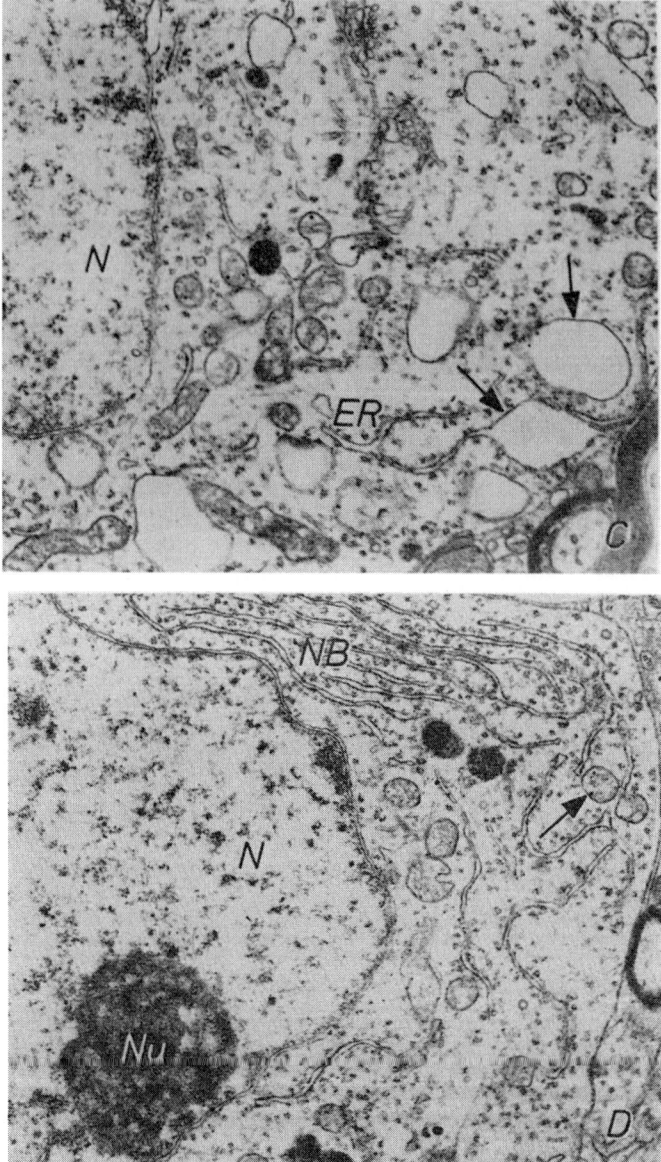

Fig. 12 C, D

increases with age and that this increase is not accompanied by any substantial shifts in the level of the blood supply of the brain. They believe that it increases because the blood volume grows in the brain. Great changes in blood supply are observed in the subcortical structures and especially in the stria-pallidum system, and also in the region of small branchings of *Arteria meningea media* (Popova *et al.*, 1976). Blood circulation in the basins of the carotid and vertebral arteries changes differently with age. An important fact is that the changes in the blood supply of the brain occur not only in people, but also in animals which are not suffering from spontaneous atherosclerosis (rats, cats).

When the blood supply of the brain worsens with age, shifts appear, compensating for those changes. For instance, neurons and capillaries are arranged more closely in the nuclei of the amygdaloid complex, the number of glia cells increases around capillaries, and astrocytes contact capillaries more frequently in old persons and animals (Kononenko, 1969).

Neural activity requires a great amount of energy. The brain, which constitutes not more than 2 per cent of the body weight, consumes up to 20–25 per cent of total oxygen, while it consumes 50 per cent of oxygen in newborns. Oxygen consumption by the cells of various parts of the brain may differ hundreds of times. During stimulation, the energy expenditures of neurons sharply grow.

The relationship between oxidative phosphorylation, glycolysis and the pentose cycle in the energy supply of cerebral activity changes with age. There are several signs which indicate that definite hypoxia of the brain occurs in old age, or at least it originates more easily in old age. This fact has been illustrated by taking the example of hypoxic and circulatory hypoxia. During ascent, the brain function is disturbed at lower altitudes in old rats in comparison with mature rats (Kolchinskaya, 1964).

The stereological investigation of the capillaries of the cerebral cortex of 34 persons 19 to 94 years old have shown that the blood supply of the cerebral cortex does not substantially decrease with age and that the capillary network can respond to a change in metabolism and blood pressure.

In persons who were more than 75 years old, the nature of capillaries (diameter, volume, the area of the specific surface, the average distance between capillaries, and the overall length per unit volume of the cortex) did not substantially differ from that in persons who were from 19 to 44 years old. In persons who were from 64 to 74 years old, the volume and the overall length per unit volume of the cortex were enlarged, while the specific surface area was reduced. In his experiments with the Sprague-Dawley male rats 6–7 and 33–34 months old, Wexler (1979) showed that the unilateral ligation of the carotid artery caused the convulsive death of all the old animals in 0.5–4 hours, but only 20 per cent of the young animals died in spite of pronounced signs of ischemia. The content of triglycerides, free fatty acids, glucose, corticosterone, and blood urea nitrogen sharply increases in old animals when their carotid artery is ligated.

Golovchenko and Potapenko (1978), our fellow workers, have shown that the administration of vasopressin, which causes the spasm of the brain vessels, does not change the content of adenyl nucleotides in mature rats and reduces the content of ATP and creatine phosphate in old rats (Fig. 13). However, there are contradictory data. According to Ferrendelli and others (1971), brain anoxia for ten seconds caused a greater drop in the ATP level (especially in the striatum) of rats 29 months old than in the level of those 4 months old. Mankovsky and Belonog (1974) observed that the shifts in the EEG were less pronounced in old persons that in young persons during short-term hypoxic hypoxia (the inhalation of a gas mixture with a low oxygen content). According to Timko

(1971), the rate at which a stimulus is propagated along the arm nerve changes more in young persons than in old persons when the arm is bound by an elastic bandage. In any case, greater resistance is observed in old persons during short-term hypoxia because the intensity of tissue respiration is reduced in them in the initial state. When hypoxia is prolonged, the insufficiency of the energy processes produces its effect and the shifts become more significant in old age.

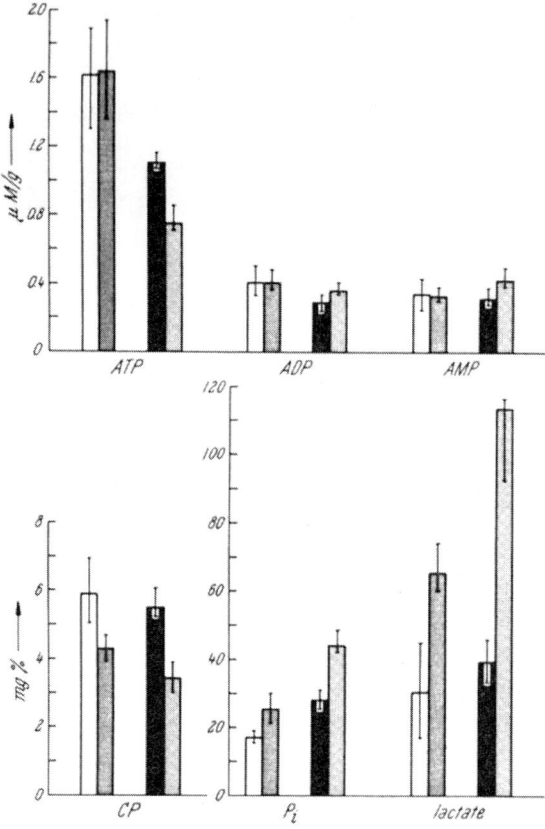

Fig. 13. Content of ATP, ADP, AMP, creatine phosphate, inorganic phosphorus and lactate in the brain of mature rats (first pair of columns) and old rats (second pair of columns) and their change under the influence of vasopressin (2.0 U/kg) (second column in each pair)

Much data show that the tissue respiration of the brain becomes less intense in old age. This decrease is expressed to a different extent in various brain structures and occurs during different age periods. For instance, the intensity of tissue respiration sharply decreases in the hypothalamus during the first four months of age, and afterwards it gradually changes. In the hippocampus and the amygdalae, this decrease is observed from three weeks to four months of age, and then after 12 months of age. Peng and others (1977) compared their own data on a change in oxygen consumption by the homogenates of the cortex, the hippocampus, the amygdalae and the hypothalamus with the other researchers' data on the number and density of neurons and concluded that the decrease in oxygen consumption with age primarily depends on the functional state of individual neurons and not on a diminution of their number.

Oxygen consumption by the brain occurs most intensively in rats 0.5–1 months old (Fig. 14A, B, C). Tissue respiration of the hemispheres, the cerebellum and the brain stem becomes less intense when they are 8–10 months old. Later, oxygen consumption by the hemispheres and the cerebellum does not change, but that by the brain stem diminishes (Potapenko, 1974). A decrease in the number of oxidative substrates somewhat reduces the intensity of tissue

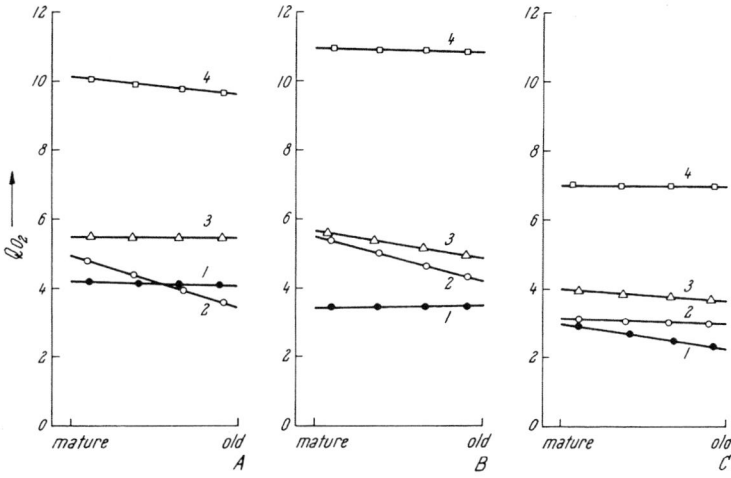

Fig. 14. Consumption of oxygen by the homogenates of various parts of the brain of rats. *A* major hemisphere; *B* cerebellum; *C* brain stem. In the absence of a substrate *(1)* and when glucose *(2)*, alpha-ketoglutarate *(3)* and succinate *(4)* are added

respiration. The addition of succinate, alpha-ketoglutarate and glucose increases tissue respiration to a different extent. Tissue respiration of mature rats does not greatly differ from that of old rats. The addition of glucose to the homogenate of the hemispheres of old rats reduces the intensity of tissue respiration (from 4.07 ± 0.09 to $3.24 \pm 0.31 \, \mu g \, O_2$/mg of dry tissue per hour). Patel (1977) has shown that less glucose is utilized by the brain in old age. The usage of various substrates is redistributed with age. Moreover, the potentialities of the system of tissue respiration are reduced and some of its mechanisms are mobilized in the initial state in old age. Hence, hypoxic states develop during intense activity and the range of tissue respiration becomes limited when substrates and hormones are given. According to Parmacek and others (1979), the intracellular utilization of oxygen becomes inadequate in old animals when the load on the energy supply system increases. The age difference is revealed in the third state of mitochondrial oxidation (during intense work with excess ADP) and not in the fourth one (the state of rest, the absence of free ADP, which has been completely converted into ATP).

The succinoxidase system is one of the most stable systems not only in the brain, but also in the heart in old age (Frolkis, Bogatskaya, 1965; McGeer *et al.*, 1971). In this respect, we proposed that succinates should be used to optimize the energy processes in old age. It has been shown that cardiac activity improves and the content of adenyl nucleotides increases in normal and pathological states when they are used (Frolkis *et al.*, 1976d). According to Dilman (1976b), the prolonged administration of succinic acid restores the function of the hypothalamic centres.

Anaerobic and aerobic glycolysis greatly attenuates, hexokinase becomes less active, the pyruvate content diminishes and the ratio between pyruvate and lactate decreases by old age (Potapenko, 1974). Fox and others (1975) did not detect any changes in the intensity of glycolysis in the brain in old age, while Aksyenova (1973) has reported that it intensifies. According to our data, the content of ATP in the brain decreases by 25 per cent and that of creatine phosphate, by 16 per cent when oxidative and glycolytic phosphorylations are reduced.

Neurons are excitable structures and the electric occurrences on the cell membranes, i. e. the active and passive transport of ions, are decisive in their functions. According to Kuprash (1974), the content of intracellular potassium in the brain decreases, while that of sodium increases in old age. A change in the activity of K^+- and Na^+-ATPase is believed to be of great importance. Potapenko (1974) has shown that the activity of K^+- and Na^+-ATPase irregularly decreases in various parts of the brain in old age (Fig. 15 A, B, C, D). A decrease in the activity of the transport ATPase can change the value of the rest potential of the cells and influence the nature of the action potentials and the lability of the nerve cells.

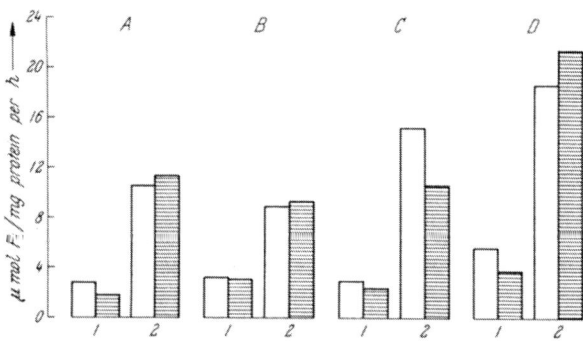

Fig. 15. Activity of Na^+- and K^+-ATPase *(1)* and Mg^{2+}-ATPase *(2)* in some structures of the brain of rats of different ages. Homogenates of: cerebral cortex *(A)*; white matter of the hemispheres *(B)*; brain stem *(C)*; microsomal fraction of cerebral cortex *(D)*. The white columns stand for mature rats and the shaded columns for old rats

We have good reasons to maintain that the shifts in energy supply are a cause of a change in the functions of the receptors in old age (Frolkis, 1970). In old animals, the reflexes of vascular chemoreceptors are not stable and are rapidly exhausted. However, they are restored when ATP and the substrates of the Krebs cycle are added to the perfusate.

According to modern concepts, the primary mechanisms of aging are connected with molecular and genetic changes, which are the main causes of the subsequent developments in the cell. There are contradictory data on the content and renewal of protein, RNA and DNA in various brain structures in old age (Finch, 1973; Rand, Ansari, 1980). The data on the total amount of DNA, RNA and protein offer little information, since they conceal contradictory shifts in the synthesis and breakdown of these substances.

The mechanisms of a change in the genetic apparatus of the nerve cells and in protein biosynthesis can be understood from the standpoint of the genoregulatory hypothesis of aging, according to which the primary mechanisms of cellular aging are connected with genome regulation (Frolkis, 1969, 1970, 1975). In old age, the content of histone proteins increases and that of non-histone ones decreases in chromatin. Histones are believed to act as repressors. At the same time, the loci of great DNA activity contain a larger amount of non-histone proteins. A change in the given relationships probably limits the activity of the genetic apparatus of the cell. As the protein-DNA bond becomes more durable, the whole genoregulatory system of the cell apparently becomes less mobile. Data on a change in genome activity in the neuron are a very important confirmation of the genoregulatory hypothesis. Cutler (1973) showed that the number of varieties of the RNA being synthesized decreases in old age, while Johnson and Erner (1972) as well as Strehler (1977) ascertained that not only the renewal of total RNA decreases, but also the synthesis of its individual fractions irregularly changes with age. The number of genes, which are responsible for rRNA synthesis, decreases by 40–50 per cent in very old age (Gaubatz, Cutler, 1978; Strehler, Chang, 1979). A shift in genome regulation, being determined by DNA-protein binding, is a cause of these changes in the brain. According to Strehler (1977), the copies of the gene, which is responsible for the production of rRNA, gradually disappear in the nerve cells. These regulatory shifts occur as the dimensions of the DNA molecules in the brain tissue remain unchanged (Ono et al., 1976), their nucleotide composition remains the same (Vanyushin et al., 1973), and the effectiveness of the reparation of unifilamental ruptures of DNA remains high (Tretyak et al., 1977). According to Herrmann (1975), however, there is twice as much cross-linked DNA in the brain of an old rat as in the liver. Moreover, macromolecules become less resistant to damaging factors (Kanungo et al., 1970; Zs.-Nagy I., Zs.-Nagy V., 1975).

In our laboratory, Muradian (unpublished data) compared the changes which occur with age in the synthesis of RNA and protein in eight structures of the rat brain (the frontal and motor regions of the cerebral cortex, the caudate nucleus, the hippocampus, the hypothalamus, the hypophysis, the brain stem, and the spinal cord). He found that the renewal of RNA and protein decreases to the greatest extent when the animals are from 4 to 8 months old, and then the renewal diminishes gradually until they are 24 months old. The relative specific radioactivity of RNA decreases most of all in the caudate nucleus and the hypothalamus. The calculation of the ratio between the relative specific radioactivity of RNA and the relative radioactivity of protein is interesting. The ratio seems to characterize the correlation between transcription and translation.

Its value gradually decreases with age for the frontal and the motor regions of the cortex, the caudate nucleus and the hippocampus, but increases for the hypothalamus. The value does not substantially change for the brain stem and the spinal cord. Hence, transcription and translation non-uniformly change with age in various parts of the brain.

Theoretically, genes which did not function earlier can be activated and new proteins, which substantially change the state of the nerve cell, can be synthesized as a result of the shifts in genome regulation. According to Cutler (1973), new types of RNA that are not found in young animals appear in the nerve cells in old age.

Thus, the changes in the regulation of the genome of the nerve cells are the main mechanism of neuronal aging, while the age shifts in the function of the nerve cells and in the brain function play an important role in the change which occurs in protein biosynthesis in other organs and tissues. Hence, the change in the regulation of the genome of neurons is the pacemaker of the organism's aging.

The age changes in protein biosynthesis can cause an extremely important change in brain activity, i. e. they can reduce the brain's ability to process and accumulate information and worsen memory. Short-term memory is connected with an active state of the reverberating chain without noticeable biochemical shifts. Long-term memory is determined by the consolidation of biochemical shifts in definite classes of RNA and protein.

The mechanisms of brain activity, interneuronal relationships and synaptic conduction are realized with the participation of the transmitter systems. The shifts in mediator metabolism are believed to be the molecular basis of a change in brain activity during aging. Hence, there has been much written on the age dynamics of mediator metabolism (Frolkis, Bezrukov, 1979). Let us discuss only some general conclusions. After comparing the general indices of the brain's development, i. e. the glioneuronal index, total protein, the content of RNA and DNA, an increase in the number of synaptosomal contacts with the growth of the concentration of monoamines in the whole brain or in its structures, and the single direction of the processes which maintain their level, many authors have drawn the conclusion that the age changes in monoamines during the early periods of development are coupled with the differentiation and maturation of the nerve structures.

Pronounced changes occur in the mechanisms of adrenergic transfer with age. The greatest shifts occur in the catecholaminergic systems as the organism ages. According to Finch (1976), the shifts in the metabolism of biogenic amines in the hypothalamus initiate the age changes in the hypo-thalamo-hypophysial-endocrine sytem. The changes in this system are largely the cause of aging and age pathology. Substantial changes in catecholamine metabolism occur in the nigrostriatal-pallidal system. They disturb fine movements and create the prerequisites for the development of parkinsonism, which is also connected with the disturbance of catecholamine metabolism. The extent of a change in this metabolism can be seen even from the fact that the activity of tyrosine hydroxylase decreases by 32 per cent in the hypothalamus and the caudate nucleus of rats (Algeri *et al.*, 1977), by 50 per cent in their

Substantia nigra (Cote, Kremzner, 1975), by 61 per cent in the amygdaloid complex, and by 41 per cent in the putamen (McGeer, McGeer, 1975). The activity of dopa decarboxylase decreases by 50 per cent in *Substantia nigra* and the hypothalamus (Cote, Kremzner, 1975) and by 35–72 per cent in the putamen and the caudate nucleus (McGeer, McGeer, 1975). Obviously, such a great change in enzymic activity influences catecholamine metabolism in several brain structures. In fact, the rate of noradrenaline renewal in the hypothalamus and the striate body diminishes by 25–50 per cent in old mice and rats (Finch, 1973; Ponzio *et al.,* 1978).

The disturbances in catecholamine metabolism create "weak" links in the central regulation systems. For instance, the disturbance of dopaminergic regulation can upset sleep in old age. According to Prinz and others (1979), falling asleep is more difficult, the duration of the fourth phase of sleep is 90 per cent shorter and the duration of paradoxical sleep is 27 per cent less, while wakefulness at night is 100 per cent longer in old persons than in young persons. Rosenberg and others (1979) showed in their experiments with rats that, with age, the total amplitude of the delta-wave activity does not change during sleep, the relative duration of the paradoxical phase of sleep decreases, the periods of sleep diminish, their number grown, and the daily rhythms of sleep are smoothed out.

Substantia nigra participates in the regulation of finger motion, which must be very exact. A change in the dopaminergic mechanisms of the hypothalamus disturbs the cyclic, ovulatory function of ovary. Attention should be especially paid to the adrenergic mechanisms of the reticular substance, which participates in the regulation of the excitability and tonicity of all the parts of the brain, including the cerebral cortex. Therefore, a pronounced change which occurs in catecholamine metabolism in the reticular formation with age can cause a change in the facilitating and inhibiting effects on other parts of the brain. Climacteric neuroses, depression and presenile psychoses develop when the adrenergic mechanisms of the brain are disturbed.

In their experiments in which young (3–4 months) and old (24–27 months) rats swam, Marshall and Berrios (1979) saw that old animals moved their legs less vigorously than young ones, and that they held their head above water with difficulty and could not keep an almost horizontal position of their body. Such disturbances could be reproduced in young animals when the dopamine-containing neurons are damaged. The disturbances in swimming were either eliminated or their extent was reduced by administering the stimulating agent of dopamine receptors, i. e. apomorphine, and the precursor of dopamine in biosynthesis, namely, *l*-dopa. According to those researchers, some of the motor disturbances occur in old age due to the age changes in the dopaminergic system. Small doses of apomorphine (0.25 mg/kg) were more effective in old animals, while large doses of it (2 mg/kg) produced the same effect in young and old animals. *L*-dopa (50 and 100 mg/kg) was more effective in old animals.

Shifts in serotonin metabolism play an important role in the molecular mechanisms of the age changes which occur in the activity of the brain. The greatest changes in serotonin metabolism occur in the limbic system and the brain stem. For instance, the activity of tryptophan 5-hydroxylase decreases by

39 per cent in *Nucleus raphe dorsalis,* the septum and the hippocampus. The serotonin content diminishes by 29–50 per cent in the hippocampus, *Nucleus raphe dorsalis* and the ventral nucleus of the pons. These shifts can probably participate in a change in sexual behaviour, sleep, memory, and the emotional aspects of stress.

Acetylcholine metabolism changes in various brain structures vary widely in old age. In the human brain, for instance, the activity of choline acetyltransferase decreases by 13–65 per cent in old age (McGeer *et al.,* 1971). Perry (1980) found that the activity of choline acetyltransferase and the amount of muscarinic receptors decrease, while the activity of acetylcholinesterase remains unchanged in various regions of the old person's brain. The activity of choline acetyltransferase and acetylcholinesterase decreases, the activity of butyrylcholinesterase increases, while the amount of muscarinic receptors remains unchanged in persons suffering from Alzheimer's disease. According to Perry (1980), the change in the cholinergic system of the brain may be an important mechanism of normal aging and Alzheimer's disease. He believes that normal aging is connected with the shifts in the nerve endings, while the shifts spread to the cholinergic processes in Alzheimer's disease. According to McGeer and others (1971), these shifts are far less in the rat brain, while no changes occur in most structures. Such a species relationship has been observed also when the activity of acetylcholinesterase was studied.

A decrease in the activity of cholinesterase in some brain structures is of definite adaptive significance when mediator synthesis diminishes. This decrease promotes the accumulation of the mediator which is needed for transmitting an impulse through the synapse. Shifts in the synthesis and breakdown of acetylcholine may influence the state of reticular formation, the regulation of the functions of the spinal cord, and so forth.

Much data indicate that the content of gamma-aminobutyric acid in the brain and the activity of glutamate decarboxylase in the brain stem and the cerebellum remain unchanged. According to Gordienko and others (1975), the content of gamma-aminobutyric acid decreases in both the whole brain and the hypothalamus in rats.

The brain functions normally only when its mediatory systems are balanced. The relationship between the mediatory systems changes with age. This change is the molecular basis of the disturbance of the brain functions.

Change in the Brain Functions with Age

Obvious and significant changes occur in the functions of the central nervous system with age. The first signs of their appearance do not need to be specially described. An aging person probably first of all notices that his mental and muscular working ability has diminished and his quick reactions have slowed down, that he has become less attentive and his memory has weakened, that it is more difficult for him to assimilate something new and his emotional background has changed, and so forth.

Aging processes as well as vitauct processes develop in the complex and diffucult field of psychic activity with age. These processes determine the appearance of the most important adaptive regulatory mechanisms which, in spite of the progressing structural and metabolic changes in the brain, make it possible to maintain a high level of creative activity for a long time and to fully perceive the surrounding environment and produce adequate reactions.

Fig. 16 A, B shows two curves which characterize the influence of age on the scientists' creative activity. They were plotted from much data on the peak of creative work and on the time when the greatest discoveries were made. Of

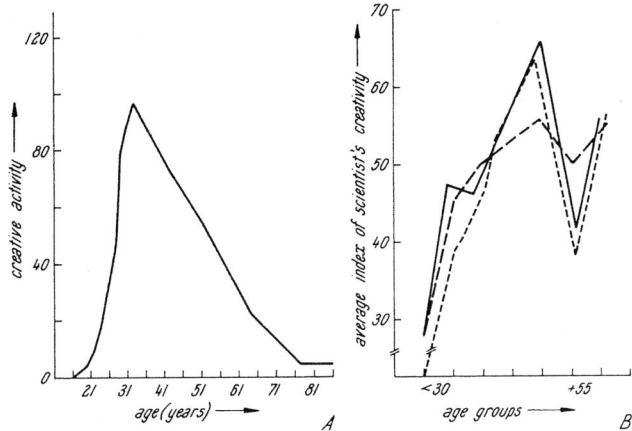

Fig. 16. Influence of age on the creative work of persons: *A* Lehman's curve as compared with creative activity at the age of 18; *B* Pelz and Andrew's curve as compared with creative activity at the age of 30. Continuous line—scientific contribution; dashed line—general usefulness; dotted line—published articles

course, such curves will differ for scientists who are engaged in different fields. However, their general regularities will remain unchanged. Lehmann (1943) maintains that creative work reaches its peak at the age of 35–39. According to Pelz and Andrew (1973), the second peak of the creative potential is observed at the age of 55–60, i. e. in persons with distinct age changes in the central nervous system. Wechsler (1961) believes that intelligence for young persons is most probably mental readiness and the ability to study and solve new problems, while for elderly and old persons, it is the ability to cope with many tasks on the basis of rich experience gained in life. Schonfeldt and Owens (1966) studied persons engaged in mental work and obtained a pattern of the intellect's stationary state from the age 20 to age 60. A longitudinal examination was made of persons 20–30 years old and was repeated 35–40 years later; however, it did not reveal any diminution of intellectual capacity (Gilbert, 1973). According to the American Psychological Association, intellectual capacities greatly diminish in elderly persons largely due to diseases, economic difficulties, social isolation and other causes which are not connected with aging.

In old age, the memory of current events becomes weaker, while the memory of the events of the distant past is retained. Mankovsky and Mints (1972) have shown that when an aspect of mechanical remembrance sharply diminishes in old age, the logical sense aspect remains and becomes especially important in a person's memory. Old persons continue to have a systemic memory, which enables them to reproduce events. Experience and knowledge allow an old person to correctly assess a situation and draw correct conclusions, while another person must make many test before he can do this. Adaptive mechanisms have been revealed in old age when a person had not only mental, but also physical working ability. Our fellow workers have described the "discontinuity phenomenon" in conformity with which the contractile forces gradually diminish in young persons when they do muscular work for a long time. In old persons, individual discontinuities of activity are observed when their working ability is still on a high level. In this case, an old person stops working even when the level of his working ability is relatively high. This "discontinuity phenomenon" is probably connected with the development of intracentral inhibition, which prevents an old person from becoming very weary.

Many works have recently been written on the age changes in mentality, higher nervous activity, the brain's integrative activity, and electro-encephalograms. Pavlov's works on the age changes in conditioned reflexes probably constitute the basis in this respect. His works are of fundamental significance in the modern neurophysiology of aging, since they correctly formulate the most important regularities of the dynamics of the basic nervous processes in old age. It has been shown in experiments with animals and in investigations involving persons that, in old age, conditioned reflexes are produced more slowly and are extinguished more gradually, differentiation is realized with greater difficulty, the restorative processes become less intense, and so forth. Internal inhibition is the first to be affected with age. It is followed by the force of excitation, mobility and the equilibrium of the main nervous processes. An important fact is that nervous processes can be optimized in elderly and old persons under definite conditions.

Modern studies of the brain's integrative activity are thoroughly reviewed in the work by Birren and Schaie (1977) and in our monographs (Frolkis, 1970; Frolkis, Bezrukov, 1979). Although much has been written on the brain's structure, metabolism and integrative activity, the neurophysiological experimental analysis of its aging is still not on a sufficiently high level.

Our fellow workers have obtained data on a change which occurs with age in the neuronal functions of some regions of the brain. According to Tanin (1977), the membrane potential (MP) of neurons does not change substantially with age. This potential of the motoneurons of the fifth and sixth lumbar segments is 58.4 ± 1.4 mV in rats 8–10 months old and 56.5 ± 1.7 mV in rats 24–26 months old. The MP of the non-identified neurons of the spinal cord, the bulk of which is made if interneurons, is 39.3 ± 0.74 mV and 40.6 ± 0.7 mV, respectively. The MP of the neurons of the motor region of the cerebral cortex of rats ranges from 14 to 72 mV, averaging 27.4 ± 1.1 mV in rats 8–10 months old and 25.9 ± 2.2 mV in rats 24–26 months old. This unchangeability of the MP of neurons conceals definite age distinctions. Neurons with low and high values of MP are frequently found in the general mass of the nerve cells in old rats. Such different values of MP are probably characteristic of atrophied and hypertrophied cells. Hypertrophy develops due to the activation of protein biosynthesis in the cell, while this activation causes the growth of the MP value.

The excitability of the neurons of the motor cortex of the brain does not change, but the excitability of the motoneurons of the spinal cord somewhat diminishes in old age. The excitability threshold of the motoneurons of the spinal cord, being determined by intracellular stimulation, is 2.5×10^{-9}–5.0×10^{-9}A, averaging $(3.0 \pm 0.3) \times 10^{-9}$A, in rats 8–10 months old and 1.0×10^{-9}–3.0×10^{-9}A, averaging $(2.0 \pm 0.2) \times 10^{-9}$A, in rats 24–26 months old.

The nature of the action potential of individual nerve cells changes in old age. The life span of the antidromic spike of motoneurons averages 1.02 ± 0.09 millisecond in young rats and 1.65 ± 0.14 millisecond in old rats ($p < 0.01$). This shift is due to an increase in the anterior front of the action potential from 0.41 to 0.65 millisecond and largely in its posterior front from 0.61 to 1.0 millisecond. The shift in the antidromic spike is followed by delayed depolarization (a small wave at the base of the spike), which is caused by the propagation of the excitation wave towards the dendrites. The antidromic responses of the motoneurons of old animals as a rule have no such wave.

Tanin has shown that the inhibiting postsynaptic potentials (IPSP) also change in old animals. These potentials are reproduced when the axon of the neuron being studied is stimulated. The duration of mainly the anterior front of IPSP changes, probably being due to a decrease in the content of intracellular potassium. The lability of neurons, i. e. their ability to generate frequent action potentials during depolarization, decreases in old animals. The motoneurons of the spinal cord respond to the intensification of the polarizing current by multiple charges with a frequency of up to 300 impulses per second in mature rats and only 80–100 impulses per second in old rats (Fig. 17).

Martynenko has shown substantial age changes in the electric properties of the nerve cell by using the neurons of the minor parietal ganglion of molluscs. In old animals, the threshold of the direct stimulation of neurons increases, impulse activity, the rate of diminution of the posterior front of the action potential and the value of trace hyperpolarization decrease, while input membrane resistance and the amplitude of the action potential remain unchanged (Fig. 18 A). Hence, there is certain similarity in the changes which occur with age in the functions of the nerve cells in animals of various species, ranging from invertebrates to higher animals.

The change in the electric phenomena in the nerve cell is due to the shifts in the basic properties of the cell membrane and in the mechanisms of active ionic transport. It is believed that there are two types of active ionic transport: (1) ion exchange between intra- and extracellular environments without any influence on the transmembranous difference of potentials (charge for charge), and (2) active "electrogenous" transport, which produces the difference of potentials on the membrane. Membranous K^+- and Na^+-ATPase is decisive in the mechanism of this transport. The activity of ATPase is selectively blocked by ouabain. The more does the electrogenous transport mechanism help to maintain the transmembranous difference of potentials, the greater is its diminution after membranous K^+- and Na^+-ATPase is blocked by ouabain.

The sensitivity of the nerve cells to hormone action changes with age. Their sensitivity to some hormones grows in old age. The hyperpolarization of the

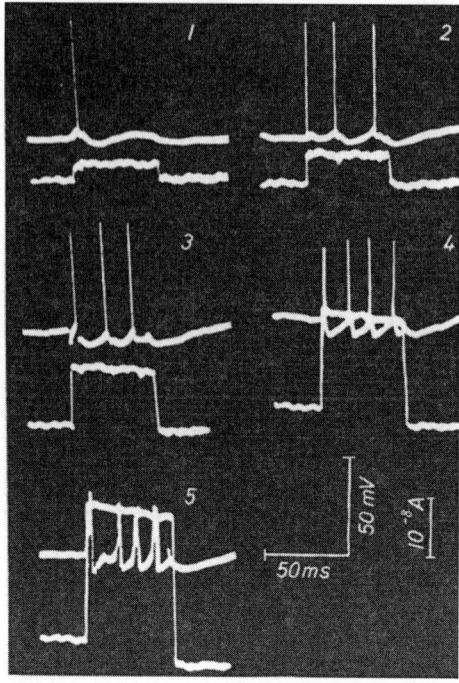

Fig. 17. Multiple discharges of the motoneurons of an old rat in the case of stimulation by rectangular current impulses. The force of stimulation *(1–5)* increases from 0.25×10^{-8} to 2×10^{-8}A. The upper lines are the responses of the cell, and the lower lines are the stimuli

neurons of the spinal cord is 2.5 times greater in old rats than in mature rats when adrenaline is administered in a dose of 3–10 μg per 100 g of weight. But when insulin or estradiol dipropionate is administered, the neurons of only mature rats are hyperpolarized (Tanin, 1977). However, the sensitivity of the neurons of the sensorimotor region of the cerebral cortex to insulin and estradiol dipropionate does not change in old age.

That change in the sensitivity of the nerve cells is connected with not only chronological age, but also the aging process itself, since the change is observed in mammals with different life spans as well as in invertebrates. According to Martynenko, the sensitivity of the neurons of the minor parietal ganglion of old molluscs to adrenaline grows, but it does not change with respect to insulin (Fig. 18B, C).

The reaction of the cells to physiologically active substances is determined by the amount and state of their receptors. There are different data on a change in neuronal receptor in old age. Obviously, their amount changes differently in the neurons of various parts of the brain. The number of beta-adrenoreceptors in the brain is believed to diminish in old age (Makman *et al.*, 1979; Weiss *et al.*, 1979). However, there are data on the unchangeability of the number of beta-adrenoreceptors in old age (Bylund *et al.*, 1977). In determining the number of receptor sites in the cerebral cortex by atropine binding, James and

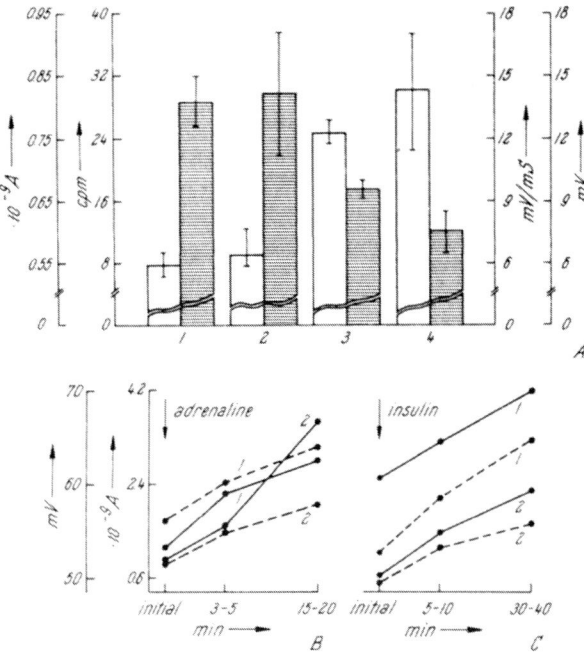

Fig. 18. A change in the threshold of direct stimulation (1), the frequency of spontaneous impulse activity (2), the rate of diminution of the posterior front of the action potential (3) and the value of the trace hyperpolarization of the action potentials (4) of the neurons of adult molluscs (white columns) and old molluscs (shaded columns). B change in the membrane potential (1) and the threshold of the direct stimulation (2) of the neurons of adult molluscs (continuous line) and old molluscs (dashed line) under the influence of adrenaline. C change in the membrane potential (1) and the threshold of the direct stimulation (2) of the neurons of adult molluscs (continuous line) and old molluscs (dashed line) under the influence of insulin

Kanungo (1976) drew the conclusion that the number of cholinoreceptors decreases in old rats.

Rogova and Khilko (1971), who work in our laboratory, used the method proposed by Turpaev (1962) and showed that the so-called "acetylcholine wave," which is observed during mercurimetric titration, originates when smaller doses of acetylcholine are added to old rats brain homogenates (Fig. 19 A, B). This fact indicates that the cholinoreceptors in the brain and the cerebellum of old animals are more sensitive to the action of acetylcholine. It has been shown that the number of corticosteroid-sensitive (Roth, 1976) and estrogen-sensitive (Kanungo, 1975) receptors diminishes in the cerebral cortex.

Our data on the specifics of the action of substances which block the appropriate groups of receptors indirectly confirm that the number of receptors in the brain decreases with age. In mature rats, the effects of the descending influences of the reticular formation of the brain stem on the spinal cord are blocked by scopolamine in a dose of 40–50 μg per 100 g of body weight, by glycine in a dose of 90–100 μg per 100 g of body weight, and by dehydro-ergotoxine in a dose of 30–40 μg per 100 g of body weight. In old animals, they

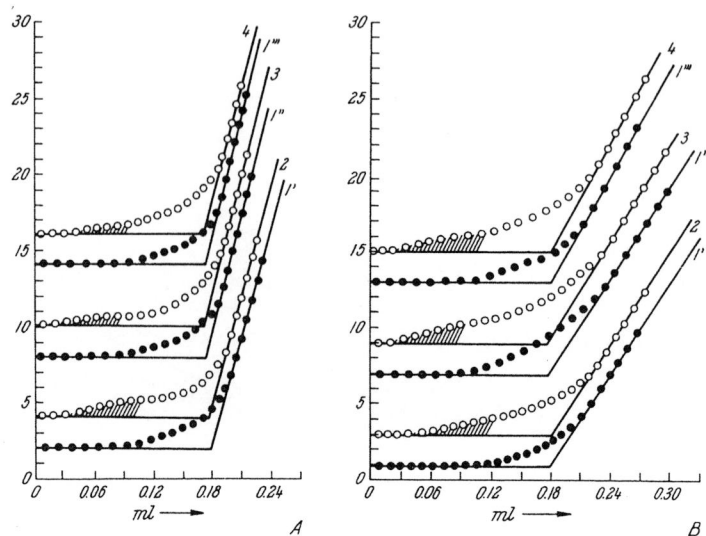

Fig. 19. Mercurimetric titration of the –SH groups of the water-soluble proteins of the cerebral cortex (A) and the cerebellum (B) of rats of different age. The ordinate is the force of the current in the microamperemeter scale division, and the abscissa is the volume of 5×10^{-4} M $HgCl_2$ (ml). A 1 control; 2 in the presence of acetylcholine in a concentration of 1×10^{-13} g/mg (rats 1 month old); 3 in the presence of acetylcholine in a concentration of 1×10^{-13} g/ml (rats 6 months old); 4 in the presence of acetylcholine in a concentration of 1×10^{-20} g/ml (rats 24–26 months old). The shaded part is the "acetylcholine wave"; the volume of the substrate is 1.5 ml. B 1 control; 2 in the presence of acetylcholine in a concentration of 1×10^{-5} g/ml (rats 1 month old); 3 in the presence of acetylcholine in a concentration of 1×10^{-5} g/ml (rats 6 months old); 4 in the presence of acetylcholine in a concentration of 11×10^{-6} g/ml (rats 24–26 months old). The shaded part is the "acetylcholine wave"; the volume of the substrate is 1.8 ml

are blocked by smaller doses (12–18 μg, 40–50 μg and 15–20 μg per 100 g of body weight, respectively).

Many hormones and mediators influence the cell through adenylate cyclase, which catalyzes the formation of cyclic adenosine nucleotide. Many researchers regard adenylate cyclase as the catalytic part of the receptor that is on the inner side of the membrane, and cyclic AMP, as the second mediator in the chain of influences on the cell. Schmidt and Thornberry (1978) found that the basal level of cyclic AMP and cyclic GMP does not change in the cerebral cortex, the structures of the limbic system and the striate body. According to Govoni and others (1977), the activity of adenylate cyclase remains unchanged in old age. However, its reaction to catecholamines and histamine is either reduced (Puri, Volicer, 1977; Makman *et al.*, 1979) or remains unchanged (Schmidt, Thornberry, 1978) in old age. Govoni and others (1977) have observed that adenylate cyclase of the retina becomes more sensitive to dopamine and apomorphine in old age. Maggi and others (1979) studied the binding of the receptors of gamma-aminobutyric acid and beta-adrenoreceptors in various regions of the brain of rats 3, 12 and 24 months old and found that the binding of the receptors of gamma-aminobutyric acid does not change with age in any of the regions which were studied, but beta-adrenoreceptors are bound less in the cerebellum and the brain stem of rats 24 months old, while this binding does not change in their cerebral cortex.

A similar decrease in the binding of the beta-adrenoreceptors in the cerebellum has been observed in persons 61–80 years old (in comparison with children up to the age of two and persons 40–60 years old). No difference has been observed in the binding of the beta-adrenoreceptors of the cerebral cortex by ^{3}H-isoproterenol. According to Govoni and others (1980), the binding of the GABA-receptors by ^{3}H-spiroperidol is substantially reduced in *Substantia nigra* and the hypothalamus of old rats, but it remains unchanged in their cerebral cortex, the cerebellum, the striatum and *Nucleus accumbens*.

Thus, the number of neuronal receptors of various physiologically active substances and the number of receptors in various brain structures change differently with age. An important correction must always be made when the shift in the number of receptors is assessed. In most cases, the number of receptors is determined not in one neuron, but in a portion of tissue, in which the number of cells varies during different age periods. The number of neurons is known to diminish by 30–50 per cent in some structures in old age, i. e. the decrease in their number is frequently more than the decrease in the calculated receptor number.

We believe that not only the number of receptors, but also their conformation changes in old age. In some cases, these changes hinder the receptor and the physiologically active substance from interacting with one another, while in others, they enhance their affinity for one another. The sensitivity of the interneurons of the spinal cord to insulin and estradiol dipropionate sharply decreases in old rats. Tanin showed that the receptors in old rats become just as sensitive as in young ones when Ionol is administered. Ionol is an effective antioxidant. By reducing the number of free radicals, it apparently helps to restore the lipid microenvironment of the receptors, return their conformation, and produce the initial reaction. In this case, the properties of the receptors, and not their number, change the receptor-hormone interaction. Golovchenko has observed that a group of cell receptors which react to very low concentrations of vasopressin appears in old age.

The reactivity of the cell decreases when the number of receptors diminishes. A change in the sensitivity of neurons to humoral factors can be determined by (a) a change in the number and conformation properties of receptors, (b) a change in the properties of adenylate cyclase, (c) a change in the arrangement of receptors on the membrane and their localization with respect to the synaptic cleft, (d) a decrease in the activity of the systems of hormone and mediator degradation and the attenuation of reuptake, and (e) shifts in the postreceptor mechanisms which regulate effects.

"What does the fact of adaptation consist in? Nothing, except for an exact link of elements of a complex system between themselves and their entire set with the surrounding situation" (Pavlov, 1951c). This fully characterizes the brain's adaptive mechanisms, which become manifested with age on the basis of the above-mentioned neuronal changes. The brain ages as a complex system in which some intracentral mechanisms become weak, while others are activated. An aging brain is a qualitatively different functional system.

The central nervous system is characterized by a programmed type of activity. The leading programme necessarily includes the analysis and synthesis of the organism's external and internal environments. Owing to the programming principle, the organism not only works according to the "stimulus-response" pattern, but also prevents possible changes by its activity and thus achieves the optimal forms of adaptation. Anokhin (1968) wrote: "A certain afferent model which can anticipate the parameters of the future results and can, at the end of action, compare this prediction with the parameters of real results is formed together with an efferent 'command' in all the cases when the brain sends stimuli through the terminal neurons to the peripheral working apparatus."

The main integrative neurophysiological mechanisms of aging are: (a) a change in the central programme caused by functional shifts in the state of various nerve centres and by differently oriented changes in the state of individual neurons; (b) the limitation of the flow of information which comes along the efferent pathways, and (c) a change in the nature of return information which goes to the centres (feed-back mechanisms). Consequently, the content of an independent programme changes, the inconsistency between the programme and the results of its realization grows, the number of incorrigible "errors" in the organism's activity increase, and the fine modulation of programmes is lost. Our analysis of the intracentral relationship shows that such mechanisms of aging of the central nervous system exist. The creation of a dynamic stereotype, i. e. a complex system of conditioned reflexes, is an example of the formation of the central programme. Buzunov (1969), our fellow worker, has compared the formations of the stereotype in persons 20–25 years old and in persons 55–60 years old. The system of successive conditioned-reflex changes in muscular working ability was incorporated into the stereotype. As Fig. 20

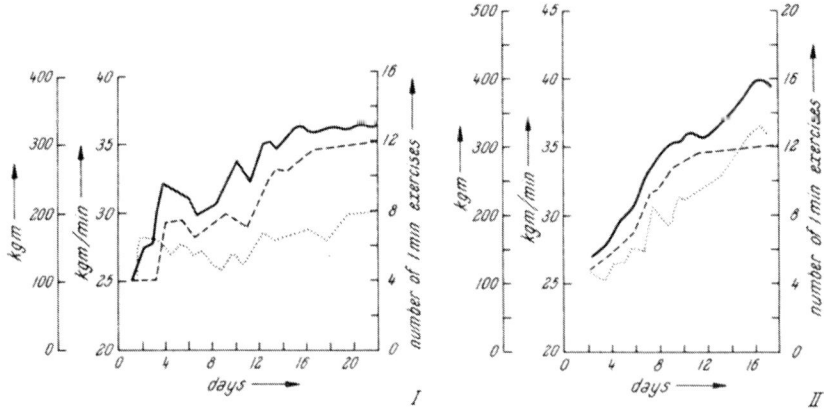

Fig. 20. Age specifics of the change in muscular working ability when the motor dynamic stereotype is being formed. *I* in persons 55–60 years old; *II* in persons 25–30 years old. Continuous line–total amount of work being done, kgm; dotted line–amount of work, kgm/min; dashed line–amount of one-minute work being done

shows, the stereotype is produced more slowly in elderly persons and, what is most important, its structure changes. In elderly persons, working ability grows mainly due to the amount of the single type of work being done, while in young persons, besides that, the amount of work done per minute increases. Work involving the typical reproduction of the rhythms of activity is the most difficult for elderly persons. According to Potvin and others (1980), many neurological functions in persons decrease linearly with age. In old age, the ability to count decreases by 29 per cent, the rapidity with which usual activities are carried out, by 30 per cent, the ability to control the muscle load on the hand, by 63 per cent, the rapidity of reactions, by 28 per cent, the rapidity of motion, by 51 per cent, and coordination, by 27 per cent.

Owing to the complex combination of vitauct and aging, diversely oriented changes in the excitability of individual brain structures occur with age. The reactions of the cardiovascular system can be produced by stimulating various brain structures. This can be done because the programme for not only certain complex acts and behavioural reactions, but also their vegetative ensurance is localized in definite centres. Fig. 21A, B, C gives Bezrukov's data on the electric thresholds of the pressor influences of various central nervous structures: they increase with respect to the sensorimotor cortex, *Medulla oblongata,* the lateral hypothalamus, and the medial nucleus of the amygdaloid complex, decrease with respect to the pyriform cortex, the central nucleus of the amygdaloid complex, and the anterior and posterior regions of the hypothalamus, and do not change with respect to the hippocampus, the reticular nuclei of the tegmentum and the pons of the midbrain, and the anterior regions of the hypothalamus. Consequently, the content of various central programmes changes differently in old age and their realization causes different peripheral effects. This is confirmed by another fact. Bezrukov (1972) studied the influence of the electric stimulation of various brain structures (i. e. those which were investigated earlier by shifts in arterial pressure) on the rhythm and depth of respiration and found that the difference in the threshold forces of stimulation in mature and old rabbits was not the same as in other cases. This indicates that a non-uniform change occurs in the influences of even the same structure on different physiological systems, namely, the systems of respiration and blood circulation, and that it is necessary to characterize the aging of a brain structure within the limits of a functional system.

The electric excitability of one brain structure substantially differs from that of another. For instance, the values of the electric current which produces pressor reactions in individual brain structures of adult rabbits range from $20 \pm 4\,\mu A$ to $410 \pm 80\,\mu A$. The excitability of some brain structures increases, while that of others decreases in old age. Consequently, the differences in intracentral excitability are somewhat evered out. In old animals, the thresholds of excitability of individual brain structures range from $40 \pm 10\,\mu A$ to $290 \pm 40\,\mu A$.

This smoothing out of the excitability gradient can probably engender irradiated and generalized reactions, disturb their strict localization, and discoordinate the peripheral effects. The fact that such a direction exists can be seen from the shifts in the coordination of motor acts, in the change in the

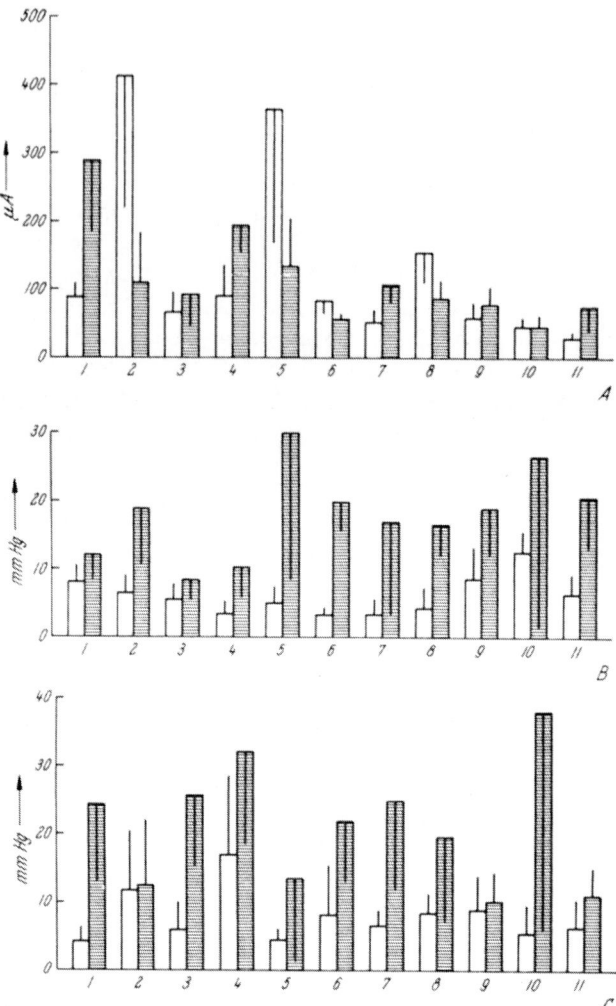

Fig. 21. Thresholds of the pressor influences of various parts of the brain (A) and the pressor reactions of arterial pressure when adrenaline (B) and acetylcholine (C) are injected in microdoses into the brain of mature rabbits (light columns) and old rabbits (shaded columns). 1, 2 sensorimotor and pyriform regions of the cerebral cortex; 3 dorsal hippocampus; 4, 5 medial and central nuclei of the amygdala; 6, 7, 8 anterior, lateral and posterior parts of the hypothalamus; 9, 10 reticular nuclei of the pons and tegmentum of the mesencephalon; 11 oblongate medulla (the fundus of the IV ventricle in the region of calamus scriptorius)

working ability of the nerve centres, in the reduction of the ability to analyze and synthesize the surrounding environment, and in the origination of the irradiated vegetative reactions.

Intracentral relationships change with age. It has been shown in our laboratory that the cortical-subcortical relationships and the subordination influences of the higher brain structures on the lower ones change with age.

Sinitsky (1976) studied the thresholds of the wakening reaction in the hippocampus (synchronization of the theta waves) and the mesencephalic reticular formation (desynchronization of the biocurrents) during the electric stimulation of the reticular nuclei of the tegmentum and showed that the reaction originated in the hippocampus when the value of the current was 0.108 ± 0.002 V in mature rats and 0.44 ± 0.004 V in old rats, and that it originated in the reticular nucleus of the tegmentum when the value of the current was 0.566 ± 0.034 V in mature rats and 0.264 ± 0.040 V in old rats. A noteworthy fact is that the excitability of the hippocampus increases substantially in old age.

Subordination influences also change with age. This fact was shown in general by Tanin (1971), who studied the development of the spinal shock. During the initial period after chordotomy, the reflex activity of the spinal cord is suppressed to a greater extent in old rats and rabbits. However, the spinal reflexes are subsequently restored more rapidly in these animals apparently because supraspinal control weakens in old age and the spinal cord slips away more rapidly from the inhibiting influence of the higher brain structures (Fig. 22).

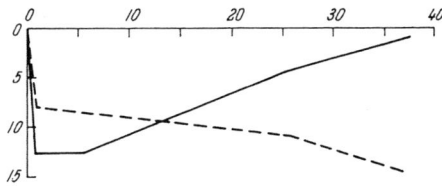

Fig. 22. Change in the excitability of the spinal cord reflexes during different lengths of time after cordotomy in animals of different age. The dashed line stands for adult rats, and the continuous line, for old rats. The abscissa is the time after cordotomy, and the ordinate is stimulus intensity (volts)

After stimulating the reticular formation of the midbrain and the pons, monosynaptic potentials were recorded and the facilitating and inhibiting effects were determined by their nature. The thresholds of the facilitating and inhibiting reticulospinal effects grow in old animals. For instance, the reflexes of the spinal cord of old rats are facilitated when the reticular formation of the brain stem is stimulated by a current which averages 0.77 (0.6–0.84) V, while inhibition occurs when the current averages 0.74 (0.64–0.84) V. In mature rats, these values are 0.46 (0.36–0.56) V and 0.42 (0.37–0.47) V, respectively. These data show that the descending facilitating and inhibiting reticulospinal effects attenuate in old age.

The values of the thresholds of the reticulospinal effects as well as the nature of the regulation of segmental polysynaptic reactions change in old animals. Thus, the threshold and subthreshold stimulation of the reticular formation causes an increase in the early polysynaptic discharge regardless of the nature of the descending influences. The mechanism of this phenomenon is probably connected with the non-uniform change in the excitability of the interneurons, which are responsible for the formation of the segmental stimulating and inhibiting postsynaptic potentials on motoneurons. That shift can help maintain reticulospinal effects in old age.

The descending influences of the sensorimotor cortex, just as the reticulospinal influences, weaken with age, but the age distinctions of their thresholds are even more pronounced. To produce the threshold inhibition of the monosynaptic potential, the cortex was stimulated by a current averaging 0.88 (0.7–1.05)V in mature rats and 1.7 (1.3–2.06)V in old rats.

Thus, substantial changes occur in the intracentral, subordinative relationships with age. The central programme may no longer conform to its realization at the periphery in old age. However, there may be situations in old age when changes in the activity of the nervous centres do not produce the appropriate effects at the periphery. Bezrukov (1967, 1969) compared the central (the electric activity of the brain) and peripheral (arterial pressure, ECG) effects after intraventricularly administering adrenaline and acetylcholine and found that shifts often occur in the EEC without the appropriate changes at the periphery in old rabbits. In other words, a central effect is produced without the appropriate peripheral component.

We have shown, together with Shchegoleva, such changes in the relationship between the central and peripheral components of the reaction when an investigation was made of the course of a convulsive seizure in animals of different age. Excitation is known to cause bradycardia during a seizure, which involves the central neurons of the vagus nerve. A seizure was reproduced by the administration of corazole. In adult rabbits, only 3 out of 14 animals had seizures which were not accompanied by bradycardia. Bradycardia originated in them in 12 out of 23 experiments when subthreshold seizure doses were administered. Bradycardia did not occur in old rabbits in 9 out of 14 experiments against the background of a seizure. In other words, the changes which occur in old age in the centres during convulsive seizures are not always realized in peripheral reactions.

Convulsive discharges which are not accompanied by a motor reaction often originate on the EEG of old animals when their hippocampus is electrically stimulated. Such changes include the "discontinuity phenomenon," which is often found when elderly persons do muscular work.

The data on the possible inconsistency of a change in the function of the nerve centres and the peripheral reaction should be taken into account when the mechanisms which realize the adaptive effects in old age are analyzed. In physiology, the central shifts are often determined by the extent of the peripheral effects. These shifts should be carefully compared in old animals and persons, since a change in the function of the centres may be inconsistent with that of the periphery. Of course, it is still difficult to see when the shifts occur during the programme's realization. They can be connected with substantial disturbances along the way leading from the centre to the effector organ (autonomic ganglia, postganglionic fibres, the peripheral synapse) and can have an intracentral origin and be blocked at the interneuronal level, which is at the very end of the way.

Data on a change in feed-back information which goes to the centres will be discussed in another chapter. This change can cause many inadequate reactions in old age.

The growing limitation of afferent signalization is typical of the aging process. It relates to information on not only the organism's external environment, but also its internal medium. An important fact is that the entry of the afferent signals into the "action acceptor" seems to change with age. For instance, the electric reactions of the brain to afferent stimulation change in old persons. According to Mankovsky and Mints (1972), the latent period of the EEG reaction to light is 0.11 ± 0.02 second in persons 17–34 years old, 0.17 ± 0.01 second in persons 40–59 years old, 0.22 ± 0.01 second in persons 60–74 years old, and 0.28 ± 0.01 second in persons 75–89 years old. In old persons, the nature of evoked potentials changes, the latent period increases, and the amplitude of the late components of the response to sonic, light and somatosensory stimulation decreases (Mankovsky *et al.*, 1978).

The action of physiologically active substances on the brain plays an important role in regulating its functions. The hormones, which act as humoral feed-back, regulate the basal level of the brain's metabolism. Mediators realize interneuronal transfer.

Many old and new works written by our fellow workers show that the reaction of the brain structures to humoral factors changes in old age. The brain may become more sensitive to several humoral factors with age. Fig. 23 A, B

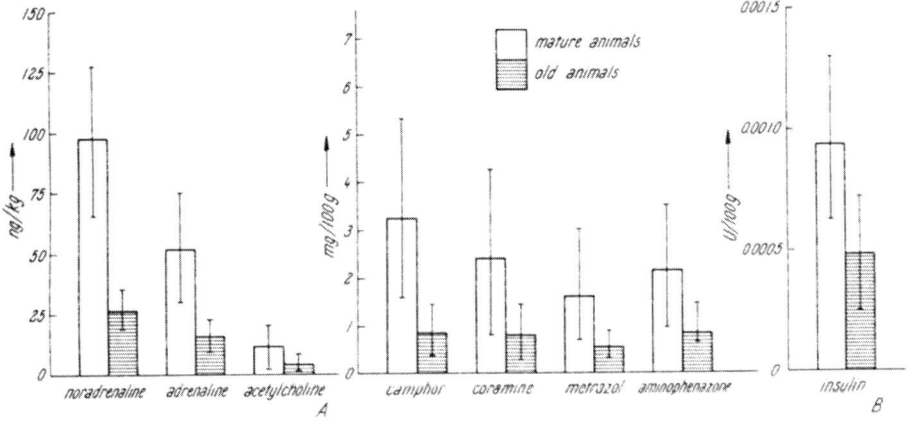

Fig. 23. Thresholds of the doses of various substances which cause changes in the electric activity of the brain of mature animals (light columns) and old animals (shaded columns). *A* rabbits, intravenous administration; *B* rats, intraperitoneal administration

shows that small doses of certain substances engender shifts in the electric activity of the brain and cause convulsions in old rabbits. Bezrukov determined the shifts in arterial pressure when adrenaline and acetylcholine were administered intracerebrally. The pressor reactions are more pronounced in old rabbits when adrenaline and acetylcholine are injected into most brain structures. Mankovsky and Mints (1972) have observed that the changes caused by adrenaline and insulin in the brain's bioelectric activity are more pronounced in elderly persons than in young persons. The changes in the brain's functional state become prolonged as a result of greater sensitivity to humoral factors in old age. When the synthesis of mediators attenuates, the growth of the sensitivity of some brain structures to them is probably of adaptive significance. This growth is caused not only by a change in the state of receptors, but also by shifts in the breakdown of mediators, as a result of which the mediators remain for a longer time within the sphere of their action.

The central nervous system becomes more sensitive with age to barbiturates (Verzar, 1963) and estrogens (Aschheim, 1976; Meites *et al.*, 1977, 1978). When barbiturates are administered intraperitoneally, rats 8–10 months old sleep for 186 minutes and rats 24–26 months old sleep for 234 minutes (Frolkis, Paramonova, 1980). A special analysis has shown that this is due not to a decrease in the detoxication of substances by the microsomal oxidative system, but to the real growth of the nervous centres' sensitivity. The centres of thermoregulation in old rabbits have become more sensitive to chlorpromazine (Lipton *et al.*, 1979). The intravenous administration of chlorpromazine in doses of 0.5–2.0 mg/kg reduces the body temperature more in old animals than in mature ones. This was observed also when the substance was administered intraventricularly in a dose of 1.0 µg/kg.

It has been observed that the nervous centres become less sensitive to estrogens and corticoids with age (Dilman, 1976a; Riegle *et al.*, 1977). Such contradictions occur because the age specifics are not delimited with respect to various substances and various doses of the same substance. An intricate pattern of the brain's reactions to humoral influences originates with age. In old age, many brain structures become more sensitive to small doses of substances; when the doses are large, a smaller reaction occurs.

The substance which is introduced into the organism has different applications in the centres and at the periphery. The mechanism of the action of substances can change in old age due to the different shifts in the sensitivity of various links of self-regulation. When papaverine acts on the vascular wall, it reduces vascular tonicity, and when it acts on the hemodynamic centre, it causes a vascular spasm and the growth of arterial pressure. The pressor reaction occurs more frequently in old persons and animals due to the greater sensitivity of the hemodynamic centre (Gromov, 1966). The direct action of sex steroids on the adrenal gland is more pronounced in old rats, while their indirect action on the hypothalamus is more pronounced in mature rats (Kopieva, 1978). When dimethylphenylpiperazinium iodide is administered, bradycardia has central genesis in mature animals and peripheral genesis in old animals, i. e. influence is directly exerted on the ganglion of the vagus nerve in the heart (Duplenko, 1965).

In a special series of experiments with old cats, Shchegoleva (1962) determined the reaction of the hemodynamic centre (a change in arterial pressure) to the humoral factor (Cardiazol, which stimulates the central neurons) and the neural factor (stimulation of the central section of the vagus nerve). Fig. 24 shows that the fewer the Cardiazol concentrations which excite the hemodynamic centre in old rabbits, the higher the force of the current that is needed to stimulate the central section of the vagus nerve. The higher the sensitivity of the hemodynamic centre to the stimulating action of Cardiazol, the lower the influence of the vagus nerve. The coefficient of regression or correlation of the influences being studied (it is determined by regression analysis) is 0.81. With age, interconnected changes occur in both the perception of humoral signals by the centres and neural afferentation, and the perception of information via various canals alters. Obviously, a different "afferent image" may then be formed in the brain and a "different idea" about the state of the organism's internal environment may be created, as a result of which an inadequate, "erroneous" reaction may be produced. We have shown that the reflexes of the mechanoreceptors of the aorta and the carotid sinus weaken with age (Frolkis, 1970). Consequently, less information on the shifts in arterial pressure enters the hemodynamic centre. When arterial pressure rises, the synthesis of the depressor agents (kinins, serotonin, histamine) is activated, and later influence the central neurons.

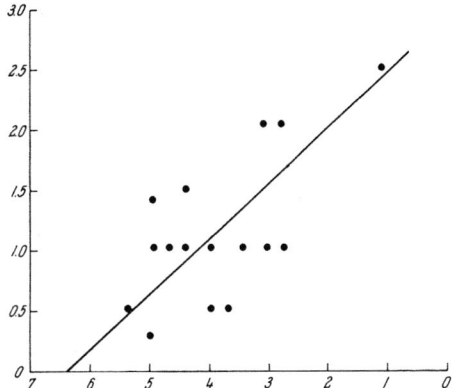

Fig. 24. Reaction of the hemodynamic centre to the action of cardiazol and the stimulation of the vagus nerve in old rabbits. The ordinate is the threshold concentration of cardiazol (mg/kg). The abscissa is the thresholds of the stimulation of the central part of the vagus nerve (volts)

Thus, the essence of the shifts which occur with age can be understood only by taking a systemic approach and analyzing all the aspects of a programme. Functional mobility, or lability, should be determined in order to assess the age changes in neural regulation. Our data show that lability diminishes in various units of the regulatory system with age. This fact can be seen from a decrease in the possible frequency of impulses in the afferent nerves (vagus, sinocarotid and aortal nerves) and efferent nerves (vagus and sympathetic nerves) of old animals (Frolkis, 1970; Shevchuk, 1979), and from the slowing down of the alpha-rhythm of the EEG of old persons and animals and the retardation of other EEC rhythms (Frolkis et al., 1972; Mankovsky et al., 1978). Hence, the most important regulatory systems function in a lower frequency range of rhythms, limiting the possibility of perceiving, transferring and recoding information in old age.

Pavlov's school made an extremely important conclusion that internal inhibition is the first system to be affected with age. It has been shown in our laboratory that the attenuation of inhibition of various types is an extremely

5*

important neurodynamic mechanism of the brain's aging, and that the thresholds of the inhibiting corticospinal and reticulospinal influences grow in old animals. In old age, reciprocal inhibition is affected in the spinal cord, as a result of which the coordination of the spinal reflexes is disturbed more easily. Reciprocal relations may be disturbed in the centres of inspiration and expiration, thus engendering the "pathological" types of respiration in old persons.

Besides its coordinative role, inhibition plays a preventive and, what is more, an active restorative role. According to Pavlov (1938) and Folbort (1969), inhibition, which terminates activity, can protect the cell from exhaustion and, what is more, can actively stimulate the restorative processes. Our laboratory data show that this active influence of inhibition on the restorative processes attenuates in old age. The influences which descend from the cerebral cortex and the reticular formation can strongly affect the functional state of the neurons of the spinal cord. In adult rats, the inhibiting reticulospinal influences help to restore the intensity of the reflexes of the spinal cord, which become weak as they are reproduced for a long time. The stimulating influence of inhibition (caused by the stimulation of the reticular formation) on the restoration of the reflexes of the spinal cord attenuates greatly in old animals. The mechanism of this phenomenon is complicated. In general, it clearly indicates that the influence of inhibition (caused by the stimulation of the reticular formation) on the restorative processes attenuates with age. The results of the experiments which were carried out in this respect show that the attenuation of the influence of inhibition on the restorative processes in old age is a mechanism that is commonly found at various levels of the central nervous system.

The restorative role of reciprocal inhibition is reduced in old age. In old animals, reciprocal inhibition does not sharply intensify the reflex after its attenuations, as is the case in adult animals. In some experiments, reciprocal inhibition in old animals sharply changed the nature of the subsequent restoration of the centres of the opposite side, i. e. restoration became phased.

A decrease in the number of inhibiting synapses and in the synthesis of the assumed inhibiting mediators that occurs in some brain structures, the shifts (according to a change in the inhibiting postsynaptic potential) on the postsynaptic membrane, and the change in ion flows are the cellular basis of a change in the inhibiting process in old age.

The weakening of the inhibiting process and the attenuation of its active influence on the restorative processes in the cells are an extremely important mechanism which increasingly limits the working ability of the nerve cells.

The basic physiological processes in the brain become less reliable and are disrupted more easily with age. This fact has been shown by us and Sinitsky by taking the example of a convulsive seizure. The seizures were simulated by skin electric shocks in rabbits of different ages and were repeated every three minutes. Young rabbits survived 80–90 seizures, while old ones died after 15–25 seizures. The tonic phase and the automatism period, and then the clonic phase decreased after a few seizures in old animals as blood circulation and respiration were increasingly disturbed.

Thus, the reliability of the brain's activity determines the duration of maintenance of the adaptive regulatory mechanisms, the organism's viability and life span. The age changes in the structure and metabolism cause the disturbance of the functions of neurons and nervous centres. They reduce the organism's adaptation to the environment, limit homeostasis, and engender secondary disturbances in other organs and tissues.

3. Hypothalamohypophysial Regulation During Aging

Regulatory Effects of the Hypothalamus

Voltaire once wrote that the more we have, the more we need. This truism applies not only to everyday life, but also to biology. The more complicated the mechanisms of homeostatic regulation, the more intensively should the adaptive mechanisms be switched on during aging.

The systems of homeostatic regulation become less reliable with age, thus causing the development of age pathology. Hence, it is natural to seek to link aging with a change in the central systems which determine the regulation of homeostasis, its preservation during constant disturbances, and homeostasis itself, i. e. the natural course of a change in metabolism, functions, and the state of the internal environment during individual development. It has been concluded that the whole organism's aging is connected with hypothalamic regulation and the changes in the hypothalamohypophysial region of the brain. However, it should be taken into account that in spite of the age changes in the cells and the tissues, the homeostatic state of several systems of the organism is maintained for a long time in old age, thus expressing the most important mechanisms of vitauct. Adaptive regulatory shifts, which help to preserve homeostasis and the vitauct processes, are connected with the age dynamics of hypothalamic activity.

Vitauct processes are of great adaptive significance, and are formed with age due to hypothalamic regulation. However, the hypothalamus itself begins to grow old with time. This is one of the main causes of the disturbance of the whole organism's functions. These opposite tendencies explain the intricate mechanism of the participation of the hypothalamus in the organism's reorganization with age. The significance of the age changes in the hypothalamus is so great that many researchers place the biological clock of the whole organism's aging in it (Everitt, 1970; Samorajski, Ordy, 1972; Denckla, 1974; Dilman, 1976b; Segall, 1979, and others).

However, biological logic and analogy are still not enough for evidence. Definite data should be obtained on the age changes in various aspects of the activity of the hypothalamohypophysial region, the effects of the changes in its functions on the whole organism, the relationship between that region and the regulatory influences of other parts of the brain, etc. Many interesting hypotheses are based largely on comparisons and the indication of similarities, and not on the direct investigation of the hypothalamic functions. Hence, there are many contradictions in the data on the specific essence of the age changes in hypothalamic regulation. According to some researchers, the hypothalamic functions are extinguished with age, thus reducing the reliability of hypothalamic regulation (Groen, 1959; Borisov, 1968; Mankovsky, Mints, 1972; Finch, 1976). Others maintain that the hypothalamic mechanisms are activated with age, and that the stimulation of the hypothalamohypophysial region causes several disturbances in the organism's metabolism and functions.

According to the elevation hypothesis proposed by Dilman (1976b), the hypothalamic region becomes less sensitive to the inhibiting influences with age, thus activating hypothalamic structures. He believes that this mechanism is common to aging and age pathology (diabetes, obesity, atherosclerosis, arterial hypertension, and cancer), and that it determines not only the unity of these processes, but also their identity.

During the last 15 years, our laboratory has obtained much data on the dynamics of the age changes in the hypothalamus (Frolkis, 1970; Frolkis et al., 1972, 1979b; Muradian, 1977a; Bezrukov, 1979; Rushkevich, 1980, and others). It is important to note that our fellow workers used direct methods to determine the electric excitability of the hypothalamic structures, record their electric activity and reactions to the intrahypothalamic administration of substances, analyze neurosecretory activity, study the shifts in the secretion of the hypophysial hormones, etc.

In man, the hypothalamic region consists of 32 pairs of nuclei. The hypothalamus is a structurally and functionally heterogenous system. When the hypothalamic mechanisms of aging are being analyzed, it should be taken into account that various functions are regulated when diverse nuclei of the hypothalamus interact with one another. For instance, dietary behaviour is determined by the interaction between the "appetite centre," which is in the lateral region of the hypothalamus, and the "saturation region," which is in its ventromedial part; thermoregulation is determined by the interaction between the structures of the anterior and posterior parts of the hypothalamus, and the reproductive function, by the interaction between the preoptic region and the nuclei of medial eminence. Therefore, the age changes in individual nuclei of the hypothalamus and their interaction should be analyzed so as to characterize it in its entirety.

Our data show that the hypothalamic functions make it possible to maintain the whole organism's homeostasis for a long time when substantial changes occur in various organs and tissues. The adaptive abilities of the hypothalamus are limited. The regulation of the hypothalamic functions is ultimately upset, thus disturbing the regulation of the organism's physiological systems and reducing the reliability of the mechanisms which regulate homeostasis. The regulation of those functions is upset because the functional state of the individual hypothalamic structures change not only differently, but also in different directions. That growing maladjustment and the disharmony in the excitability of hypothalamic structures and in their sensitivity to humoral factors disturb the integral function of the hypothalamus and its ability to control the organism's complex adaptive reactions. The maladjustment of the hypothalamic functions is promoted by a phenomenon which we call "hypothalamic misinformation." The essence of the phenomenon is that the sensitivity of the hypothalamic structures to nervous impulses, hormones and mediators changes in different directions with age, producing "errors" in the information on the state of the organism's internal environment and in the realization of the hypothalamic programme for regulating the given environment.

It has already been mentioned that the disharmony in the entry of "neural" and "humoral" information into the nerve centres is just as important to the whole system of self-regulation as the shifts are at the stage of a direct link: the attenuation of nervous control over the effectors and a change in their sensitivity to humoral factors. A change in the neural and humoral cycles of self-regulation (direct and inverse relationships) is, in old age, one of the main causes of the prolonged, generalized metabolic and functional reactions, which are occasionally very "costly" for the organism. We have shown that the above-mentioned maladjustment makes it easier to disturb the hypothalamic mechanisms of aging and to promote pathology in old age. A change in such extremely important manifestations of aging as the disturbance in reproductivity, in the rhythm of sleep and wakefulness, and in dietary and other types of behaviour, the shifts in regulating metabolism, protein biosynthesis, blood circulation, and so forth, are connected with the shifts in hypothalamic regulation.

Differently expressed changes in various hypothalamic structures develop with age. This is evident from the data on the neuronal loss in various hypothalamic structures. According to Hsu and Peng (1978), neurons are lost mostly in the medial preoptic region (30 per cent), the anterior hypothalamic region (23 per cent), and the arcuate nucleus (23 per cent). The regulation of the reproductive function is connected with exactly those parts of the hypothalamus. Neuronal density decreases differently in various nuclei. It decreases by 7.3 per cent in the lateral mamillary and perifornicate nuclei of rats (Mezhiborskaya, 1970), by 25 per cent in their supraoptic nucleus, by 21 per cent in their paraventricular nucleus, and by 37 per cent in their ventromedial nucleus (Hsu, Peng, 1978). Buttlar-Brentano (1954) did not observe any loss of neurons in the supraoptic and paraventricular nuclei of old persons. Lamperti and Blaha (1980), who studied nine nuclei of the hypothalamus morphologically (the medial preoptic nucleus, the supraoptic nucleus, the paraventricular nucleus, the ventromedial nucleus, the dorsomedial nucleus, the arcuate nucleus, the subventricular part of the arcuate nucleus, the suprachiasmatic nucleus, and the mamillary medial nucleus) in young (4–6 months) and reproductively senescent (15–18 months) female golden hamsters, did not detect any substantial age distinctions in the number of neurons and the diameter of the hypothalamic nuclei.

Irregular changes occur also in the accumulation of lipofuscin. Much lipofuscin is deposited in the preoptic and supraoptic nuclei, but less of it in the paraventricular nucleus (Machado-Salas et al., 1977). The destruction of neurons is preceded by their structural changes: the bodies swell, the dendrites shorten, tigrolysis increases, and the nerve cells wrinkle, deform and degenerate.

The shifts in the neurosecretion of the hypothalamic nuclei play a great role in the mechanisms of neurohormonal regulation. Neurosecretory processes become less active with age (Bogdanovich, 1974; Stepanov, 1974).

Our data show that the dimensions of the cellular nuclei in the paraventricular and supraoptic nuclei of the hypothalamus are reduced in old rats (they are 525 μm^3 in mature rats and 482 μm^3 in old rats) and their nucleoli are smaller (they are 8.2 μm^3 in mature rats and 7.5 μm^3 in old rats). The accumulation of the neurosecretory substance due to the retardation of its secretion prevails in many regions of the neurosecretory system of old animals. Degenerated neurons of elongated form with a poorly outlined pyknotic nucleus are observed.

Borisov (1968) concluded from logical constructions and literary data that the age changes in neurosection are the main mechanism of both the destruction of the neurosecretory neurons and the diminution of the hypothalamic functions. However, Andrew (1971) did not notice any increase in the number of disintegrating nerve cells in the nuclei of the anterior hypothalamus in old age. The data presented by Hsu and Peng (1978) show that the neurosecretory elements are very reliable. In their experiments with female rats 8–26 months old, Davies and Fotheringham (1980) showed that the volume of most of the cellular and subcellular components of the supraoptic nucleus of the hypothalamus did not change with age. However, the volume occupied by the hormone-containing granules and lipofuscin increased with age. It is believed that the hormone-secreting cells are somewhat "protected" from aging and can possess some properties of the "pacemaker" cells.

The age changes in the neurosecretory process are especially manifested when stress situations develop. In our experiments, stress was reproduced by either pain stimulation (100 V, 20 stimuli in 30 seconds) or adrenaline administration (30 μg/100 g). Neurosecretory shifts are more pronounced in mature rats in the case of reflex stimulation and in old rats in the case of adrenaline administration. We found that the shifts are less pronounced in the neurosecretory response of the paraventricular and supraoptic nuclei also when the nuclei of the amygdaloid complex are stimulated (Frolkis, 1970).

Neurosecretion is an extremely important link in the complex neurohormonal chain which is responsible for the realization of stress reactions. In our investigation of its individual links, we also showed that the shifts in the functions of the adrenal cortex are more pronounced in mature rats in the case of the "reflex type" of stress, but they are more pronounced in old animals when several humoral agents (catecholamines, vasopressin) are administered.

In stress situations, the hypothalamohypophysial mechanisms are largely switched on by the action of the "initial mediators of stress," i. e. catecholamines. In the case of the reflex pain stress, the content of noradrenaline increases more in mature rats than in old ones. When adrenaline is administered, stress is more pronounced in old rats. Thus, the participation of the hypothalamus in the organism's adaptive reactions in old age is largely limited at the stage when its mechanism is switched on.

In a special series of works, Bezrukov (1979) compared the age changes in the electric excitability and electric activity of various structures of the hypothalamus. He found that the electric excitability of various hypothalamic structures changes differently: the excitability of the anterior hypothalamic nucleus and the rostral part of the supraoptic nucleus increases, the excitability of the caudal part of the supraoptic nucleus and the medial preoptic area does not change, and the excitability of the lateral hypothalamic area decreases.

Bezrukov's data indicate somewhat that the age changes in various nuclei of the hypothalamus are not of a single type. He compared the changes in the electric activity of the supraoptic, ventromedial and medial mamillary nuclei and of the lateral hypothalamic area (Fig. 25 A, B).

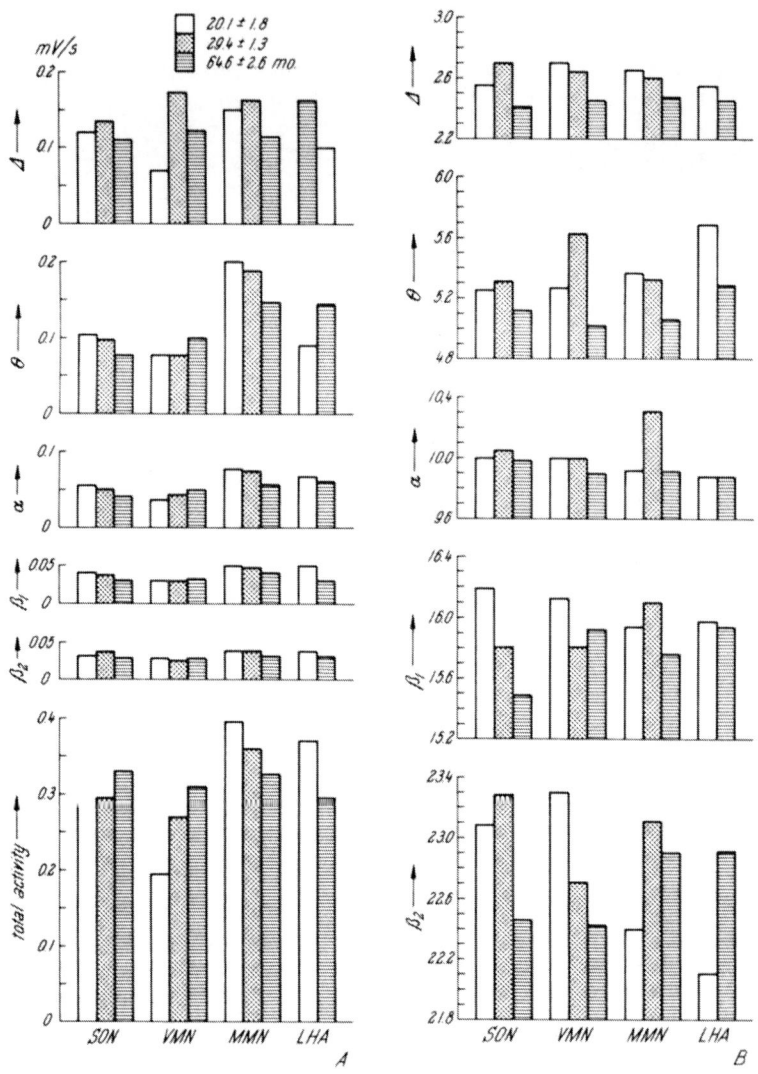

Fig. 25. The power of the rhythms, the total power *(A)* and frequency (Hz) of individual rhythms *(B)* of the background electrogram of the nuclei of the hypothalamus in rabbits of different age. *SON* supraoptic nucleus; *VMN* ventromedial nucleus; *MMN* medial mammillary nucleus; *LHA* lateral hypothalamic area; Δ, Θ, α, β_1, β_2 are the frequency ranges of rhythms

The frequency of most rhythms in various regions diminishes somewhat with age. The theta rhythm in the ventromedial and mamillary nuclei and the beta rhythms in the supraoptic and ventromedial nuclei slow down in old animals in comparison with younger ones.

The total energy (power) of the electrograms of various parts of the hypothalamus changes differently with age (Fig. 26). The total energy of the electrogram of the mamillary medial nucleus greatly diminishes, that of the electrogram of the lateral hypothalamic region tends to decrease, the energy of the ventromedial nucleus somewhat increases, while that of the supraoptic nucleus does not change. The total energy of various nuclei of the hypothalamus differs in mature rabbits. When old age is reached, the values of the total energy of the electrogram of various hypothalamic nuclei are "levelled out" as a result of the different age changes, which are expressed to a different extent in various parts of the hypothalamus. The changes in the energy of individual rhythms are mainly of the same nature: the energy of various rhythms in the mamillary medial nucleus and the lateral hypothalamic region decreases, but increases in the ventromedial nucleus and does not change in the supraoptic nucleus. Thus, the energy of the appropriate rhythms in various nuclei of the hypothalamus is levelled out in old age.

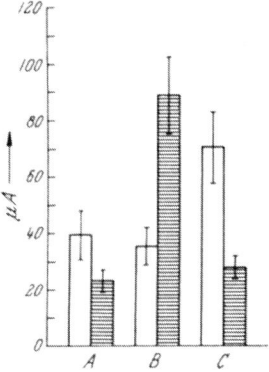

Fig. 26. Electrical thresholds (μA) of the origin of the EEG effects when the anterior medial (A), midlateral (B) and posterior medial (C) parts of the hypothalamus are stimulated in adult rabbits (light columns) and old rabbits (shaded columns) in acute experiments

In a special series of experiments, an investigation was made of the threshold electric current that produces electrographic reactions of the hypothalamus and other structures of the brain. The electric excitability of the posterior hypothalamus is much greater, while that of the lateral hypothalamus is less in old rabbits than in mature ones. The threshold of the excitability of the anterior hypothalamus was somewhat less in old rabbits than in mature ones (Fig. 26).

Synchronized theta-like activity, being especially clearly expressed in the sensorimotor cortex and the posterior medial hypothalamus, was recorded in the cortical and hypothalamic leads during the threshold stimulation of the hypothalamic nuclei. When the stimulating current sufficiently intensified, "desynchronized" activity was electrographically recorded in the cortical and hypothalamic leads. When it greatly intensified, convulsive activity originated in various regions of the cortex and the limbic and reticular complex.

According to Bezrukov, who based his work on the threshold of influence which some central nervous structures exert on others, the functional links between some structures weaken to a greater extent with age (e. g. the influence of the mamillary medial nuclei on the cerebral cortex, the influence of the supraoptic nucleus on the mamillary nuclei, the influence of the supraoptic nucleus on the cortex, and the influence of the ventromedial nucleus on other hypothalamic nuclei). A complex of nuclei usually participates in intricate behavioural and vegetative reactions. The above-mentioned changes in internuclear relations and their misalignment can alter the specifics of homeostatic regulation in old age.

The different changes in the excitability of the ventromedial hypothalamus and the lateral hypothalamus can upset the regulatory relationships between these formations. This should be reflected in dietary behaviour and carbohydrate and fat metabolism. A decrease in the excitability of the ventromedial hypothalamus can play a great role in both the diminution of the organism's adaptive abilities and the attenuation of the reaction of the hypothalamohypophysial adrenal system to stress influences. Inadequate "stagnant" vegetative reactions can originate when the specifics of the electric excitability of the hypothalamic structures are levelled out to a definite extent. The irregular changes in the functions of individual nuclei of the hypothalamus are based on the different destruction of neurons in them, different glycolysis, and mediator metabolism, which have been described by various authors.

In this respect, the stability of important metabolic cycles in several hypothalamic structures should also be taken into account. For instance, no distinctions were found in the content of RNA and DNA in the preoptic region of mice and the supraoptic nucleus of rats of different ages (Chaconas, Finch, 1973). According to our data, there are no age distinctions in the content of DNA and RNA in the anterior, posterior and lateral regions of the hypothalamus. The incorporation of leucin into the total proteins of the hypothalamus does not change in old age (Gordon, Finch, 1974).

Fig. 21 A, B, C gives our data on a change in the level of arterial pressure when adrenaline and acetylcholine are injected into various hypothalamic structures. It can be seen that greater changes occur in the circulatory reactions of old animals, but they are expressed differently when the agents are injected into various hypothalamic structures. This growth of the sensitivity of several hypothalamic structures to catecholamines and acetylcholine is of adaptive significance when the intensity of catecholamine and acetylcholine synthesis changes. In old mice, for instance, the activity of catechol-O-methyltransferase decreases and the activity of monoamine oxidase increases (Algeri et al., 1977), but the level of catecholamines does not change (Anisimov et al., 1977). The greatest changes occur in the rate of catecholamine metabolism, i. e. the dopamine content decreases by 33 per cent, while the intensity of dopamine uptake by the synaptosomes of the hypothalamus diminishes by 30 per cent (Jonec, Finch, 1975; Finch, 1976). According to Anisimov and others (1977), the content of noradrenaline in the hypothalamus of rats 13–15 months old decreases only by 14.2 per cent as compared with rats 2–3 months old, while the amount of serotonin remains unchanged. Zhubrikova and Gordienko (1980) have observed that the content of serotonin and noradrenaline changes inconsiderably in the hypothalamus of old rats, while the content of dopamine in them grows somewhat. The distinct discrepancy in the data on the age dynamics of the content of biogenic amines in the hypothalamus may be due to the possible difference in experimental conditions (circadian rhythms, seasonal changes, and the link with the physiological activity of other systems).

It has been shown that the basal level of cyclic AMP and the sensitivity of adenylate cyclase to catecholamines do not change with age (Schmidt, Thornberry, 1978). Makman and others (1979) indicate that the basal activity of adenylate cyclase remains unchanged in the hypothalamus and that its ability to be activated is reduced under the action of dopamine, noradrenaline and histamine.

Our data show that not only the extent, but also the nature of the efferent influences of the hypothalamus on the cardiovascular system changes with age. In most cases, the researchers recorded only the shifts in arterial pressure when they stimulated the hypothalamus. However, new aspects of the hypothalamic regulation of blood circulation are revealed when the general hemodynamic changes are studied. According to our data, the hemodynamic structure of the reactions changes in old rabbits when their hypothalamus is stimulated. The same level of arterial pressure is attained during different age periods due to the different relationships between cardiac output and vascular tonicity. In old age, pressor reactions occur more frequently as cardiac output grows (Fig. 27 A, B).

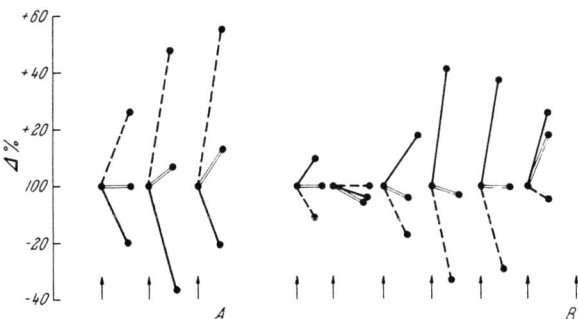

Fig. 27. Hemodynamic effects of hypothalamic stimulation in mature rabbits (A) and old rabbits (B) when the stimulation of the hypothalamus is gradually intensified. Double line stands for arterial pressure, the dashed line stands for total peripheral resistance, and the continuous line, for cardiac output

The efferent influences of the hypothalamus on respiration change greatly with age. Bezrukov (1975) showed that the current which caused tachypnea in old rabbits during hypothalamic stimulation was $60 \pm 10\,\mu A$ for the anterior hypothalamus, $120 \pm 10\,\mu A$ for the lateral hypothalamus, and $60 \pm 10\,\mu A$ for the posterior hypothalamus. In adult rabbits, the figures were 50 ± 10, 60 ± 10 and $100 \pm 10\,\mu A$, respectively. The influences which caused bradypnea were also different.

According to our data (Frolkis *et al.*, 1979a), hypothalamic influences regulate the activity of the genetic apparatus and the intensity of protein biosynthesis. Hence, plastic processes become adapted to the organism's general requirements and an adequate adaptive shift occurs in protein biosynthesis. This extremely important mechanism of regulation is realized due to the hypophysial influences on the glands, whose hormones are the direct inductors of the genetic apparatus. Our data show that the synthesis of various classes of RNA and various protein enzymes changes when the hypothalamus is stimulated. We believe that one of the most important mechanisms of the whole organism's aging is determined by a change in both the hypothalamic regulation of the genetic apparatus of the cells and protein biosynthesis. In old animals, the syntheses of individual classes of RNA and the inductive syntheses of glucose-6-phosphatase, fructose-1,6-diphosphatase, tyrosine aminotransferase, and tryptophan pyrrolase change when the ventromedial nucleus of the hypothalamus is stimulated (Bezrukov, Muradian, 1974; Frolkis *et al.*, 1979a, b). Fig. 28A, B shows that the inductive synthesis of enzymes is less

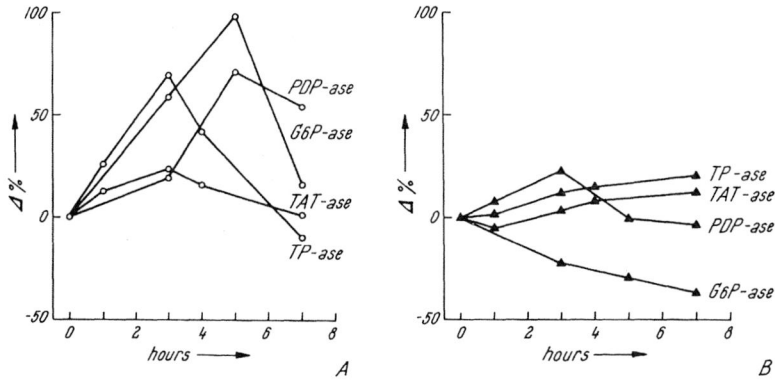

Fig. 28. Influence of the single stimulation of the hypothalamus on enzymic activity in mature rats *(A)* and old rats *(B)*. Enzymic activity in sham-operated animals is taken as the basis. The time after stimulation (hours) is indicated horizontally

pronounced in old animals than in mature ones when the hypothalamus is stimulated. The differences are especially great in the regulation of protein biosynthesis when the hypothalamus is stimulated for a long time. The inductive synthesis of enzymes and the rate of RNA renewal rapidly diminishes in old animals. Shimazu and others (1978) have shown that the activity of glycogen synthetase and phosphorylase of the liver changes more faintly in old rats than in young ones (2 months old) when the ventromedial hypothalamus and the lateral hypothalamus are electrically stimulated. It will be shown by an analysis of the whole system (hypothalamus–hypophysis–adrenal cortex–tissues) in another chapter that the limiting link is localized in the hypothalamic structures. A situation originates in which the genetic apparatus of the cells can still react adequately, but the central and hypothalamic mechanisms can no longer do so. The hypothalamic mechanisms are activated during the organism's intense activity and also in stress situations, when the energy and plastic processes occur intensively. The hypothalamic changes in the regulation of protein biosynthesis limit the plastic ensurance of the functions, thus making them inadequate in old age. Hence, the molecular and genetic mechanisms of cellular aging are determined by a change in their supracellular (central, i. e. hypothalamic) regulation.

Hypothalamohypophysial Influences

Important efferent influences of the hypothalamus on the tissues are realized through the hypophysial hormones. There are many works on a change in the hormonal function of the hypophysis during aging, on the possible role of activation or suppression in the genesis of aging, and on the possible synthesis of substances, which actively suppress the organism's metabolism and functions, in the hypophysis.

The disturbance of genome regulation in the hypophysial cells releases the genes which were suppressed earlier and which are responsible for the production of certain inhibiting agents (Denckla, 1974). A peptide with a molecular weight of 15,000 (not seen in adult animals) has been found in the hypophysis of old rats (Wilkes et al., 1978). There are much data on a change in the secretion of the hypothalamic releasing hormones and the hypophysial hormones, but they are very contradictory. The content of the somatotropin-releasing factor decreases in the hypothalamic tissue of old rats. The secretion and content of the growth hormone (GH) do not change in human blood plasma (Dudl et al., 1973). GH release, being caused by adequate arginine stimulation or by insulin hypoglycemia, either does not change (Kalk et al., 1973) or somewhat diminishes (Dudl et al., 1973). The activity of the somatomedin-like substances, through which the growth hormone of the hypophysis acts, is reduced in old rats. The corticotropin-releasing activity of the hypothalamic extracts diminishes in old animals. The basal level of corticotropin does not change in human blood (Blichert-Toft, 1975), but it increases in the blood of rats (Tang, Phillips, 1978). According to our laboratory data, the thyrotropin content increases in rats 18–24 months old and decreases in rats 28–32 months old (Valueva, Verzhikovskaya, 1977). Some researchers maintain that the content of the thyrotropin-stimulating hormone (TSH) in human blood plasma grows somewhat, others hold that it diminishes, and still others believe that it does not change.

Great interest is taken in the secretion of the gonadotropins, since the reproductive functions ends with age. Some researchers hold that the content of the gonadotropin-releasing factor grows in the hypothalamus of old rats (Clemens, Meites, 1971; Baranov et al., 1972), while others believe that it diminishes (Riegle et al., 1977). The level of the follicle-stimulating hormone (FSH) grows in women during the postmenopausal period. The content of FSH and the luteinizing hormone (LH) grows in men with age. The content of LH in the blood plasma of male mice and rats decreases with age (Finch et al., 1977). According to Kopieva (1978), the content of FSH is 1.25 ± 0.11 ng/ml in rats 8–10 months old and 1.57 ± 0.12 ng/ml in rats 26–28 months old. The figures for LH are 1.38 ± 0.12 and 1.15 ± 0.11 ng/ml, respectively, and those for corticotropin are 98.3 ± 7.6 and 14.3 ± 9.7 ng/ml, respectively.

Thus, the secretion or, to be more exact, the content of various hypophysial hormones in the blood changes differently with age. The hormone content depends on not only hormone secretion, but also metabolism, which can change with age. Since the data on the content of the hypophysial hormones are contradictory, some researchers believe that the hypothalamohypophysial region is activated, while others hold that it is suppressed. As we have already seen, the basal level of this content in old age cannot be regarded as an indicator of hypophysial hormone secretion. The content of hormones depends on the intensity of their breakdown, which changes in old age. The breakdown of some hormones (insulin, aldosterone, etc.) greatly decreases in old age. In old age, the secretion of aldosterone decreases more than its blood content. This fact is apparently due to the attenuation of the hormone disintegration processes. Therefore, the unchangeable or somewhat elevated basal level of the content of hormones may be due to the attenuation of their secretion in old age. The age changes in the degradation of the hypophysial hormones have not been adequately studied yet.

The relationship between various links of the hypothalamohypophysial endocrine system changes with age. The combination of the processes of both aging and vitauct makes it possible to keep the whole system at a definite level when its abilities are curtailed. The system is adapted to a narrower range of reactions.

The secretory activity of the adenohypophysis is regulated by releasing factors, which are synthesized in the hypothalamic nuclei and which enter the hypophysis through the portal system. Interestingly the content of the releasing factors in the hypothalamus (the corticotropin-releasing factor, the thyrotropin-releasing factor, and probably the gonadotropin-releasing factor) decrease when the blood level of tropic hormones is normal or even elevated. This phenomenon is probably connected with the growth of the sensitivity of the hypophysial structures in old age to the hypothalamic releasing factors. When the thyrotropin-releasing factor (TRF) is administered in small doses (100 μg), the thyrotropin level grows more in old persons, and when it is administered in a dose of 300 μg, it grows more in young persons (Ohara et al., 1974). We obtained similar results in the experiments involving the administration of TRF and the determination of TSH synthesis in the hypophysis of rats. In old age, the sensitivity of the hypophysis to TRF grows, but the possible amplitude of the response and the reactivity of the hypophysial cells diminish. Age differences have not been observed in the reactions of the hypophysis to TRF (Finch et al., 1977). The luteinizing hormone is surged to the same extent in mature and old rats when they are given the same doses of the exogenous gonadotropin-releasing factor (Watkins et al., 1975).

Substantial changes occur also at the next stage of the realization of the hypothalamic effects, i. e. in the hypophysis and the endocrine glands. We carried out investigations in this respect by taking the example of the hypophysial regulation of the functions of the adrenal cortex and the thyroid and sexual glands.

Fig. 29 A, B gives Magdich's data on the influence of various doses of corticotropin on the secretion of aldosterone, which was determined radio-immunologically in the blood which flows out of the adrenal gland. It can be seen that the secretion of aldosterone is more pronounced in old rats when corticotropin is administered in a small dose and in mature rats when it is administered in a large dose. When its dose is large, secretory activity is suppressed in old animals and the "disengagement phenomenon" occurs in them. Such relationships originate also during a load involving potassium, which is a specific stimulant of aldosterone secretion.

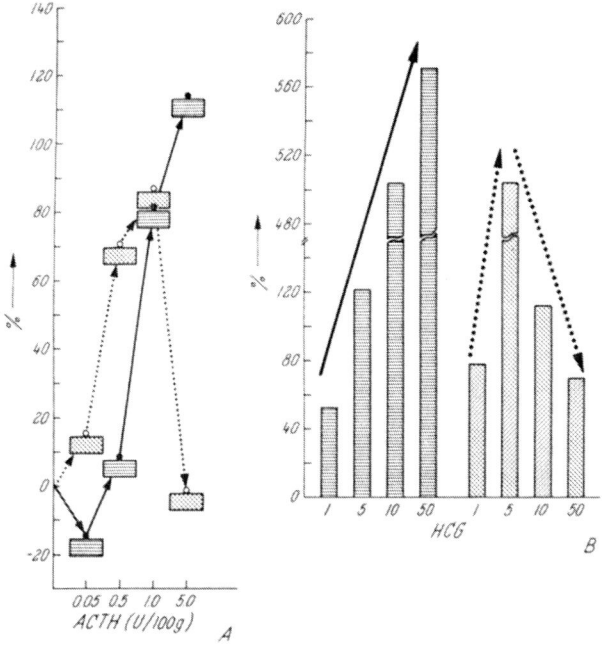

Fig. 29. Influence of various doses of corticotropin on the rate of aldosterone secretion *(A)* and human chorionic gonadotropin on the serum testosterone *(B)* in the rat (continuous lines stand for mature animals and the dotted lines for old animals). Chorionic Gonadotropin doses are 1.0–50.0 U/kg

There is an important circumstance which is common to all the studies of the mechanisms of humoral regulation in old age. The direction which the reactions take with age can be correctly understood only when greatly varying doses are administered and the dose-dependent reactions are taken into account. Many contradictions originate because this extremely important condition of gerontological researches is hardly taken into consideration. For instance, if one medium hormone dose is used, it can be concluded that the reaction does not change in old age; when the dose is small, the reaction may be considered enhanced, and when it is large, it may be considered weak.

The conclusion that the reaction range diminishes with age was confirmed by Becker (unpublished data) during an investigation of a change in the content of glucocorticoids when corticotropin was administered. When the doses of a tropic hormone are small, the reaction is more pronounced in old rats.

We have shown together with Valueva and Verzhikovskaya (see Chapter 6) that when the thyrotropin doses are small, the tissue respiration of the thyroid gland is activated more strongly and the content of thyroxine in the blood grows more intensively in rats 24–26 months old, and when the doses are large, this occurs in rats 8–10 months old. Moroz (unpublished data) administered various doses of choriogonin and showed that the content of testosterone in the blood grows more in old rats when the hormone doses are small (1, 5 and 10 U/100 g) and in mature rats when they are large (50 U/100 g). An interesting fact is that the tropic hormones which are administered to old animals cannot only promote, but also suppress the activity of the glands. This distortion of the hormonal effect may be of definite significance in the mechanism of the hypothalamohypophysial regulation of other endocrine glands in old age. In specific situations, this may be the cause of the suppression of the gland's functions in old age.

Thus, the possible reaction range decreases with age as regards the hypophysis and the endocrine gland. At the same time, smaller doses of the tropic hormone make the gland cells unstable. Such a regularity (which will be thoroughly analyzed in other parts of this book) is observed also at the hormone-tissue stage. Thus, the possible range of the changes in the functions of the hypothalamohypophysial systems decreases with age. This fact undoubtedly affects the course of the most important adaptive reactions which occur with that system's participation. However, the growth of sensitivity in various links of that system is of adaptive regulatory significance, since the organism adapts itself (even though to a limited extent) to its conditions. Great hormonal "disturbances" may be destructive for the organism when the abilities of tissue metabolism are limited. The hypothalamus may exert its influence on the endocrine glands via the nerve tracts, which change considerably with age. The hypothalamus takes part in regulating the function of the beta cells of the pancreas. These activating influences are realized through the vagus nerve

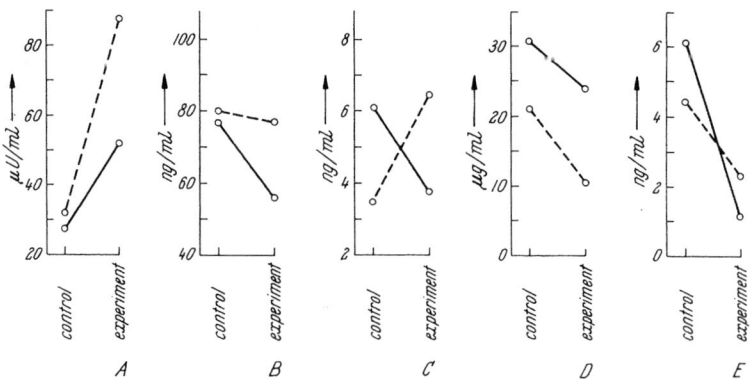

Fig. 30. Change in the content of hormones in adult rats (dashed line) and old rats (continuous line) after the ventromedial nucleus of the hypothalamus is damaged. *A* insulin; *B* corticosterone; *C* plasma somatotropin, *D* hypophysial somatotropin; *E* plasma thyrotropic hormone

system. This nerve pathway of hypothalamic control of the beta cells becomes less effective in old age, as can be seen from (1) the data presented by Bezrukov (1979) on the less pronounced insulinemia after the destruction of the ventromedial nucleus of the hypothalamus in old rats (Fig. 30), and (2) the less pronounced insulinemia during the initial phase of the sugar load, being associated with the neurogenous influences on the gland. Shifts in the peripheral cholinergic neural apparatus may be of definite significance in the mechanism of the formation of that changed reaction (Frolkis, 1970).

The hypothalamus influences the thyroid gland through the hypophysial thyrotropic hormone also by means of sympathetic neural regulation. The thyroid gland is innervated by postganglionic fibres which stem from *Ganglion cervicale superius*. According to our laboratory data (which will be given in the next chapter), structural changes occur, excitability, lability and acetylcholine synthesis diminish, and other phenomena take place in that ganglion in old age. All that obviously affects the realization of the sympathetic influences on the thyroid gland.

Mechanisms of Vasopressin Regulation

Vasopressin is produced mainly in the cells of the supraoptic nucleus of the hypothalamus and is delivered to the posterior lobe of the hypophysis through the hypothalamohypophysial tract. Vasopressin in negligible amounts is known to produce antidiuretic effects due to the resorption of water by the epithelium of the distal parts of the nephron.

In large doses, vasopressin causes great changes in the functions of the cardiovascular system and sharply increases vascular tonicity, including the tonicity of the coronary vessels (Cowley et al., 1980; Mohring et al., 1980). There are now enough data which show that in physiological and especially pathological situations, the concentration of vasopressin in the blood is above the threshold level for the reaction of the heart and the vessels. The concentration of vasopressin in the blood increases 20–30 times under the conditions of experimental and clinical stress (Golovchenko, 1973, 1976, 1979; Chebotareva, 1978; Felsch et al., 1978). Vasopressin is especially interesting because it simulates coronary insufficiency, arterial hypertension, arrhythmia, and cerebral ischemia.

It has been shown that the sensitivity of the cardiovascular system to vasopressin grows with age (Frolkis, Shchegoleva, 1963; Golovchenko, 1973, 1976; Frolkis, 1975, 1977; Frolkis et al., 1976a–d). In old rats and rabbits, small hormone doses produce objective signs of coronary insufficiency and a change in hemodynamics. No changes occur in the ECG when vasopressin is administered in a dose of 0.005 U/100 g to mature rats, but the T wave grows in 65 per cent of the cases and the S-T segment is displaced upwards in 40 per cent of the cases when the hormone is administered in the same dose to old rats. The administration of vasopressin in a dose of 0.1–0.2 U/100 g reduces cardiac output by 41.3 ± 3.1 per cent in old animals and by 27.8 ± 4.1 per cent in mature animals. Total peripheral resistance also increases in old rats.

6*

It has been shown directly in experiments with dogs (which had an intact thorax) involving the perfusion of the coronary vessels that small doses of vasopressin cause a greater growth of perfusion pressure in old dogs (Fig. 31 A, B). Golovchenko (1973) showed in her experiments with aortic strips that old animals have a group of receptors which are especially sensitive to vasopressin (the threshold dose is 1.7×10^{-12} M of vasopressin in old rats and 2.8×10^{-9} M of vasopressin in mature rats). The properties of various groups of receptors with respect to vasopressin change differently with age.

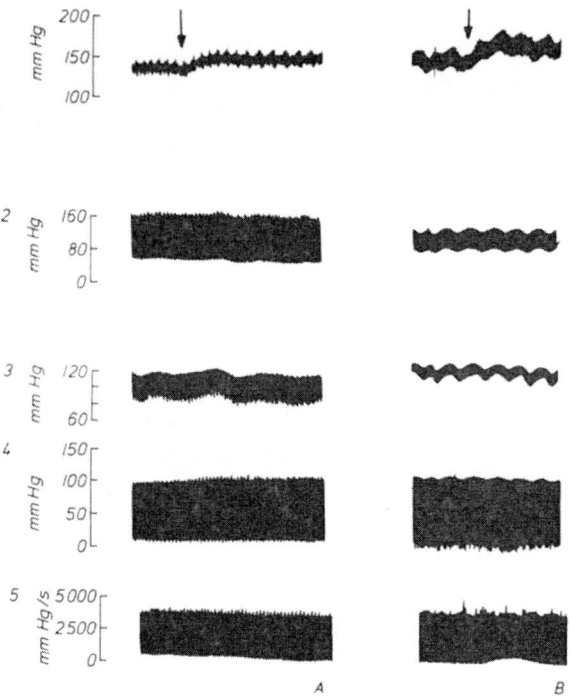

Fig. 31. Influence of the intracoronary administration of vasopressin (0.03 U, marked by an arrow) on the parameters of the hemodynamics in a mature dog *(A)* and an old dog *(B): 1* perfusion pressure in the coronary vessels; *2* systemic arterial pressure in the femoral artery; *3* perfusion pressure in the femoral vessels; *4* blood pressure in the left ventricle of the heart; *5* rate of a change in left ventricular pressure

The fact that the cardiovascular system becomes more sensitive to vasopressin in old age has been illustrated also in experiments involving the simulation of arterial hypertension (Pugach, 1970). When vasopressin is administered in a dose of 0.2 U/kg daily for 30 days, arterial pressure does not change in mature rabbits (it is 110 ± 8.5 mm Hg), but arterial hypertension develops in old rabbits (173 ± 12.5 mm Hg).

It has been shown that shifts become more pronounced in the energy metabolism of the brain and the myocardium under the action of vasopressin (Golovchenko, Potapenko, 1978). The content of adenyl nucleotides, creatine phosphate and glycogen changes more in the brain and the myocardium of old rats than in those of mature rats.

As we have seen, sensitivity to vasopressin grows in old persons and animals. Moreover, an increase is observed in the content of it in the blood, which Golovchenko (1979) determined by a biological method in which the antidiuretic effect of vasopressin is used (Fig. 32 A, B, C). We used not only biological, but also radioimmunological methods (kits of the Labomed, FRG) to show that the concentration of vasopressin increases in the blood of elderly persons. In persons 18–25 years old, the concentration of vasopressin in the blood is 2.4 ± 0.3 pmole/ml, while in persons 65–75 years old, it is 13.2 ± 1.8 pmole/ml. There are good reasons to believe that this growth of the content of vasopressin is due to not only the intensification of its synthesis, but also the attenuation of its breakdown. Moreover, the hemodynamic effects of

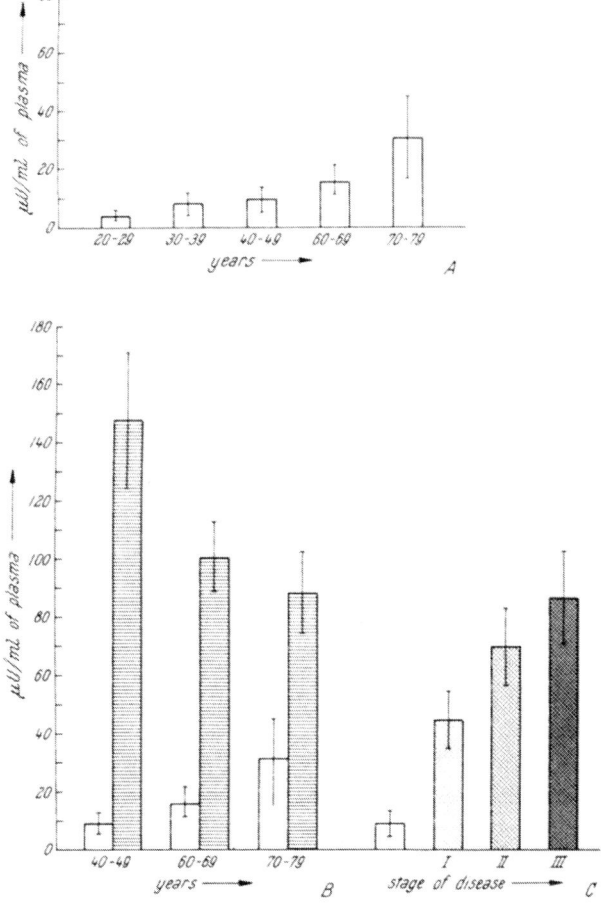

Fig. 32. Concentration of vasopressin in the blood of persons of different age. *A* virtually healthy persons (light columns); *B* persons suffering from hypertension at the first and second stages (slanting shading); *C* persons suffering from chronic ischemia (cross-hatched shading)

vasopressin are characterized by tachyphylaxia, i. e. a decrease in sensitivity to the repeated injections of a hormone. Tachyphylaxia with respect to vasopressin attenuates in old age (Medved, 1980). When the hormone is administered to adult animals a second time, the amplitude of the T wave of the electrocardiogram grows by less than one-third of that when the hormone is administered initially. In old animals, these shifts do not greatly differ from one another.

In old age, prerequisites are probably created for the participation of vasopressin in the development of myocardial and cerebral ischemia and arterial hypertension. These prerequisites include: (a) the greater sensitivity of the heart and the vessels to vasopressin; (b) the higher concentration of vasopressin in the blood, and (c) the attenuation of tachyphylaxia with respect to vasopressin, which intensifies its action. The content of vasopressin is higher in the blood of persons suffering from arterial hypertension and cardiac ischemia than in healthy persons (Fig. 32 A, B, C).

Since the possible participation of vasopressin in the mechanism of pathological development is acknowledged, it is quite correct to treat patients experimentally with cardiovascular pathology by administering hormone antagonists. We studied, together with Golovchenko, the influence of the natural metabolite of vasopressin, i. e. desglycineamide vasopressin (DGVP), on the hemodynamic effects of vasopressin. DGVP has the signature R, which is the same for vasopressin and which allows the receptor to recognize stimuli. According to Chipens and Papsuevich (1971), the specific vasoconstrictive action of vasopressin is determined by the tail part of the molecule (signature S) that is changed in desglycineamide vasopressin. Hence, DGVP should compete with vasopressin for the cellular receptors and should not produce vascular effects. DGVP was produced by hydrolyzing vasopressin with trypsin, followed by separation in the Dawex 50 × 2 column. We studied the influence of DGVP on the development of coronary insufficiency, which was simulated by vasopressin. The administration of DGVP in a 5 : 1 ratio prevented signs of coronary insufficiency (the growth of the T wave, the displacement of the S-T segment, etc.) from developing. DGVP reduces the hemodynamic effects of vasopressin and weakens its action on the vascular strips. After the administration of DGVP, the maximum contraction of the aortic strips due to vasopressin decreased by 45.8 per cent.

Thus, we believe that vasopressin play a great role in arterial hypertension and myocardial and cerebral ischemia in old age. Atherosclerosed vessels are more sensitive to vasopressin. According to Korkushko (1969), the capillaries of old persons react to much smaller amounts of pituitrin. Hence, it is expedient to look for the antagonists and inhibitors of vasopressin in order to use them therapeutically.

It has been shown in the studies of the urinary system that the mechanism of the action of vasopressin on the cells consists in its attachment to the receptor by ionic, hydrogen and hydrophobic bonds and in the subsequent activation of adenylate cyclase with the formation of cyclic AMP. Medved (1980) has shown in our laboratory that the content of 3′,5′-AMP decreases in the myocardium when vasopressin is administered in a dose of 0.05 U/100 g. In this respect, the content of cyclic AMP decreases more in old rats (by 40.2 per cent) than in mature rats (by 28.3 per cent). Cyclic AMP decreases in the myocardium in experiments *in vivo* due to the vasopressin influences which are connected with the spasm of the coronary vessels and the action of the vagus nerve on the heart. Actually, the content of cyclic AMP in the myocardial tissue grew in experiments *in vitro*. It grew more in old rats than in mature rats.

Feed-backs in the System of Hypothalamohypophysial Regulation in Old Age

The hypothalamohypophysial regulation of the organism's homeostasis is highly reliable due to the system of correlation, which is realized via the reflex and hormonal pathways. Some of these systems give information on the ultimate adaptive effect which had been produced, while others give information on the concentration of the hormone which had produced the effect. Zavodovsky (1931) was among the first to point out the role of these relationships. He proposed the concept of the "plus-minus" and "minus-plus" relationships between the endocrine glands. The second type of relationships is usually analyzed when the age changes in hypothalamohypophysial regulation is discussed.

There are contradictory data on the nature of a change which occurs in feed-backs with age. According to Dilman and Anisimov (1980), the tonic centre of the hypothalamohypophysial complex becomes less sensitive to estrogen suppression with age (a larger dose of estrogens should be administered intraperitoneally and injected into the third ventricle of the brain in order to suppress the hypertrophy of the ovaries when hemicastration is performed). The diminution of the level of catecholamines in the hypothalamus with age, the smaller uptake of estrogens by the anterior hypothalamus and the mediobasal hypothalamus, a decrease in the activity of the epiphysis, and a change towards mainly using free fatty acids to provide the organism with energy in old age play an important role in the mechanism of that change. The sensitivity of the hypothalamus to estrogen suppression was normalized in old rats when *l*-dopa, phenphormin, dilantin, an epiphyseal extract and succinic acid were administered to them.

According to the electric activity of the neurons, the neurons of the preoptic region and the arcuate nucleus become less sensitive to estradiol with age (Babichev, 1973). Unfortunately, the animals used in this respect were not old. The sensitivity of the hypothalamohypophysial system to factors which realize the negative feed-back does not change in old age (Odell, Swerdloff, 1968; Wise *et al.*, 1973). Aschheim (1976) had drawn the conclusion that the sensitivity of the hypothalamus to sex steroids grows with age. According to Kratin and Propp (1963), estradiol propionate produces opposite effects on the electroencephalograms of rabbits: the effects are activated in old rabbits and inhibited in mature rabbits.

Kopieva (1978), our fellow worker, thoroughly studied the changes in the feed-backs on the hypothalamus in old age. Various steroids (testosterone, estradiol dipropionate, dexasone) were administered to mature and old rats and the content of corticotropin was radioimmunologically determined in their blood. The contradictions in the data on a change which occurs in negative feed-back with age were overcome by using a complex approach and by taking account of the polyhormonal character of reaction. The data obtained show that the nature of a change in negative feed-back does not correspond to any scheme. Testosterone caused an increased blood content of corticotropin. It was noted that administration of large and small doses of the hormone resulted in a more marked shift of the corticotropin content in old rats. Estradioldipropionate also caused a more noticeable alterations of the corticotropin level in old rats. Quite different interrelationships were observed with dexasone: the administration of 100 μg/kg produced a more marked fall of the corticotropin content in mature rats, whereas in old animals it was found at a dose of 500 μg/kg.

We carried out a series of experiments to study the state of feed-back on the basis of thyroid regulation (Frolkis et al., 1978) and found that small doses of thyroxine suppress the synthesis of the thyrotropic hormone more in old rats, while large doses of it suppress this synthesis more in mature rats. We have already shown that shifts in arterial pressure are more pronounced in old rabbits when adrenaline and acetylcholine are injected into the hypothalamus (Fig. 21A, B, C). Thus, the nature of hormonal feed-backs to the hypo-thalamohypophysial region and the reaction of its various structures change differently with age; sensitivity is greater to some hormonal effects and less to others, while reactivity decreases in the case of one type of feed-backs and increases in the case of another. Age changes at the stage of feed-back in the system of hypothalamohypophysial regulation where shown in our experiments, which were carried out together with Bezrukov. In them, the electric activity of individual hypothalamic nuclei were recorded. Electrodes were inserted into the ventromedial, medial mamillary and supraoptic nuclei and the lateral hypothalamic area of two groups of rabbits 12–16 and 52–60 months old. A few months after the operation, the changes in the electric activity of the hypothalamic nuclei of mature and old rabbits were compared after administering various doses of adrenaline, insulin and estradiol dipropionate. The threshold doses of adrenaline and insulin that produce noticeable shifts in the electrogram of the hypothalamic structures were much lower in old animals than in adult ones. The nature of the EEG changes depended on the hypothalamic structure, the dose of a substance, and the initial electric activity of the hypothalamus. For instance, adrenaline in a dose of 0.01 μg/kg caused greater changes in the theta rhythm of old animals, while in a dose of 10.0 μg/kg (intravenous administration), it caused greater changes in this rhythm of mature animals (Fig. 33). Adrenaline influenced also the electrographic effects of the ventromedial and mamillary nuclei and the lateral hypothalamic region in the case of light and sonic rhythmic stimulation. The suppressing reaction of the hormone to the effects of stimulation were more pronounced in old animals.

In our experiments, insulin was administered in doses of 0.001, 0.01, 0.1, and 1.0 U/kg. Old rabbits reacted to the administration of insulin by accelerating the theta rhythm (Fig. 34). This age difference was especially pronounced when the hormone doses were small (0.001 U/kg). Estradiol

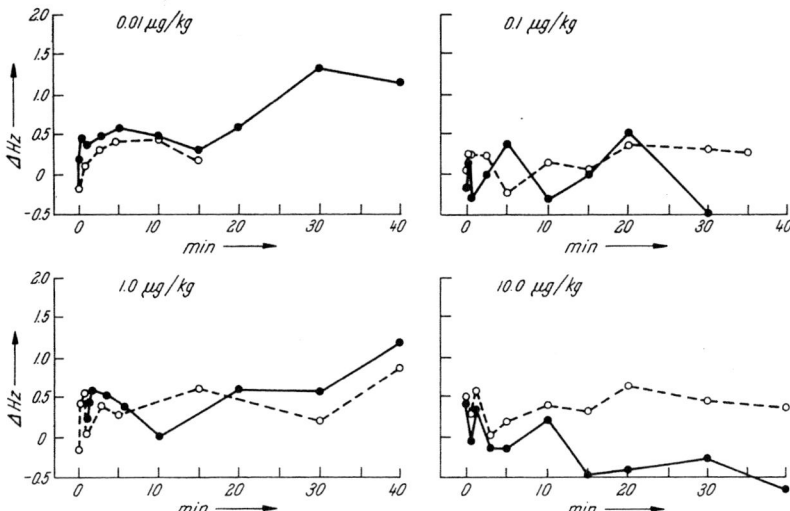

Fig. 33. Change in the theta rhythm in the nuclei of the hypothalamus when various doses of adrenaline are administered intravenously to adult rabbits (dashed line) and old rabbits (continuous line). The rhythmic shift (Hz) is indicated vertically, and the time after the administration of adrenaline (minutes) is indicated horizontally

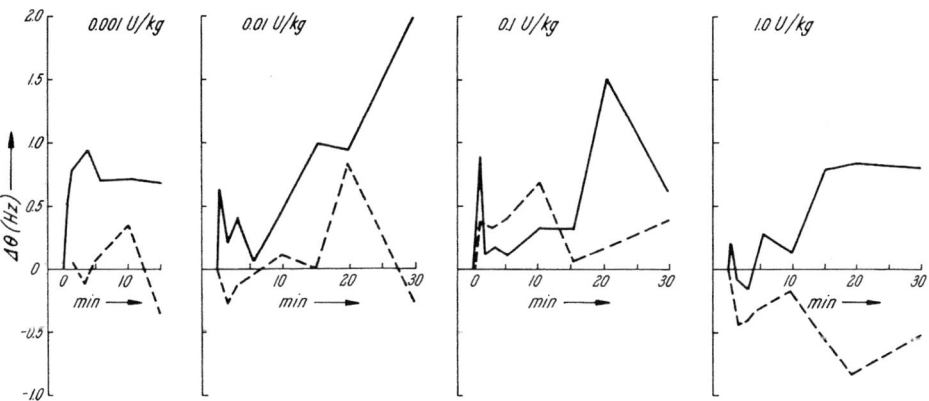

Fig. 34. Change in the theta rhythm in the nuclei of the hypothalamus when various doses of insulin are administered intravenously to adult rabbits (dashed lines) and old rabbits (continuous line). The rhythmic shift (Hz) is indicated vertically, and the time after the administration of insulin (minutes) is indicated horizontally

dipropionate (50 μg/kg) produced roughly the same changes in the electric activity of the hypothalamic nuclei in mature and old rabbits.

A special series of experiments were carried out to determine the electric excitability of various nuclei of the hypothalamus against the background of hormone action. Insulin, like adrenaline, influences the electric excitability of various hypothalamic structures to a different extent with age (Fig. 35). Thus, a

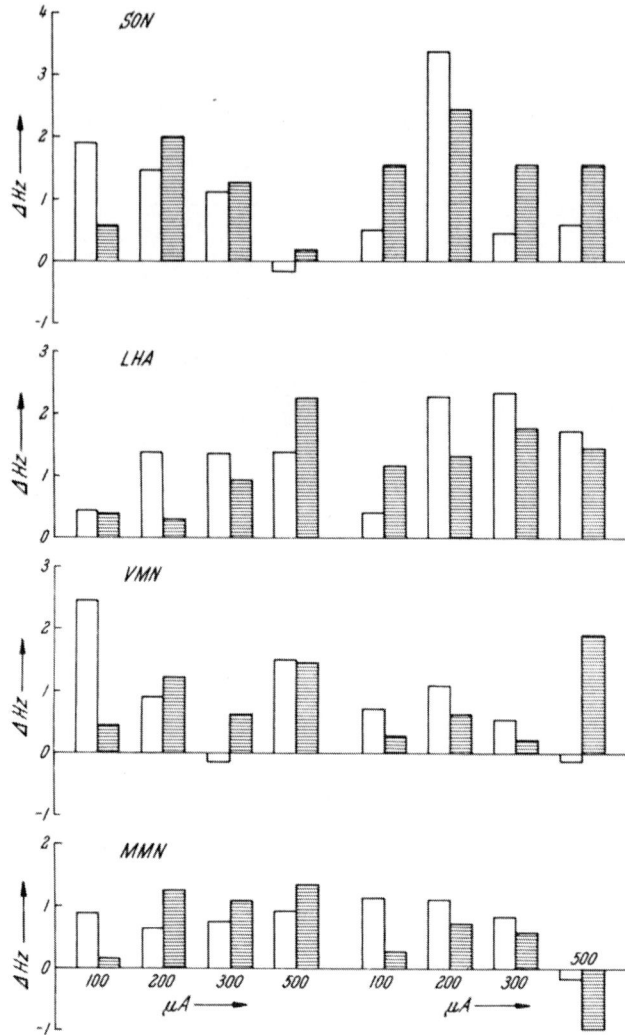

Fig. 35. Change in the basic EEG rhythm when the nuclei of the hypothalamus of animals of different age are stimulated before (light columns) and 20 minutes after the intravenous administration of insulin in a dose of 1 U/kg (shaded columns). First four pairs of columns–adult animals, last ones–old animals. The abbreviations are the same as in Fig. 25

study of the influence of hormones on the electric activity of the hypothalamic nuclei has revealed that (1) sensitivity to some hormones grows, but does not change to others with age, and (2) the reaction of various nuclei changes differently with age.

Hypothalamic feed-backs are realized not only through the blood hormones, but also through the system of information about the final result of the adaptive effect, i. e. metabolic shifts and the reflex influences of the receptors. Our data show that the reflexes of the mechanoreceptors of many organs attenuate, while the sensitivity of the chemoreceptors grows in old age (Frolkis, 1969, 1970, 1975; Shevchuk, 1979). The significance of the changes in the influence of these feed-backs on the hypothalamic structures is evident from the role of the hypothalamus in regulating blood circulation, respiration and digestion. These changes can lead to prolonged functional reactions. Many reflexes of the interoreceptors attenuate with age, thus giving rise to "hypothalamic misinformation." Information which comes via the "canals" of neural and humoral control is redistributed with age.

Thus, a vicious circle originates with age: negative and positive feed-backs, which should promote the realization of the central programme, can cause its divergence and lead to greater inconformity between the programme and the peripheral effects, and to programme "errors" and the development of pathology. Thus, the changes in the hypothalamic functions and in the perception of hormonal shifts, which are characteristic of every stage of the sexual cycle, upset the periodicity and structure of this cycle during the premenopausal period. FSH and LH play a definite role in ovulation and the formation of the yellow body. These hormones supplement one another in their action. Therefore, the sexual cycle is upset when their relationship is disturbed. The different dynamics of their age changes and the different shifts in the sensitivity and reactivity of the appropriate gonadotropin-synthesizing cells can be a cause of the disturbances of the sexual cycle.

The changes in the perception of return information are connected with the shifts in the hypothalamic receptors. The amount of the hypothalamic and hypophysial receptors of androgens (Chouknyiska, Vassileva-Popova, 1977) and the amount of the estradiol-binding receptors (Peng, Peng, 1973) diminish with age. The hypothalamus becomes more sensitive to thyroxine due to the activation of the deiodination processes (Frolkis *et al.*, 1973).

Adaptive Reactions of the Hypothalamus in Old Age

Claud Bernard once wrote that the organism's ability to preserve the relative constancy of its internal environment is a prerequisite of life. This property, which was evolutionarily acquired and which allows the organism to adapt itself and maintain a high level of viability in spite of the great changes in the environment, is largely determined by the mechanisms of hypothalamic regulation. The reliability and perfection of hypothalamic regulation and the development of the vitauct processes in regulating the internal environment are extremely important factors which determine the life span of a species.

There is much biological data on the great variability of the life span within some species, depending on environmental conditions, the state of the population, etc. We have already cited similar examples. The more highly organized animal and the greater its adaptation to the environment, the more perfectly it maintains homeostasis and homeorhesis under various conditions. The course of homeorhesis is determined by hypothalamic mechanisms.

Although the organism's internal environment is considered to be "relatively stable," it continually changes and disturbances occur in it under ordinary conditions and especially in extreme situations. Thus, hypothalamic regulation is characterized not by the stability of the mechanisms, but by constant dynamics. Extremely important is the fact that the mechanism of regulation is perfected and the vitauct processes are formed during constant changes in the state of the organism's internal environment. In our laboratory, we compared the mean life span of three groups of rats: (a) animals which were kept under ordinary conditions; (b) animals which were maximally protected from stimuli and stress situations, and (c) animals which were subjected daily to short-term stress influences of various types (Frolkis *et al.*, 1976b). The mean life span was 938 ±19 days in the first group of animals, 835 ±17 days in the second group of animals, and 1,120 ± 34 days in the third group of animals. Thus, the life span is reduced when the organism is protected from the environment and from tensions and emotional disturbances.

In analyzing the age dynamics of hypothalamic regulation, researchers quite correctly try to link the causes of the organism's aging with it. However, no account is taken of the fact that the vitauct processes, which make it possible to maintain the organism's great viability for a long time and preserve some extremely important homeostatic parameters (even under the conditions of reduced reliability) until old age, are connected with hypothalamic regulation. Thus, several functional systems preserve their viability in spite of the substantial metabolic and structural changes. Many important metabolic cycles, the electric activity of the hypothalamic nuclei, and the basal level of the secretion of many hypophysial hormones can be stably maintained for a long time. However, the hypothalamic mechanisms of regulation become less reliable with age.

Rushkevich (1980), our fellow worker, studied the dynamics of a change in the functions of the cardiovascular system and the structural changes in the myocardium when the hypothalamus was stimulated for a long time (up to 3 months). He showed that great shifts occur in cardiovascular activity some time after the beginning of the experiment. A substantial increase in arterial pressure was recorded on the 25th day of stimulation in old rabbits being higher in comparison with mature animals (Fig. 36). In this respect, distinct electrocardiographic signs of the disturbance of coronary blood circulation appear in most rabbits. In old animals, these shifts are accompanied by a diminution in the heart rate, which can occasionally drop to a very low level. Somewhat later during the experiment, the arterial pressure of such rabbits diminished and they died within a few days. By the middle of the second month of hypothalamic stimulation, 67 per cent of old animals and 33 per cent of mature animals died. A morphological investigation of the myocardium of the rabbits which died has revealed many necrotic changes that occurred at different times and that were rather great in some cases. Thus, the regulatory mechanisms of the hypothalamus become less reliable in old age when it is electrically stimulated for a long time.

The manifestations of vitauct at the hypothalamic level include the greater sensitivity of the hypophysis to several releasing factors and the greater sensitivity of the hypothalamic structures to adrenaline when the electric excitability of some nuclei is reduced and some regulatory influences on the hypothalamus are weakened.

Of course, it is difficult to work out distinct objective age criteria for assessing the extent to which various brain structures grow old. However, an analysis of the morphological and metabolic shifts shows that the age shifts are more pronounced in some brain structures (the neocortex, the striapallidal system) than in the hypothalamus. When age disturbances inevitably and naturally occur in the hypothalamus, that phenomenon becomes an extremely important mechanism of the whole organism's aging.

As we have already seen, the limitation of the hypothalamic regulation of the genetic apparatus of the cells and protein biosynthesis is of great significance. It affects virtually the most important process in the organism, i. e. the plastic ensurance of the organism's functions and adaptive reactions. This inconformity between functional ensurance and plastic ensurance ultimately makes the functions of some of the organism's systems inadequate. That occurrence is an important mechanism of the organism's aging.

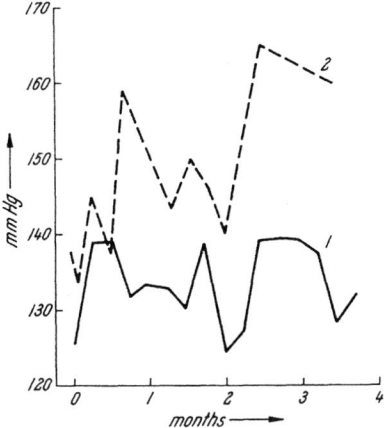

Fig. 36. Influence of the prolonged stimulation of the hypothalamus on the arterial pressure of mature rabbits *(1)* and old rabbits *(2)*

The loss organism's reproductivity occurs due to age changes in hypothalamic mechanisms. At this stage, life is divided into genetically informative and genetically uninformative parts. Many researchers associate the beginning of aging with the loss of reproductivity. This is erroneous, since its loss is not the beginning, but the inevitable consequence of the organism's aging.

The content of the gonadotropin hormones grows during the post-menopausal period, bit it greatly decreases 20 years after the beginning of the menopause (Chakravarti *et al.*, 1976). The change in the hypothalamic function is believed to be of paramount importance in the development of the menopause (Baranov *et al.*, 1972; Dilman, 1976a, b). According to Dilman (1976a, b), this change is due to both the progressive diminution of the sensitivity of the hypothalamus to negative feed-back and the growth of gonadotropic activity. Another widely held view is that the diminution of both the hormonal function of the ovaries and the secretion of estrogens and progesterone (as a result of which hypothalamic activity compensatively increases) is of paramount importance in the development of the climacteric (Adamopoulos et al., 1971).

According to Everitt (1976), the menopause in rodents is mainly hypothalamic in nature, but it is peripheral, or estrogenous, in humans. Aschheim (1976) showed that when ovaries of old rats are transplanted to young animals the cyclic changes are recommenced in them, though this is not a case when young ovaries are transplanted to old rats. Cooper and Linnoila showed in their experiments on 17 month-old female rats that the systematic administration of l-tyrosine together with food restored the vaginal cycle and ovulation; l-leucine was ineffective in this respect. These substances were ineffective when they were introduced through an implanted cannula into the medial preoptic region. The ovarial cycles were restored when l-dopa was administered intrahypothalamically or systemically.

It is believed that the decrease in serotonin and an increase in catecholamine metabolism in the brain are among the mechanisms with which the precursors of catecholamines in the hypothalamus restore the function of the ovaries in old anovular female rats. Reproductivity is lost due not simply to the attenuation or activation of the secretion of the gonadotropic hormones and the decrease in the gonad functions, but to the disturbance in the relationship between the follicle-stimulating hormone, luteinizing hormone, estrogens and androgens, and to a change in the reactions during their forward or backward occurrence. Hence, normal cyclic activity passes over to "chaos" and eventually "calm," thus upsetting the sequence of the chain reaction, including the central (gonadotropic hormones) and peripheral (sexual steroids) mechanisms.

The greatest structural disturbances occur and the largest number of neurons are lost in the arcuate nucleus and the preoptic region, i. e. regions which are responsible for regulating the synthesis of the gonadotropic hormones (Hsu, Peng, 1978). Owing to the intrahypothalamic relationships, these changes in some structures affect the functional state of other nuclei, too. An interesting fact is that the greatest disturbances occur in the ovaries with age.

What attracts attention is the appearance of possible genetic anomalies in the sex cells together with the disturbances in the endocrine mechanisms which stop human reproductivity. The extent of the genetic risk increases from 0.1 per cent for persons under 35 years of age to 3.54 per cent (by 35 times) for women who are older than 45 (Frota-Pessoa, 1978). Among women 38–40 years old, 5 per cent of the fetuses are with trisomy, while the figure is 20 per cent among women 44 years old and more (Sachs et al., 1977).

Aneuploidy occurs very frequently in the progeny of old women (Dejmek, Preiss, 1974). The number of births with an abnormal karyotype (47XXY, 47XXX) increases as the parents' age grows (Carothers et al., 1978). The number of aneuploid embryos increases in old mice (Fabricant, Schneider, 1978). It has long been known that a relationship exists between a mother's age and the frequency of Down's syndrome. Demographic data on several industrialized countries show that the frequency of trisomies and anomalies of a dominant nature decreased by 20–40 per cent in the last two decades due to the parents' younger age (Natsunaga, 1972).

   The climacteric stage, especially in women, is biologically significant because it prevents the disturbances in the genetic apparatus (which occur in the undividing ova) from being hereditarily transmitted. The number of hereditary anomalies is much higher in elderly mothers than in elderly fathers, whose spermatozoa are formed during mitosis (Evans, 1979). This probably explains the different occurrence of the climacteric stage in men and women. To understand the biological essence of the climacteric, its effects on life should be known.

   What are the mechanisms (including hormonal reorganization) which cause the loss of reproductivity when the disturbances of the genetic apparatus of the sex cells accumulate? What is the source of the information which includes that about the complex neurohumoral age reorganization and which protects the progeny and species from great hereditary disturbances? There is apparently a connection between the disturbance in the ova and a decrease which occurs in the hormonal activity of the ovaries with age. The evolutionary and embryogenic similarity of these factors determines the relationship between the structural changes in the ova and the hormonal shifts which disturb the organism's reproductive function. Hypothalamic shifts are first of all compensative, and then they acquire a "damaging" nature. A species would inevitably and naturally die if neurohumoral reorganization (which leads to the loss of the organism's reproductivity) did not occur at a definite stage of aging and if the sexual function remained on a high level when the sex cells are greatly damaged. Therefore, the loss of reproductivity with age is of definite adaptive significance. Account should also be taken of the possible effects of the disturbances caused by pregnancy and delivery on an elderly organism.

   The organism's reaction to the stress influences of the most diverse nature, including the pain stress, the cold stress, the hypodynamia, and adrenaline secretion, greatly changes as a result of the hypothalamic shifts which occur with age (Frolkis, 1963; Finch, 1973; Kaack et al., 1975; Riegle, 1976). The adaptive syndrome is phased and occurs in the following manner: alarm, the stability phase, which passes over to the phase of restoration or exhaustion, depending on the course of the occurences in the organism. Our data (Frolkis, 1970) show that the phases are displaced when the stress situations are reproduced in old age. The organism's protective properties increase less in old animals during the phase when the general adaptive syndrome is stable. The exhaustion phase occurs when the conditions are still optimum for mature animals. An interesting fact is that stress is more pronounced when reflex stimuli are produced in young and mature rats and when humoral stimuli are produced in old rats.

   The hypothalamic mechanisms of aging determine the diminution of the organism's ability to adapt itself to a temperature change (Verzar, 1963; Finch et al., 1969; Segall, Timiras, 1975) and to dietary changes (Everitt, 1970; Jakubczak, 1976). The relationship between the hypothalamic centres of "appetite" and "satiety" changes with age. It has been shown (Bezrukov, Epstein, 1977; Bezrukov, 1979) that the growth of the body mass and the blood insulin content is less pronounced in old animals when the ventromedial nucleus of the hypothalamus is lesioned (Fig. 37A, B, C). This fact, just as the shifts in

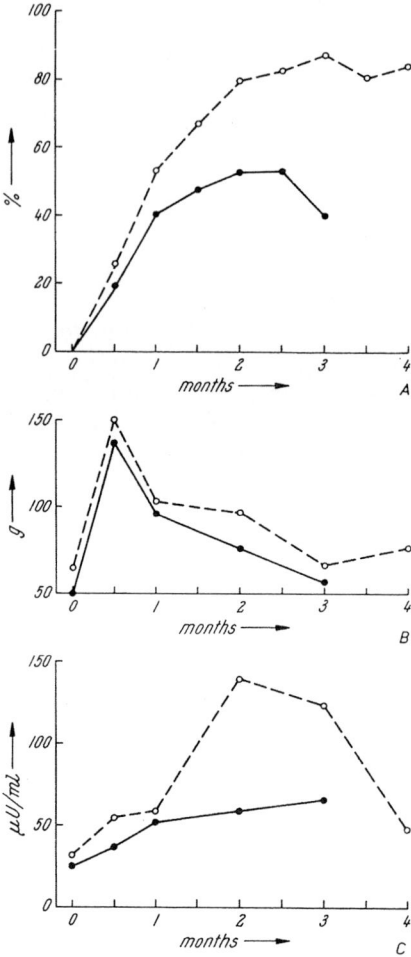

Fig. 37. Specifics of a change in the body mass (A), daily food consumption (B) and the level of insulin in the plasma (C) of mature rats (dashed line) and old rats (continuous line) during different lengths of time after the ventromedial hypothalamus is electrolytically damaged

thermoregulation, shows that the control of energy homeostasis weakens in old age.

Thus, the shifts in the adaptation of the aging organism, the most important shifts in protein biosynthesis, in energy homeostasis, in reproductivity, in dietary behaviour, in the regulation of blood circulation, and so forth, are connected with a change in the hypothalamic mechanisms. These shifts create the prerequisites for the disorder which occurs with age.

Biologically, the hypothalamus integrates individual functional and metabolic cycles and regulates the organism's activity. The hypothalamus allows individual components to combine into the "organism's internal environment," a complex biological system which produces an adequate reaction and which is adapted to the organism's external environment. Therefore, the above-mentioned "maladjustment" and "hypothalamic misinformation" are an extremely important mechanism of the whole organism's aging at a definite stage. They disturb the integration of homeostatic reactions and the production of a single general systemic adaptive effect. The words "general systemic" mean an adequate relationship between various vegetative changes, their emotional expression and behavioural reactions. The extent of the age changes in every link of the hypothalamic reaction may not be very great, but their different directions may disturb the integrity of the reaction. A situation may arise in which the activation of the vitauct processes in a certain structure may promote maladjustment. This situation is the source of unity and struggle between opposite tendencies of development that inevitably reduce the system's reliability.

While acknowledging the decisive importance of the hypothalamus in the whole organism's aging, it should be taken into account that all its changes occur as it interacts with other brain structures. Much data show that substantial changes occur in the structure and metabolism of *Locus ceruleus* with age (Brody, Vijayashankar, 1975). However, noradrenergic neurons are known to be directed to the hypothalamus exactly from there. This fact seems to engender a situation which is similar to the age changes in the striapallidal system, in whose aging a great role is played by the changes in *Substantia nigra,* which is the "source" of the mediators whose metabolism is affected in old age. Further investigations will reveal the real relationships which are formed between various brain structures with age.

The age changes in hypothalamic regulation should be considered together with the shifts in other structures of the limbic system, especially the hippocampus and the nuclei of the amygdaloid complex. These formations are very closely connected with the hypothalamus by afferent and efferent morphological bonds. The hippocampus and the amygdaloid complex influence the hypothalamic nuclei in a modulating manner. Many influences of the hippocampus and the amygdaloid complex on the vegetative system and various types of behaviour are realized through the hypothalamic nuclei. They include the influence of the amygdaloid complex on dietary and sexual behaviour, on emotional and vegetative reactions and on the endocrine balance, and also the influence of the hippocampus on the vegetative system during complex forms of behaviour and reflex activity. It has been shown that substantial morphological and metabolic shifts occur in these structures of the limbic system in old age.

In a special series of experiments which were carried out together with Bezrukov, a study was made of the influence exerted by the stimulation of the hypothalamic nuclei on the electric activity of the hippocampus and the amygdaloid complex and, conversely, the influence exerted by the hippocampus and the amygdala on the hypothalamic nuclei.

Acute experiments have revealed irregular and even differently directed shifts in the thresholds of the influences of various nuclei on the limbic structures. It was learned from the experiments that the supraoptic and mamillary medial nuclei should be stimulated by a weaker current, while the lateral hypothalamic region, by a stronger current in old animals as compared with mature animals so that initial shifts could appear on the electrogram of both the hippocampus and the nuclei of the amygdaloid complex.

The influence of the hippocampus on the electrogram of the hypothalamic nuclei virtually does not change with age. However, the thresholds of the influence of the medial amygdaloid nucleus on the hypothalamus increase, but those of the influence of the central amygdaloid nucleus on it decrease in old animals.

Data show that the direction of the age shifts is not clearly dependent on a structure's phylogenetic "age." The excitability of an older hippocampus does not change substantially, that of the central amygdaloid nucleus increases, and that of the younger medial amygdaloid nucleus decreases in old age.

Both hypothalamic and limbic formations participate in the regulation of various types of metabolism and various systems. Therefore, those changes in the links of the given central nervous structures can greatly influence homeostatic regulation. For instance, the attenuation of the modulating influences of the medial amygdaloid nucleus on the anterior and medial hypothalamic regions may be an important factor which worsens the regulation of the reproductive function. The intensification of the influences (at least, the reduction of their threshold) of the central amygdaloid nucleus on the hypothalamic mechanisms of regulation can greatly promote the origination of the affective behavioural reactions. The diminution of the poststimulatory hypothalamic effects as the hippocampus is stimulated can worsen the vegetative ensurance of muscular reactions, while the attenuation of the hypothalamic influences on the hippocampus can be an important cause of the worsening memory of some types. The age changes in the relationship between hypothalamic and limbic formations can be the basis of many functional disturbances in old age.

4. Adrenergic Mechanisms of Regulation During Aging

In 1937, the tradition-loving British were stocked when King Edward VIII fell in love with Miss Simpson, a movie actress, and abdicated. Somewhat later, Bogomolets said in his opening speech at a conference that a Miss Simpson may soon appear in endocrinology, taking away the crown from adrenaline. Indeed, the researches carried out in the subsequent decades and the rapid development of the concept of stress and universal reactions may seem to have produced a new competitor for the leading role in endocrinology: glucocorticoids. As physiology developed, everything seemed to fit into the right place and the polyregulatory nature of most of the organism's complex reactions (in whose initiation catecholamines play a big role) seemed to have been established.

The regulatory effects of the central nervous system are largely realized through the adrenergic mechanisms. Adrenergic influences control some of the most important links of cell metabolism, the energy processes in the cell, and the processes of protein biosynthesis. In the case of adrenergic influences, the metabolic shifts are so great that they change the function of the cell. The biological role which the sympathoadrenal system plays in realizing the organism's most important adaptive reactions was clearly defined in the works by Cannon (1929), Orbeli (1935) and Gellhorn (1943).

The changes in the organism's internal medium, which take place during motor activity, fear, hunger, eating behaviour, sexual behaviour, and so forth, occur mainly through the sympathoadrenal system. The activation of the sympathoadrenal system provides the metabolic and autonomic basis of the tensions in activity and is of great adaptive and regulatory significance. It is a component of vitauct, as it ultimately ensures a high level of the organism's vital activity, which is aimed at preserving the organism under the rigid conditions of the external environment. This is exactly how we should assess, for instance, the shifts in hemodynamics, glycemia and lipolysis, which occur during sympathoadrenal influences in the organism when there is intense muscular activity and emotional stress. Great tensions and the most important adaptive reactions virtually cannot be realized without them, when the organism's internal medium is quite "calm."

The rapid headway in the investigation of the autonomic nervous system and researches in the field of the morphology and function of the sympathetic system has created a great impression. As early as 1922, Dogiel, who did a great deal of research in the morphology of the sympathetic nervous system, had concluded that the age changes in the sympathetic nervous system are cardinal in the genesis of the intact organism's aging. Of course, this was a one-sided, limited idea of the essence of aging, but it somewhat expressed the growing interest taken by researchers in the neurohumoral mechanisms of aging.

Effects of the Adrenergic Influences in Old Age

The functional effects of the adrenergic influences are very diverse. The most important functions and metabolic cycles of the complex organism, i. e. hemodynamics, respiration, glycemia, digestion, lipemia, and so forth, are regulated with the participation of the adrenergic mechanisms.

In our laboratory, we carried out many researches which showed that substantial changes occur in the adrenergic mechanisms of regulation during aging. We have good grounds to maintain that sympathetic neural control over the activity of several organs attenuates in old age. In our opinion, firstly, these shifts in sympathetic neural control changes the course of the most important autonomic reactions and thus limit the adaptive abilities of the aging organism. Secondly, the decrease in sympathetic neural control, while disturbing the most important metabolic processes in the tissues, may be an important cause of aging of the effectors. Moreover, the content of catecholamines in the blood and the reaction of the cells and tissues to the action of adrenaline and noradrenaline change as the organism ages.

Many contradictions in the description of tissue reactions to catecholamines in old age arise because the effects are compared when the catecholamine doses are different. Large catecholamine doses are used not only in age physiology, but also physiology in general. We suppose that this is the result of pharmacological influence on physiology. At the same time, the influence of catecholamines on the organism should obviously be studied within a wide range of doses while necessarily using doses which approximate the threshold or physiological values, i. e. doses which cause physiological changes in metabolism and functions, and not necessarily doses which are large and which approximate extreme values. This is exactly what we did in our laboratory. In our experiments, we determined the sensitivity of the tissues to catecholamines as well as their reactivity. Sensitivity was determined by the minimum amount of the substances which produce the appropriate effect, i. e. the criteria of sensitivity coincide with the threshold of excitability. Reactivity was determined by the dose of the substance which produces the maximum reaction.

The range of the reactions to the action of catecholamines narrows down with age as the reactivity of the tissues diminishes, while the sensitivity of the tissues to the hormone and the transmitter grows. This concept was confirmed even when various cellular, organic and systemic reactions were realized. Fig. 38A, B gives the data presented by Shevchuk (1966) on a change in the level of blood sugar in adult (10–12 months) and old (60–62 months) rabbits. Hyperglycemia was distinct in old rabbits when smaller doses of adrenaline were administered, while it was more distinct in mature animals when larger doses were administered. Such an increase in sensitivity and a decrease in reactivity were shown by taking the example of another systemic reaction: the shift in arterial blood pressure (Bezrukov, 1971). It was shown that the threshold dose

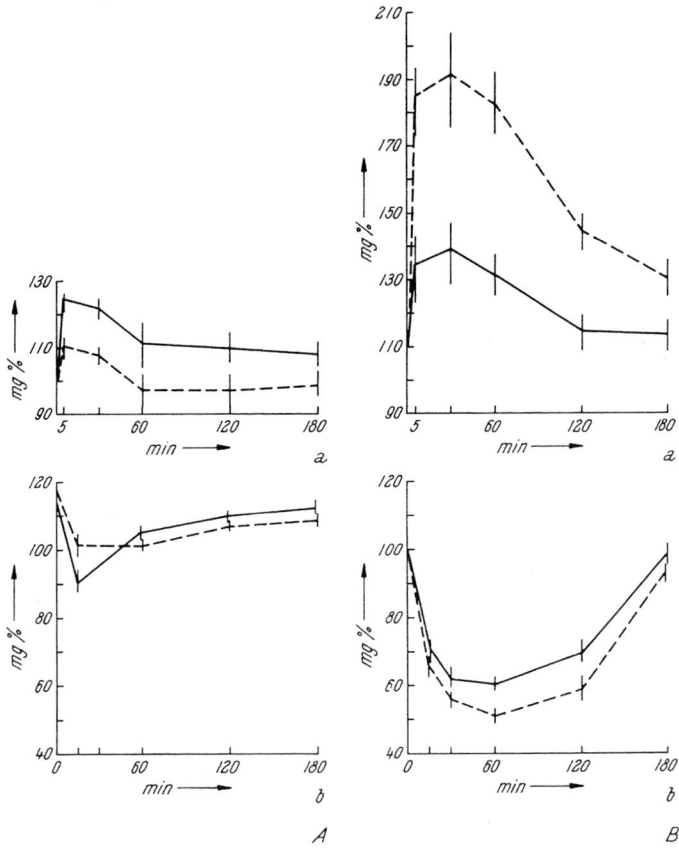

Fig. 38. Age differences in the hormonal regulation of the blood sugar level. The dashed line stands for mature rabbits, and the continuous line, for old rabbits. *A* intravenous administration of adrenaline: *a* 5 μg/kg; *b* 50 μg/kg. *B* intravenous administration of insulin: *a* 0.025 U/kg; *b* 1.5 U/kg

of adrenaline which causes the growth of arterial blood pressure in old rabbits is 16.0 ±1.65 ng/kg, while in mature animals, it is 114.3 ±14.3 ng/kg; the threshold doses of noradrenaline are 33.7 ± 3.0 and 183.6 ± 23.5 ng/kg, respectively. The maximum growth of arterial pressure, being attained when the dose of noradrenaline is enlarged, is greater in mature animals (206.0 ± 4.6 mm Hg) than in old ones (187 ± 6.0 mm Hg). An increase in sensitivity to catecholamines, which was shown by studying systemic reactions, has been observed also in the investigation of persons of different age (Korkushko, 1969). When 0.5 ml of 0.1 per cent adrenaline solution is administered, arterial pressure does not change in persons 20–29 years old, but it grows from 117.9 ± 3.5 to 138.8 ± 6.3 mm Hg in persons 80–89 years old. Hoffman and others (1975) have shown that noradrenaline, adrenaline and isoprenaline cause greater changes in the heart rate of elderly persons. According to the data presented by our laboratory (Verkhratsky, 1962), smaller doses of

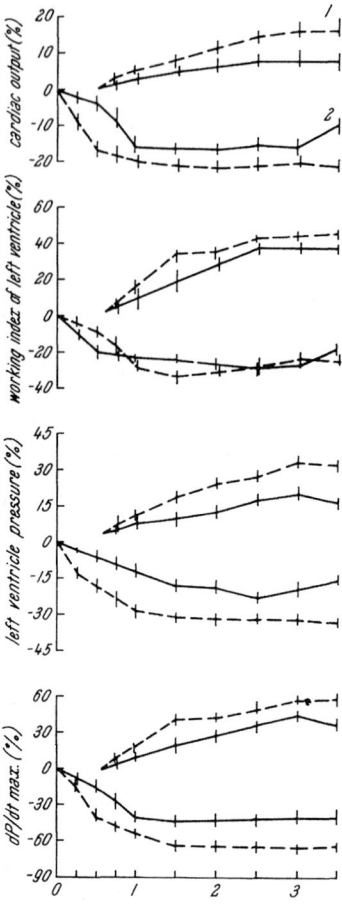

Fig. 39. Change in the hemodynamics and contractile ability of the myocardium in animals of different age when the sympathetic and vagus nerves are stimulated. *1* sympathetic nerve; *2* vagus nerve. The dashed line stands for mature rabbits, and the continuous line for old rabbits. Abscissa: intensity of stimulation (volts)

adrenaline cause the spasm of arterioles and capillaries in old persons as compared with young people.

The nictitating membrane of the cat eye is a classical object for comparing neural and humoral adrenergic influences. Verkhratsky (1972) has shown that in order to cause the contraction of this membrane in old cats, it is necessary to stimulate the sympathetic nerve by an electric current which is 1.5–1.8 time greater than that used for stimulating the nerve in adult cats. Such an effect was produced when not only the preganglionic fibres, but also the postganglionic fibres of the nerve were stimulated. Smaller doses of adrenaline and noradrenaline had to be administered to old animals in order to cause the contraction of the nictitating membrane. The weakening of neural adrenergic control in old age (Fig. 39) has been demonstrated by Shevchuk and Lakiza. They have established that the changes in myocardial contractility and the shifts in cardiac output originate in old rats, rabbits and dogs when the stellate ganglion and the sympathetic nerve are stimulated by a stronger electric current.

Sympathetic innervation is known to play a certain role in regulating vascular tonicity. In the research work carried out by Frolkis together with Verkhratsky and Zamostyan (1967), the changes in the vascular tonicity of various regions (the posterior exremity, the intestine and the kidneys) were recorded under the conditions of resistographic perfusion, and the threshold intensities of the

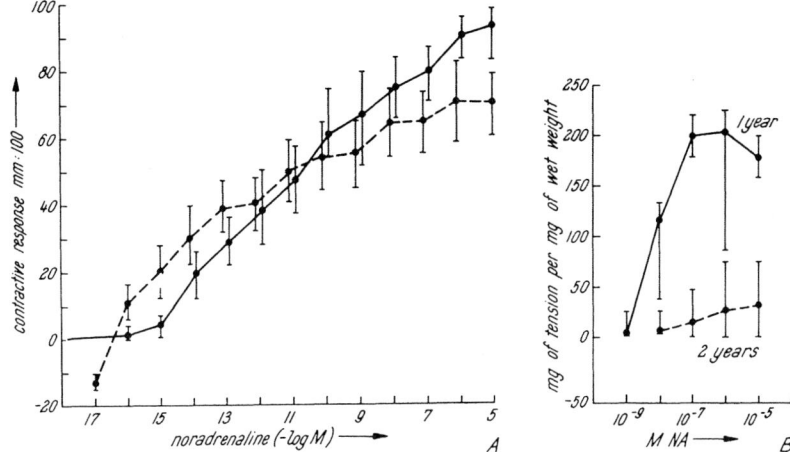

Fig. 40. Influence of noradrenaline on the contractile ability of an aortic strip of rats of different age. *A* Lakiza's data; *B* Tuttle's data. The continuous line stands for mature rats, and the dashed line, for old rats

stimulation of the sympathetic chain that lead to vascular constriction were determined. To constrict the vessels of an extremity, the sympathetic chain must be stimulated by a stronger current in old rats than in mature ones (0.59 ± 0.05 V and 0.38 ± 0.05 V, respectively; $p < 0.05$). There are no age differences in the effects of the action of the sympathetic nerves on the kidney vessels, while the thresholds of the sympathetic neural influences on the intestine vessels diminish in old age. In our *in vitro* experiments on individual vascular strips, we showed that the reaction of the vessels to the action of catecholamines changes (Lakiza, 1979; Fig. 40 A). Sympathetic neural influences on vascular tonicity ultimately occur due to a change in the electric activity and contractility of the smooth muscle cells. The frequency of the action potentials grows and the level of the membrane potential and the values of cell membrane resistance change under the influence of catecholamines. The smooth muscle fibres were steadily depolarized for a long time when the concentration of noradrenaline was increased.

The changes in the electric activity of the smooth muscle cells of the wall of the portal vein were recorded in adult and old rats in a special series of experiments involving the use of the microelectrode method (I. V. Frolkis, 1976 c). In adult rats, the shifts in the electric activity of the smooth muscle cells of the portal vein and their contractile abilities had originated when the concentration of noradrenaline was 1×10^{-9}, while in old rats, they originated when it was 1×10^{-11} (Fig. 40 A, B). This growth of the sensitivity of individual smooth muscle cells explains why vessels react to smaller doses of catecholamines in old age.

The attenuation of neural sympathetic influences and the enhancement of the sensitivity to catecholamines are determined ultimately at the cellular level and depend on the reactions of individual cells to adrenergic effects. In this respect, we carried out a special series of researches in order to analyze the age specifics of the reactions of the cells to sympathetic neural stimulation and the action of catecholamines. The change in the value of the membrane potential of the cells is an important indicator of a cellular reaction. The hyperpolarization of individual muscle fibres of *Musculus gastrocnemius* is more pronounced in mature rats when the sympathetic chain is stimulated (I. V. Frolkis, 1973). Hyperpolarization is more pronounced in adult rats. In old animals, small doses of noradrenaline cause the growth of the membrane potential of these cells (Turaeva, 1978). However, the possible amplitude of the growth of the membrane potential under the action of catecholamines diminishes with age. The reaction of the kidneys to catecholamines changes in old age. According to Faizulin (1979), sympathetic neural influences on the acinar cells of the parotid gland attenuate in old rats. Kalinovskaya (1978) has shown that adrenaline in a dose of 2.5 µg/kg reduces the plasma and blood flows by 50—60 per cent in 15 minutes in old persons, but it virtually does not reduce them in young persons. The nature of the ionic shifts is also in full conformity with this fact (Turaeva, 1979). According to Kostikova and others (1974), the activating effect of adrenaline and corticotropin on the lipolytic enzymes decreases with age. Chaika (1977) studied the effect of adrenaline of greatly varying doses on the lipolytic activity of the epidimymal fat of young and adult rats and showed that lipolytic activity greatly increases under the influence of small doses of the hormone in old rats. Reactivity, i. e. the maximum value of the reaction, is greater in young animals. All the given functional effects obviously have a definite metabolic basis. We have shown earlier in our laboratory that the shifts in the content of glycogen, in the activity of phosphorylase, in oxidative phosphorylation and in macroergic phosphorus compound metabolism originate in the myocardium of old rats under the action of smaller doses of catecholamines (Frolkis, 1970). The given age dynamics of adrenergic regulation is characteristic of not all the systems and organs. This fact was demonstrated by Faizulin (1978), who studied the adrenergic regulation of the electric activity of the acinar cells of the parotid gland. It was learned that the reaction of the cells to catecholamines is more pronounced in mature animals. Interestingly the reaction of the acinar cells to the sympathetic neural influences is not stable, and the rapid exhaustion of reactions is seen in old age. In mature rats, higher sensitivity to catecholamines is combined with a decrease in the effects of stimulation of the sympathetic nerve. This is obviously a manifestation of the general regularity of the link between the state of adrenoreceptors and the nature of the impulses which pass through the synapses.

That type of age change in the reactions to catecholamines is common in the animal kingdom. It is found among the species of animals which phylogenetically differ greatly from one another. The experiments carried out by Martynenko, who studied the reactions of the giant neurons of the small parietal ganglion of the pond snails of different age, are an example of this. Hyperpolarization developed and the thresholds of the direct stimulation of the cell through the microelectrode as well as the frequency of spontaneous activity increased in both adult and old animals under the influence of adrenaline. An important fact is that these shifts in the electric properties of the neuron membranes originated in old animals (22–24 months) under the influence of adrenaline administered in doses which were one-half of those administered to adult animals (0.5 μg/ml and 1.0 μg/ml, respectively).

The data on a change in sensitivity to catecholamines in old age differ. For instance, Erisson (1973) showed that the relaxing effect of isadrine decreases in old rats. Berkowitz (1976) observed that the contractile reaction of the isolated abdominal aorta to noradrenaline is the greatest in animals 3–5 weeks old, but it is the slightest in animals 35–38 weeks old. A decrease in the reaction of the aorta to catecholamines has been observed by Fleisch (1971), Tuttle (1976) and Pandya (1977). At the same time, Hruza and Zweifach (1967) have shown that the sensitivity of the cardiovascular system to adrenaline grows in old age. Freji (1966) discovered qualitative differences in the reactions to noradrenaline, depending on age. The strips of the vessels of young rabbits responded by relaxation with ensuing contraction, while those of old ones responded only by contraction.

These contradictions are largely due to the different selection of the age groups of animals for experiments and the use of limited doses of substances. The methods used also often have their disadvantages. For instance, Tuttle (1976) recorded the contraction of a strip under conditions which did not allow him to ascertain the threshold reactions. But if a device is more sensitive, the relationships in the reaction of the strips of the aorta of adult and old rats differ from those observed by Tuttle.

Thus, the adrenergic regulation of the cells, organs and tissues changes with age. This was shown in the investigations involving animals of different species, i. e. pond snails, rats, rabbits, cats and dogs, and in those involving man. An important fact is that the extent of the age changes in the adrenergic regulation of different organs is not always the same. Consequently, qualitative differences are created in the "organization" of complex adaptive reactions. Some of the most important adaptive reactions, which are regulated by adrenergic mechanisms, weaken with age. This direction of the changes in adrenergic regulation largely determines the age limitations of the adaptive reactions of the organism. The attenuation of autonomic reactions, their prolonged latent period and the diminution of their possible range are some of the reasons why working ability decreases with age. However, there is another important fact. The attenuation of adrenergic neural control and the substantial destruction of many sympathetic terminals can be a cause of the great metabolic, morphological and functional disturbances in the tissues being innervated. Of course, analogy is not evidence. However, it should be noted by way of example that shifts similar to the changes which occur with age are observed during the sympathetic denervation of the salivary glands, the bone, the heart, etc. For instance, adrenergic stimulation is known to regulate the intensity of the secretion of protein with saliva. According to the data obtained in our laboratory (Faizulin, 1978), more protein is secreted in adult animals than in old ones under the influence of prolonged adrenergic stimulation.

Intense adrenergic stimulation activates not only the synthesis of protein which is to be taken outside, but also protein which meets the plastic requirements of the cell. Therefore, not only functional synthesis of protein, but also its plastic synthesis apparently abates during adrenergic stimulation in old age. This may be the cause of the great structural changes in the gland cells and of even their death.

Very distinct natural age changes occur in osseus tissue (osteoporosis). Similar changes occur during the sympathetic denervation of the bone, being more pronounced in old animals.

The structural disturbances of the sympathetic nervous system affect the state of vascular tonicity and the structure of the vascular wall. Indeed, the disturbances of the wall structure in the vessels of the muscle type (with their pronounced sympathetic innervation) become very considerable with age. Such disturbances of the sympathetic terminals have been observed also in other organs (the heart, the salivary glands, the urinary bladder).

Thus, all the changes in the sympathetic nervous system not only alter the adaptive reactions of the organism in old age, but also become a cause of the age changes in the structure and metabolism of the organs being innervated.

Many researchers, including the members of our laboratory, have recently been taking great interest in the significance of the brain structures in the genesis of aging when the adaptive reactions are involved. An important fact is that the changes in the efferent, centrifugal link of the transfer of information play a definite role in this respect. These changes cause the above-mentioned phenomenon, i. e. the activation of the brain structures in old age is often not realized in the appropriate peripheral effects. Another important fact is that the tonic adrenergic neural influences on the tissues change and the basal level of their trophism greatly alter with age. These disturbances of the centrifugal pathways are often among the main causes of the change in the neural regulation of the tissue with all its consequences.

Thus, the whole system of adrenergic regulation is characterized by a narrower range of reactions and a diminution of the amplitude of this regulation in old age. In many cases, these features are combined with greater sensitivity to catecholamines. A smaller outgoing signal upsets the system. This signal does not grow considerably when the incoming signal, i. e. the incoming information, increases. The system is adapted, as it were, to limited tensions. We believe that the greater sensitivity to catecholamines is of adaptive and regulatory significance, being a manifestation of vitauct. As a result of this shift, the cells react to adrenergic stimulation by ejecting a smaller amount of the mediator and are drawn into the general adaptive reaction in spite of the diminution of the content of blood catecholamines. Hence, adaptive shifts may originate when the loads on the organism are slight. Such a situation may originate when the organism's abilities and reserves are limited in old age. An increase in sensitivity to several humoral factors, including catecholamines, changes the nature of the reactions. Their latent period increases and they become prolonged. At the same time, the possible range, amplitude and reliability of many adaptive reactions decrease as reactivity diminishes.

Thus, the adrenergic shifts which occur with age are characterized not only by disturbance and extinction, but also by internal contradictory changes.

Of course, there is a definite link between the attenuation of the adrenergic neural effects on the tissue and the growth of sensitivity to humoral factors. In principle, this link was clearly formulated by Cannon and Rosenblueth (1951) in the law of denervation. The law states that if a unit is destroyed in a series of efferent neurons, excitability with respect to the action of chemical agents increases in an isolated structure or structures, the effect being the maximum in the directly denervated regions. We want to emphasize that the attenuation of neural influences plays a definite role in the development of the age changes in sensitivity, but it is not the essence of this phenomenon. It will be shown further that several metabolic shifts, including those in the exchange of the mediators during aging and denervation, may not be identical. For instance, a decrease in sympathetic neural control is known to increase both the number of adrenoreceptors and the response of the adenylate cyclase system. At the same time, the number of adrenoreceptors falls with age.

Chemical adrenergic denervation (even partial) can be caused by a group of substances which deplete the reserves of catecholamines in the vesicles of the sympathetic terminals. One such substance is reserpine, which substantially reduces the content of noradrenaline, particularly in the vessels and the heart of animals of various species, such as cats, mice, rabbits and dogs. The action of reserpine is believed to pass through three phases. The first phase is connected with the depletion of the labile fraction of catecholamines in the brain. The second phase, which has been studied most thoroughly, originates in about four hours after the administration of reserpine and is connected with the depletion of the labile fraction of amines in the heart and the vessels. The third phase is connected with the depletion of the stable, nucleotide-dependent fraction of catecholamines.

An increase in the sensitivity of the adrenoreceptor apparatus to catecholamines is an important feature of pharmacological desympathization caused by reserpine (Ramires et al., 1976; Ahn, Makman, 1977). Lakiza from our laboratory studied the changes in the hemodynamic effects of noradrenaline in animals of different age before and after the administration of reserpine and showed that the thresholds of the sensitivity of the cardiovascular system to noradrenaline decrease in adult rats four hours after the administration of reserpine, while the thresholds do not change in old animals. Hence, pharmacological denervation in itself produces unexpected results in mature and old rats.

The data produced by Weiss and others (1979) are interesting in this respect. They showed that the prolonged administration of reserpine increases substantially the number of adrenoreceptors in the cerebral cortex of young and mature rats, but it almost does not change their number in old animals.

The attenuation of neural influences and the growth of sensitivity to humoral factors in old age have also been structurally consolidated to a certain extent. Dolgo-Saburov and others (1960) have described the so-called axovasal synapses, i. e. nerve endings which terminate on small vessels, in the brain. The mediator separated into the blood stream is believed to be carried to the appropriate group of cells. According to Govyrin (1967), the sympathetic nerve influences on the skeletal muscles, being interpreted by Orbeli as adaptive trophic ones, are realized through noradrenaline which is released from the sympathetic terminals on the vessels. Noradrenaline is carried by blood flow to the muscle fibres. Axovasal synapses have been shown to exist in the heart, the adrenal glands and the skeletal muscles (Kulchitsky, Badaeva, 1972). The number of these axovasal synapses, particularly in the heart, grows in old age (Kulchitsky, Badaeva, 1972). This fact is probably a peculiar adaptive phenomenon which results from the attenuation of neural influences on the tissue. The attenuation of neural influences and the growth of sensitivity to humoral factors are a natural, but not a universal phenomenon which occurs with age.

Since aging is characterized by an increase in sensitivity and a decrease in reactivity, we always take account of the following points:

1. The attenuation of neural influences, an increase in sensitivity and a decrease in reactivity to humoral factors are expressed to a different extent in various tissues and in various cells of the same tissue. We have already indicated that the reactions of the vessels of various organs to neural and humoral influences change differently. Data have already been given on the non-uniform, differently oriented shifts in excitability and sensitivity to the chemical influences of various nervous structures, glands, etc. There can be no common ratios of a change in the reaction of various effectors to regulatory influences.

2. The sensitivity of several organs and some groups of cells virtually does not change with age. Verkhratsky, for instance, showed that the threshold doses of acetylcholine and adrenaline, which cause the contraction of the intestine in rabbits of different age, virtually do not differ from one another. According to Faizulin (1978), the acinar cells of the salivary glands are more sensitive to alpha-adrenostimulation in mature rats than in old ones, while their sensitivity to beta-adrenostimulation virtually does not change in old age.

3. In old age, sensitivity does not change with respect to some substances, but it diminishes with respect to others. To cause shifts in the function of the neural and muscular apparatus of old rats, larger doses of Listenone, ephedrine, sodium fluoride and some other substances are to be administered to them.

4. In advanced old age, the growth of sensitivity to humoral factors may be followed by its progressive diminution.

Thus, the existence of a definite regularity of the reaction of the effectors to catecholamines in old age does not mean that it mechanically applies to all the substances and to the reaction of all the tissues. Otherwise, the essence of an extremely complex biological process would be greatly simplified, its mechanism would be explained in a one-sided manner, and the direction in which we are exerting our efforts would be undermined.

Sympathetic Ganglia During Aging

Sympathetic nervous ganglia are an extremely important link in the realization of adrenergic influences. Their age changes can themselves upset adrenergic control.

In evolutionary and age physiology, diverse data have been obtained on both the phylogenesis and the early stages of the ontogenesis of the ganglionic apparatus (Sheveleva, 1977; Yarkin, 1977, and others). Until recently, we knew far less about the functional changes in the sympathetic ganglia at the last stages of ontogenesis. In our laboratory, we carried out systematic research in this respect. Our experiments involved cats, rabbits and dogs of different ages.

In the case of the preganglionic stimulation of *Ganglion cervicale superius*, excitability is reduced in old animals. The thresholds of electric stimulation that cause the contraction of the nictitating membrane are 0.11 ± 0.041 V in cats 1–4 years old and 0.30 ± 0.045 V in cats 10–12 years old (the duration of the impulse is 0.5 millisecond and the frequency is 20–40 Hz).

The value of the membrane potential of the neurons of *Ganglion cervicale superius* does not, on the average, change substantially with age: it ranges from 50 to 85 mV in adult and old cats. According to Skok (1970), it ranges from 40 to 70 mV in adult rabbits, averaging 57 mV in them. However, neurons with a low value of the membrane potential (20–30 mV) are more frequently found in old age. This fact is probably in accord with the appearance of atrophied, degenerated neurons in the sympathetic ganglia.

According to Sheveleva (1977), the value of the membrane potential of the neurons of *Ganglion cervicale superius* increases from 19.5 ± 0.9 mV in newborns to 77.3 ± 2.2 mV in adult animals in postnatal ontogenesis. The mechanisms which maintain a definite value of the membrane potential are changed in old age. For instance, when sodium fluoride (which blocks glycolysis) was used in a concentration of 0.001 ml/mole, the value of the membrane potential decreased by 12 mV in old animals and by 7 mV in adult ones. Spontaneous electric activity of the neurons was observed more frequently in old animals.

One of the most important characteristics of the functional state of autonomic ganglia is their lability. Many changes in the functional state of autonomic ganglia, ranging from optimal to pessimal reactions, may occur in conformity with both the frequency of the impulses which pass along the preganglionic fibres and the state of synaptic transfer.

Tonic impulsation in individual postganglionic sympathetic neurons is low, being 2–4 impulses per second (Bronk, 1939). Impulse frequency grows sharply in the case of reflex influences. According to Skok (1970), the optimal frequencies of the stimulation of the preganglionic sympathetic neurons are 20–25 impulses per second.

A decrease in the lability of the sympathetic ganglia and the origination of rarer rhythms of optimal and pessimal frequencies are among the most important functional features of these ganglia during aging. In studying the function of *Ganglion cervicale superius* of old and adult cats, the preganglionic trunk was stimulated and the contraction of the nictitating membrane of the eye and the electric activity of the postganglionic nerves were recorded (Duplenko, 1965). The total difference of potentials drawn off all the axons in the common postganglionic trunk was then recorded. Therefore, the transformation of the rhythm of the impulses even in a part of the ganglionic neurons was expressed in a decrease in the amplitude of the potentials. This transformation became more pronounced as more cells lost their ability to react simultaneously with the stimulation rhythm. Potentials of sufficiently high values were recorded in the postganglionic fibre by carrying out preganglionic tetanization with a frequency

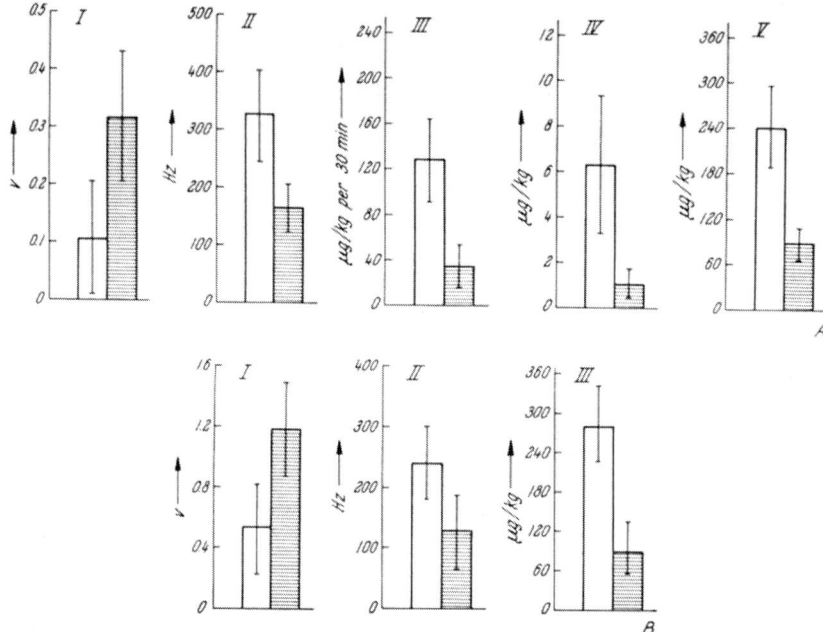

Fig. 41. Age differences in the functional state of *Ganglion cervicale superius* (A) and the parasympathetic ganglia of the heart *(B)* of cats and rabbits. *I* thresholds of the excitability of the preganglionic trunks in cats; *II* pessimal frequencies of preganglionic tetanization in cats; *III* activity of cholinesterase in the ganglionic tissue of rabbits; *IV* threshold acetylcholine doses which stimulate the ganglia in cats; *V* threshold benzohexonium doses which suppress the ganglionic transmission of excitation in cats. White columns stand for adult animals, and the shaded columns, for old animals

of 40 impulses per second. The potentials decreased until they fused with the noise as the stimulation rhythm increased to 80 impulses per second. The transition to rarer stimulation rhythms restores the amplitude of potentials and the extent of muscle tetanus (typical replacement of the optimal reaction by a pessimal one according to Vvedensky's principle). A decrease in the extent of muscle contraction with the simultaneous reduction of the amplitude of the action potentials in the postganglionic fibre confirms the well-known concept of the localization of the pessimum in the ganglionic apparatus.

The pessimum in *Ganglion cervicale superius* originated in old animals when the frequencies were smaller than in adult animals. In the case of superthreshold preganglionic tetanization, the pessimal reaction originated at a frequency of 108.5 ±11.37 impulses per second in old cats and at a frequency of 226.7 ± 47.73 impulses per second in adult cats. The value of the pessimal frequency of stimulation changes as the force of the stimulation of the preganglionic sympathetic nerve increases. When the impulses doubled in comparison with the tetanization threshold, the pessimum originated at a frequency of 150.8 ±16.62 impulses per second in cats 10–20 years old and at a frequency of 315.6 ± 35.57 impulses per second in cats 1–2 years old (Fig. 41).

With age, a decrease in the lability of autonomic ganglia and in the frequencies of their optimal and pessimal stimulations affect their functional state. These shifts are probably important in the formation of an inert type of vegetative reactions as well as reactions with a prolonged period of restoration of the initial level of the function in old age. When the organism grows old, the shifts in the optimal frequencies of ganglionic stimulation together with the changes in central efferent signalization largely determine the intensity of the reactions of various effectors and various internal organs.

Another important regularity of the age changes in the functional state of autonomic ganglia can be defined in the following way: the sensitivity of sympathetic ganglia to the action of several humoral factors grows as the lability and excitability of autonomic ganglia decrease during preganglionic stimulation. In other words, smaller amounts of several chemical agents stimulate and suppress ganglionic transfer in old animals. In these animals, smaller amounts of the activating and blocking agents of ganglionic transfer influence sympathetic ganglia. In old cats, *Ganglion cervicale superius* was activated by acetylcholine chloride in a dose of 1.1 ± 0.19 μg/kg, but in adult cats, it was activated by a dose of 6.3 ±1.35 μg/kg (Fig. 41).

The sensitivity of ganglia to substances which block ganglionic transfer also grows with age. This transfer can be blocked by influencing either the secretion and destruction of acetylcholine or the H-cholinoreactive systems of the ganglionic neurons directly.

It has been shown in experiments with cats that smaller doses of benzohexonium administered intravenously upset ganglionic transfer in old animals. The threshold doses of benzohexonium which reduced excitability in the case of preganglionic stimulation of *Ganglion cervicale superius* averaged 241.7 ± 24.48 μg/kg in adult cats and 86.5 ± 7.81 μg/kg in old animals (Fig. 41). In old cats, smaller doses of benzohexonium also reduced the lability of *Ganglion cervicale superius*. Ganglion blockers change the electric properties of the cells of sympathetic ganglia. The value of the membrane potential of neurons decreased to a greater extent in old animals when the dose of benzohexonium administered to them was the same as that administered to adult animals. It has been shown that the impulse frequency in the postganglionic neuron diminishes more in old animals under the action of benzohexonium.

The sensitivity of sympathetic ganglia to not only blocking agents, but also activating agents (nicotine, DMPP) grows with age (Duplenko, 1965). This great sensitivity of sympathetic ganglia to the agents which block ganglia was shown not only in model experiments, but also in clinic physiological studies involving healthy persons of different age. In our laboratory, Dukhovichny

(1974) recorded hemodynamic changes in persons 17–29 years old and 60–64 years old when various doses of benzohexonium were administered (0.3–0.5–1.0 ml of 2.5 per cent solution). Unlike young persons, arterial pressure in elderly persons decreased already when 0.3 ml of the benzohexonium solution was administered (12.0 ± 2.4 mm Hg). When 0.1 ml of the preparation was administered, systolic pressure decreased inconsiderably in young persons, but it dropped by 22.6 ± 2.7 mm Hg in elderly persons.

All these functional changes in autonomic ganglia are connected with the shifts in the metabolism of transmitters and with structural disturbances. Cholinergic mechanisms are known to play a definite role in realizing conduction in sympathetic ganglia. According to Duplenko (1965), acetylcholine synthesis becomes less intense with age; in old rats, the activity of choline acetylase in *Ganglion cervicale superius* is 47 per cent lower than in one-month-old rats and 24 per cent lower than in ten-month-old rats. Acetylcholine hydrolysis also becomes less intense. The activity of true choline esterase is lower by 30 per cent and that of pseudocholine esterase, by 38 per cent in rats 24 months old in comparison with adult rats.

Thus, the hydrolysis of the mediator attenuates as its synthesis decreases. Under the conditions which are created with age, the attenuation of acetylcholine hydrolysis may be an adaptive mechanism which promotes the accumulation of the necessary amount of the mediator in spite of the attenuation of its synthesis. The lability of ganglionic neurons decreases when the hydrolysis of the mediator becomes less intense.

Many works have been written on the specifics of extramural and intramural ganglia which develop with age. Some morphologists maintain that the dimensions of the nerve cells and the number and thickness of the processes change, pigment deposition increases, the mutual arrangement of the structural aspects of a ganglion alters, i. e. continuous fields or groups of nerve cells separated by bundles of nerve fibres and connective tissue appear, the vascular walls undergo changes (hyalinosis), etc. Some authors believe that the ganglion cells become smaller and wrinkle with age, while others maintain that the cells become larger with age. Changes in fibres are observed in the form of varicose, beaded and spindle-like thickenings along the axons, and the fibres may even disintegrate.

Vitauct processes, including the hyperfunction of individual cells, the activation of RNA synthesis in them, and an increase in the number of synapses on the body of the nerve cell are observed together with the obvious structural disturbances in sympathetic ganglia.

Functional and structural changes in autonomic ganglia can obstruct the transmission of impulses from the centres to the periphery. Moreover, the death and degeneration of the neurons of sympathetic ganglia influence the trophism of the tissue being innervated. The irregularity of the age disturbances at the periphery can to a certain extent be the outcome of the non-uniform death and destruction of ganglionic neurons. The cellular structures which are being innervated by the dying neurons will apparently be subjected to greater age shifts.

Catecholamine Metabolism

The investigation of the functional and metabolic effects gives an idea how adrenergic regulation changes in old age, but the study of catecholamine metabolism shows why it changes. An analysis of the change in the content of catecholamines in the blood and urine of persons and animals of different ages gives a definite idea about the general direction of the age changes in catecholamine metabolism, an idea which is important to clinical physiology. The data obtained in this respect can probably enable us to assess the shifts in the activity of the sympathoadrenal system. Blood catecholamines are an important way of realizing generalized reactions when the system is being activated. Euler and Lishajko (1961) as well as Morozova (1971) and others have found that less catecholamines are excreted with urine in old age.

Table 2. *Change in the content and excretion of catecholamines with age*

Age	Content in blood (μ g/lit)	
	Adrenaline	Noradrenaline
Persons		
20–35 years	0.470 ± 0.025	0.916 ± 0.034
60–75 years	0.545 ± 0.019*	0.148 ± 0.032***
Rats		
0.5–1 month	0.340 ± 0.097	2.000 ± 0.174
8–10 months	0.697 ± 0.023***	1.115 ± 0.111***
24–26 months	1.035 ± 0.086***	0.154 ± 0.072***

	Excretion with urine				
	Adrenaline	Noradrenaline	Dopamine	DOPA	Vanillylman-delic acid
Age	mg/day	mg/day	mg/day	mg/day	mg/day
Persons					
20–35 years	3.63 ± 0.43	11.68 ± 1.50	300.14 ± 51.87	33.73 ± 3.16	4.03 ± 0.33
60–75 years	2.60 ± 0.62	4.88 ± 0.80**	334.33 ± 27.50	18.77 ± 3.95*	1.79 ± 0.15***

* $p < 0.05$;   ** $p < 0.01$;   *** $p < 0.001$.

The content of blood catecholamines and their excretion with the urine of persons and white rats of different ages were thoroughly studied by Voronkov (1975), who worked in our laboratory. His data are given in Table 2. As the Table shows, the content of adrenaline and noradrenaline in the blood is approximately halved in old age. This occurs because · the amount of noradrenaline substantially decreases as the amount of adrenaline somewhat increases. As a result of such a shift, the ratio between noradrenaline and adrenaline decreases by almost two-thirds. An important fact is that this dynamics of a change in the content of catecholamines is biologically natural, i. e. it is observed when both rats and human beings grow old.

Such a differently oriented change in the content of catecholamines shows that the relationships between the sympathetic and adrenal parts of the sympathoadrenal system substantially change in old age. Blood noradrenaline is secreted mainly in the adrenergic terminals. A substantial diminution of the content of noradrenaline is in accord with the data on the attenuation of sympathetic neural influences on the tissue in old age.

The excretion of catecholamines with urine also substantially changes in old age. The content of dihydroxyphenylalanine in the urine of persons 60–75 years old decreases by 45 per cent in comparison with its content in the urine of persons 20–35 years old, but the content of dopamine does not greatly change. Vanillylmandelic acid (VMA), which is excreted with urine, is the main metabolite of catecholamines. Its content is halved in old age.

An interesting fact is that, in old age, the excretion of VMA with urine is greater than the excretion of unchanged adrenaline and noradrenaline (the ratio between VMA and adrenaline + noradrenaline diminishes only by 12 per cent in persons 60–75 years old in comparison with persons 20–35 years old). This may indicate that the catabolism of catecholamines becomes less intense with age. The ratio between noradrenaline and dopamine diminishes even more with age. This ratio makes it possible to determine the relative intensity of the synthesis of noradrenaline and dopamine. The ratio is 3.9 in young persons and 1.5 in persons 60–75 years old.

The change in the content of catecholamines in the blood and urine of persons 90–100 years old is especially interesting. The changes in the indices under consideration are less pronounced in such persons than in persons 60–75 years old. As Table 2 shows, the content of adrenaline and noradrenaline in the blood and urine and the content of VMA in urine change less sharply in them. This confirms the concept that long life is connected with the quantitatively and qualitatively changed aging rate and with the specifics of vitauct.

The high level of dopamine and the low level of adrenaline and noradrenaline in the urine of elderly persons suggest that the transition of dopamine to noradrenaline is obstructed. This is evident from the data presented by Gey and others (1965), who showed that the activity of dopamine β-hydroxylase, which catalyzes the formation of noradrenaline from dopamine, sharply diminishes with age. Therefore, the content of catecholamines in urine and the blood of elderly persons is almost halved when dopamine excretion is adequate. The content of VMA decreases especially sharply in these persons. In old persons, not only the synthesis, but also the catabolism of catecholamines is affected.

The functional effects of blood catecholamines, while being applied to everything, depend largely on the duration of their circulation. A brief increase in their circulation or their prolonged stay in the blood will cause various reactions. Fig. 42A, B gives Voronkov's data (1975) on the elimination of catecholamines from the blood after their single administration. The difference in the elimination of adrenaline and noradrenaline from the blood is interesting. The elimination of adrenaline from the blood of old animals is greatly retarded, but the elimination of noradrenaline from the blood of these animals remains unchanged as compared with adult animals. A big role in the cessation of the action of noradrenaline is played not only by its enzymic breakdown, but also by the active removal of the mediator as a result of its reuptake by the adrenergic terminals (Kopin, 1965; Iversen, 1967; Axelrod, 1969). The lesser reuptake of noradrenaline is probably a cause of its slow elimination from the blood of old animals. Adrenaline is also metabolized more actively than it is captured by the tissue (Axelrod, 1966). An interesting combination originates: the content of blood noradrenaline decreases, but less mediator is eliminated from the blood in old age. Blood noradrenaline, which is secreted from the sympathetic terminals, seems to promote the irradiation of the adrenergic effect. In old age, definite prerequisites are created for this. When less mediator is formed, retarded elimination can play a definite adaptive role and the mechanisms which prolong the attenuated neural effect are mobilized.

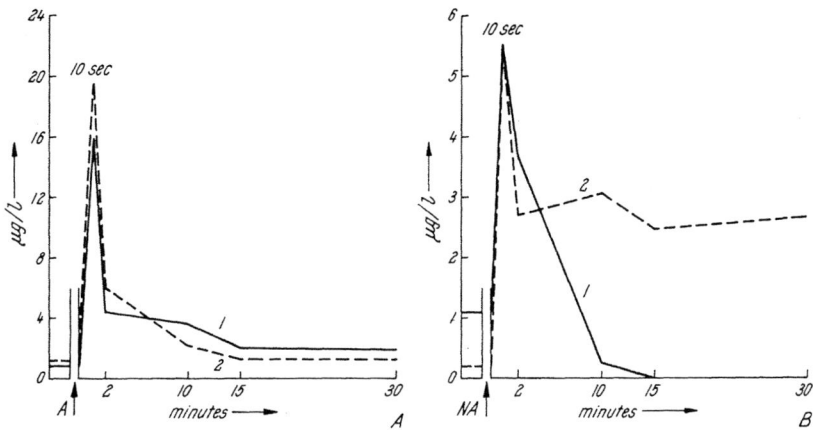

Fig. 42. Influence of the intravenous administration of 50 μg/kg of adrenaline (A) and noradrenaline (B) on the content of catecholamines in the blood of mature rats (1) and old rats (2)

Sympathoadrenal mechanisms cause the most important adaptive systemic reactions due to the generalized excitation of the sympathetic nervous system, the release of adrenaline into the blood, and the release of noradrenaline. Therefore, in order to assess the developing adaptive reactions, it is very important to evaluate the shifts in blood catecholamines during various functional loads. Voronkov (1975) studied the changes in the content of blood catecholamines of adult and old animals during a muscle stress load, i. e. during running in a treadmill (12 rps) for 5 minutes. Slight changes in the content of blood catecholamines occurred in old animals, but they were substantial in adult animals. The level of blood adrenaline more than doubled in adult animals, indicating that the hormonal link of sympathoadrenal regulation became substantially involved in the stress reaction. Such a difference in the growth of blood catecholamines will obviously give rise to differences also in the functional responses which are involved in the reaction. Hence, it is clear why the shifts in the systems of the vegetative processes of the organism are expressed more faintly during various reactions in the organism in old age. This limitation of the involvement of the sympathoadrenal system in the vegetative reaction narrows down the range of also the organism's adaptive reactions. It should be emphasized once more that the increase in the sensitivity of some cells and tissues to catecholamines is of adaptive significance when their concentrations in the blood are insignificant. Tissues become adapted to a smaller amplitude of the shifts in blood catecholamines, thus causing an adaptive reaction, which may not be very strong.

Regulatory influences of the hypothalamus play a special role in complex reactions, particularly emotional, behavioural and stress ones. In our experiments, we compared the shifts in the content of blood catecholamines after stimulating the ventromedial nucleus of the hypothalamus for 10 minutes with the exchange of polarity every 0.5 minute. In rats 8–10 months old, the content of blood adrenaline grows sharply, but that of blood noradrenaline virtually does not change. In old animals, slight shifts occurred when stimulation was effected in the above-mentioned way.

Thus, the same age differences are observed in the content of blood catecholamines when the hypothalamus is stimulated as when a motor stress load is applied. The ventromedial nucleus of the hypothalamus is known to be connected with the regulation of satiety, the sex function, the regulation of blood circulation, etc. The autonomic ensurance of these reactions will be greatly affected due to the shifts in the sympathoadrenal mechanisms.

The attenuation of adrenergic neural influences, a decrease in the reactivity of the tissues with respect to the action of catecholamines, a change in the basal level of blood catecholamines, and the slight change in the content of catecholamines during stress situations clearly show that adrenergic control decreases in old age. The diminution of these control neurohumoral mechamisms results in a decrease of adaptive reactions and causes secondary metabolic and structural disturbances in the tissue.

To describe the state of adrenergic regulation, definite information is obtained by determining the content of catecholamines in various organs. The content of noradrenaline in the heart decreases considerably in old age (Gey *et al.*, 1965). Verkhratsky (1971, 1972) systematically studied the shifts in the content of catecholamines during aging. The total amount of catecholamines and the ratio between adrenaline and noradrenaline change non-uniformly in various organs. For instance, their content in the heart and the spleen diminish, but it does not change in the skeletal muscle and the liver. The dynamics of the change in the content of catecholamines may be non-uniform in the same organ. Interestingly the maximum content of noradrenaline is observed in the auricles, and the minimum content, in the left ventricle. Such topography is in accord with the extent of the sympathetic innervation of various sections of the heart. A decrease in the content of noradrenaline in the heart conforms to the above-mentioned attenuation of adrenergic neural influences on the heart. Another comparison is also interesting. The content of catecholamines in the kidneys does not change with age; at the same time, sympathetic neural influences on the renal vessels, which are densely innervated by the fibres of the sympathetic nervous system, do not change.

There is functional evidence which shows that the reserves of catecholamines in the sympathetic terminals diminish in old age. As we have already seen, reserpine depletes the reserves of catecholamines and causes the sharp diminution of the number of adrenergic vesicles. Reserpine becomes bound with a protein of the vesicular membrane, thus disturbing the reuptake of noradrenaline (Trendelenburg, 1976) and preventing the mediator from being preserved in the sympathetic vesicles. Moreover, reserpine influences noradrenaline synthesis. Under the influence of reserpine, the synthesis of the mediator is restrained as a result of both dopamine formation and the inhibition of the activity of tyrosine hydroxylase (Slotkin, 1974).

In our laboratory, Lakiza (1979) determined the changes in the hemodynamics of animals of different ages 4 and 24 hours after the administration of reserpine.

Reserpine causes greater changes in the hemodynamics of old animals than in that of adult animals, i. e. it reduces the heart rate, cardiac output, the cardiac index, and the working index of the left ventricle. The changes in hemodynamics after the administration of reserpine are connected with pharmacological desympathization. As the noradrenaline reserves decrease in old age, it apparently becomes easier to cause this desympathization and to switch off sympathetic neural control in old animals, thus making the shifts in hemodynamics more pronounced.

There are several noradrenaline pools in the sympathetic terminals. It has been shown that the main reserves of catecholamines are depleted under the influence of reserpine. A part of the mediator, however, is resistant to the action of reserpine, but it is quickly released when the sympathetic nerves are electrically stimulated (Altshuler and Granik, 1976). In Lakiza's experiments, the reserves of catecholamines were depleted by reserpine (5 mg/kg) and then the thresholds of the electric stimulations of the sympathetic nerve that cause shifts in hemodynamics were determined four hours later. The thresholds increased by more than four times (from 2.5 to 12 V) in adult rats, but they virtually did not change in old rats. The mediator fraction which resists the action of reserpine probably decreases in old age, i. e. not only the total amount of the mediator, but also the relationship between its fractions changes in old age.

Tyrosine is the product which starts catecholamine biosynthesis. According to Lebedeva (1965), the concentration of tyrosine in women's blood decreases by the time they reach old age. Gey and others (1965) have discovered that the concentration of tyrosine in the blood of old rats is the same as that in the blood of rats which are one month old. Tyrosine is hydroxylated with the formation of 3,4-dihydroxyphenylalanine (DOPA) under the influence of tyrosine hydroxylase. The activity of this enzyme decreases substantially in old age (Ponzio et al., 1978). The next stage of noradrenaline biosynthesis is the decarboxylation of DOPA with the formation of dopamine under the influence of decarboxylase of aromatic L-amino acids. The transformation of DOPA into dopamine in the heart becomes less intense with age (Gey et al., 1965). If the activity of DOPA decarboxylase in the heart of one-month-old animals is taken as 100 per cent, it is 40 per cent in animals 8–10 months old and 52 per cent in animals 24 months old. The activity of dopamine β-hydroxylase, which determines the transformation of dopamine into noradrenaline, decreases substantially in old age. It has been shown that the activity of DOPA decarboxylase decreases in old age (McGeer, 1971). According to Gey and others (1965), a decrease in the hydroxylation of dopamine is one of the main causes which limit noradrenaline biosynthesis in old age.

Thus, noradrenaline synthesis decreases with age, because the basic enzymes which catalyze this process become less active. The diminution of noradrenaline synthesis is the molecular basis of the given attenuation of neural sympathetic influences on the organs and tissues in old age. Thus, the functional effects are exhausted more rapidly during prolonged sympathetic stimulation in old animals. Unlike acetylcholine, noradrenaline remains in its sphere of action for a rather long time, later diffusing and penetrating into the blood. Therefore, the effects of the action of noradrenaline largely depend on the specifics of its catabolism.

Noradrenaline is then transformed under the influence of two basic enzymes: monoamine oxidase (MAO) and catechol-o-methyltransferase (COMT). COMT acts on the bulk of noradrenaline, forming normetanephrine. Noradrenaline undergoes oxidative desamination under the action of MAO with the formation of 3,4-dihydroxymandelaldehyde. According to Utevsky (1967), there is one important way of transforming noradrenaline, namely, by quinoid oxidation. Moreover, catecholamines can undergo N-methylation, demethylation, N-acetylation and dehydroxylation, and they can become bound with sulphuric and glucuronic acids. In the organism, these processes result in the formation of many substances which are biologically less active than noradrenaline and adrenaline, but which possess various other physiological properties.

According to Gey and others (1965), the activity of COMT in the rat heart does not change with age. Verkhratsky (1971) has discovered that MAO becomes more active in the heart in old age. Thus, various ways in which catecholamines are catabolized change irregularly with age. There are grounds to believe that oxidative deamination is becoming cardinal. Verkhratsky showed that the oxidation of noradrenaline is greatly suppressed when MAO is blocked in old animals. In his experiments *in vivo*, he used pyrogallol, which is a COMT blocking agent, and iproniazid, which is a MAO blocking agent. Greater shifts in the noradrenaline content occur when MAO is blocked in old animals and when COMT is blocked in mature animals. According to Kopin and Axelrod (1961), COMT mainly inactivates noradrenaline which enters the synaptic cleft, but MAO is an intraneuronal mediator. If this scheme is accepted, the relationship between various mediator pools really changes in old age.

There is now enough evidence which shows that the action of noradrenaline stops as a result of not only its degradation, but also its elimination from the sites of contact with the receptors by means of a special transport mechanism which exists in the adrenergic synapses. Sympathetic terminals can uptake noradrenaline which has been secreted as well as noradrenaline which has been administered even when the concentration of the hormone is several thousand times greater in the terminals than in the external liquid. This mechanism probably plays a decisive role in regulating the circulation of catecholamines. It makes their use economical and limits both physiological effects and the origination of generalized reactions.

The reuptake of noradrenaline lessens with age. If the same amount of noradrenaline (25 μg/100 g) is administered to adult and old rats, its content in the myocardium grows by 79 per cent (from 1.37 ± 0.11 to $2.44 \pm 0.21 \mu$g/g, $p < 0.001$) in adult animals and only slightly (from 1.06 ± 0.05 to $1.33 \pm 0.8 \mu$g/g) in old animals.

In a special series of experiments, Verkhratsky and Leonteva used Falck's (1962) hystochemical method modified by Govyrin to determine the capture of intravenously administered noradrenaline (25 μg/100 g) by various sections of the heart in rats of different age. It was learned that the terminals of old animals were less capable of uptaking noradrenaline.

The reuptake of noradrenaline is an energy-dependent process in which glycolysis plays an important role. Sodium fluoride and monoiodoacetate block the reuptake of the mediator. In old animals, these disturbances originate when the given inhibitors of glycolysis are administered in doses which are smaller than those administered to adult animals. In their investigations, Hruza (1973) and Limas (1975) have shown that old animals become less capable of depositing adrenergic granules and, consequently, terminating the physiological action of a mediator.

When the uptake of noradrenaline by the sympathetic terminals of old animals attenuates, the mediator which has been administered and secreted may be capable of staying for a longer time in the sphere of synaptic action, thus producing a prolonged adrenergic effect. Moreover, the uptake of catecholamines is an extremely important source from which the mediator reserves in the sympathetic terminals are replenished. When the uptake of noradrenaline by the sympathetic terminals attenuates in old age, they may exert less influence and the sympathetic mechanisms may lose their effect more rapidly. Indeed, our experiments have shown that when the sympathetic nerve of old animals is stimulated for a long time, it loses its influence on the acinar cells of the salivary glands more rapidly (hyperpolarization develops), while its influence on vascular tonicity becomes less stable. When the stellate ganglion of old animals is stimulated for a long time, the adrenergic stimulation of cardiac activity attenuates more rapidly. It should also be taken into account that when *Ganglion cervicale superius* of old cats is frequently stimulated for a long time, the contraction of the nictitating membrane of the eye attenuates. All these facts show that the synthesis of the mediator in the adrenergic terminals becomes less reliable. Consequently, several sympathetic neural effects on the tissue may attenuate.

Dale (1936) believed that there were two types of adrenoreceptor. Adrenaline excites an organ when one of them is influenced, but it suppresses the organ's function when the other is influenced. At present, wide use is made of the classification proposed by Ahlquist (1948), who singled out α- and β-adrenoreceptors on the basis of different sensitivity to sympathomimetic amines. β-Adrenoreceptors can be easily differentiated into β_1 and β_2 receptors. It is believed that β_1 adrenoreceptors activate lipolysis and cardiac activity, while β_2 adrenoreceptors promote the relaxation of vessels and bronchodilatation.

α-Adrenoreceptors are more sensitive to noradrenaline and less sensitive to isadrine, and they are blocked by phentolamine. β-Adrenoreceptors are very sensitive to isadrine and are blocked by propranol. Adrenoreceptors not only react to an adrenergic stimulus, but also regulate the secretion of noradrenaline from the adrenergic neuron into the synaptic cleft. According to Manukhin (1978), α-adrenoreceptors are localized not only on the effector cell, but also on the membrane of the adrenergic axon, regulating the extrusion of noradrenaline. Hedqvist (1974) observed that a greater amount of noradrenaline is released into *Vas deferens* when α-adrenergic blocking agents are added.

There are various models of adrenoreceptors. An adrenoreceptor is believed to be a protein or an alveolus of the protein lattice. Moreover, it is assumed that the functions of α- and β-adrenoreceptors are performed by one molecule. However, there are other views. Recent investigations have given rise to the assumption that the adrenoreceptor has a protein nature and, like many other enzymes, can have an allosteric centre together with an isosteric one.

Various methods are now used to assess the state of adrenoreceptors; for instance, their amount is directly determined by the binding reaction and their state is chemicopharmacologically analyzed. As we have already seen, there are many works on the change in the number of adrenoreceptors in various structures of the brain (these works have been discussed in Chapter 2). Chemicopharmacological data also show that the number of adrenoreceptors changes. In our laboratory, Shevchuk (1973) determined the threshold doses of phentolamine (an α-adrenergic blocking agent) and Obsidan (a β-adrenergic blocking agent), which cause shifts in hemodynamics and block catecholamine effects. In old animals, smaller doses of Obsidan, firstly, cause hemodynamic changes and, secondly, prevent catecholamine hemodynamics from being influenced. Hemodynamic effects are produced when Obsidan is administered in a dose of $100\,\mu g/kg$ to adult rabbits and in a dose of only $25\,\mu g/kg$ to old rabbits. Phentolamine, which blocks α-adrenoreceptors, removes the adrenergic effects on the cardiovascular system in adult and old animals when it is administered in the same doses to them. Hence, the amount of α- and β-adrenoreceptors changes differently with age. Lakiza (1979) got basically the same results also in experiments involving an aortic strip.

Fig. 40 A shows the results of Lakiza's experiments with an isolated aortic strip of mature and old rats. In them, the curve of the dose-effect and the influence of noradrenaline on the contractility of the aorta were determined. The noradrenaline doses which produced a contractile effect were smaller in old animals than in mature ones, but the maximum reaction was greater in mature rats.

Applying the principle of calculations based on the dose-dependent reactions of arterial pressure (Manukhin, 1968), Bezrukov showed the change which occurred in adrenoreceptive reactions. Calculations have revealed that the theoretically maximum reaction of the cardiovascular system (arterial blood pressure) in adult rabbits is 206 ± 4.5 mm Hg, while the dissociation constant of the adrenaline-adrenoreceptor complex (K) is $1.65\,\mu g$ per cent. In old rabbits, the figures are 187 ± 6.0 mm Hg and $0.96\,\mu g$ per cent, respectively. The value which characterizes the affinity of adrenoreceptors for catecholamines (1/K) is 1.7 times greater in old rabbits than in adult animals.

Thus, the amount of active adrenoreceptors is greater in adult animals, but their sensitivity to catecholamines is greater in old animals.

This change in the amount and sensitivity of adrenoreceptors explains: (a) the origination of many functional and exchange effects that are produced in old animals by catecholamine doses which are smaller than those in adult animals; (b) a decrease in reactivity and the narrowing down of the possible range of reactions in old animals when large doses of adrenaline and noradrenaline are administered to them.

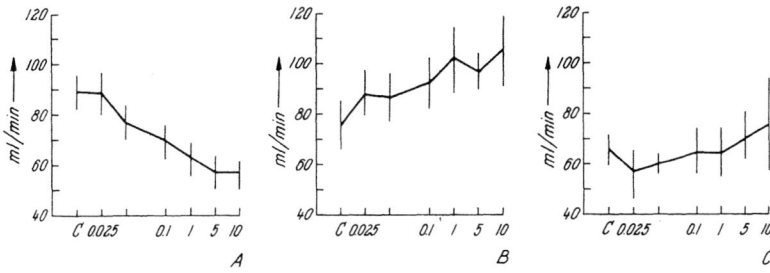

Fig. 43. Influence of actinomycin D on the enhancement of the sensitivity of the heart to noradrenaline after the administration of reserpin. The abscissa shows the concentration of noradrenaline, μg/kg, the letter C standing for control. The ordinate shows cardiac output, ml/min. A administration of noradrenaline; B administration of noradrenaline against the background of reserpin (5 mg/kg); C administration of noradrenaline and reserpin against the background of actinomycin D (1 mg/kg)

According to Lefkowitz (1976), sympathetic denervation caused by the section of the sympathetic nerves or by the administration of reserpine increases the number of receptors on the cell membrane. Adrenoreceptors, protein structures, synthesize apparently according to the principle of genetic induction. The growth of sensitivity to noradrenaline after pharmacological denervation in mature animals is probably connected with the appearance of new active adrenoreceptors. In old animals, however, this growth is absent or greatly retarded. We believe that the age changes in the biosynthesis of receptor proteins are among the principal mechanisms of cellular aging and of the change in the reaction of the cell to neurohumoral influences. This hypothesis is confirmed by another fact. Actinomycin D blocks protein biosynthesis, acting on the synthesis of DNA-dependent RNA. In our experiments, it was administered to an animal in a dose of 500 μg/kg. It does not change the hemodynamics by itself. Afterwards, reserpine was administered and sensitivity to noradrenaline was determined. When protein biosynthesis is blocked, pharmacological denervation produces the same result in adult animals as in old ones: sensitivity to noradrenaline does not grow (Fig. 43 A, B, C). A decrease in the number of adrenoreceptors in old age is probably due to the inadequate synthesis of protein structures as well. This explanation is in accord with the genic regulatory hypothesis of aging, which proves the primary role that the changes in genome regulation play in the mechanism of aging. The number of adrenoreceptors as well as their state and conformation may change with age. Consequently, the adrenoreceptor-catecholamine complex will be formed less.

It is known that adrenoreceptors are linked with the adenylate cyclase system and that adrenergic effects are realized through 3',5'-AMP. Moreover, it is assumed that adenylate cyclase is a catalytic subunit of adrenoreceptors. We have every reason to believe that sensitivity to catecholamines grows because of this link of adrenoreception. According to Kulchitsky, the content of 3',5'-AMP grows more in old rats when the sections of the tissue of the liver,

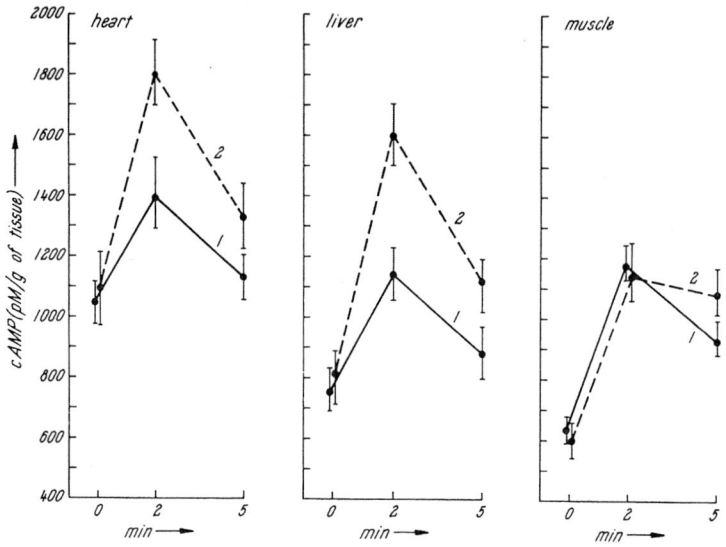

Fig. 44. Influence of adrenaline (150 μM) on the content of cyclic AMP in the tissue of the heart, the liver and the muscle in mature rats *(1)* and old rats *(2)*

the heart and muscles are incubated with adrenaline in a dose of 50 μM (Fig. 44 A, B, C). I. V. Frolkis (1978) has shown that the content of 3',5'-AMP in the portal vein does not change with age. Experiments carried out *in vivo* and *in vitro* have revealed that the content of cyclic AMP grows more in old animals than in mature ones under the influence of noradrenaline (Fig. 45 A, B, C). According to Kranz and Wollenberger (1976), the activity of adenylate cyclase grows more intensely in the vascular walls of old animals under the action of catecholamines.

Hence, tissue reactivity is limited in old age, since the number of adrenoreceptors decreases and their synthesis is inadequate. Sensitivity grows because of the conformational changes and the shifts in the adenylate cyclase system. Sympathetic neural control attenuates due to the destruction of the sympathetic terminals and autonomic ganglia and to a decrease in the synthesis of noradrenaline and its reuptake by the nerve endings.

The relationship between opposite tendencies, namely, vitauct and aging, is clearly revealed when adrenergic regulation, catecholamine metabolism and the

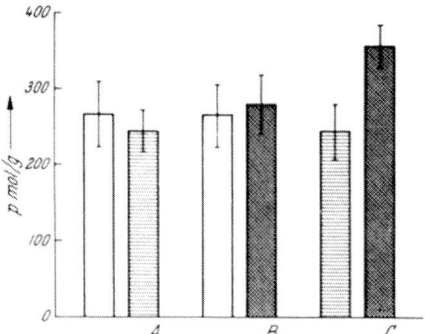

Fig. 45. Initial content of cyclic AMP *(A)* in the wall of the portal vein of mature rats (white columns) and old rats (shaded columns) and its change after the intraperitoneal administration of noradrenaline (30 μg per 100 g of an animal's weight) to mature rats *(B)* and old rats *(C)*. Black colums stand for the content of cyclic AMP in the vascular wall after influence is exerted

state of the receptors are analyzed. These tendencies are revealed diversely in various organs and tissues, changing their reaction to adrenergic stimulation differently. An important fact is that the primary disturbances in the sympathoadrenal system can cause secondary trophic disturbances in the tissues.

5. Cholinergic Mechanisms of Regulation During Aging
Acetylcholine Metabolism

Timiryazev, a Russian scientist, wrote that "a physiologist cannot be satisfied with merely an analysis of life phenomena, as he needs to know the history of organisms."

The basic factors of the formation of cholinergic regulation originated at the early stages of the organisms' historical and individual development. In their day, Orbeli (1935) and Koshtoyants (1951) noted the similarity between the factors which determine the neural mechanisms of regulation and the factors which existed at the nerveless stages of development in evolution and ontogenesis. This applies also to the system of actylcholine metabolism. In their works, Buznikov (1971) and Deeb (1972) have shown that acetylcholine and biogenic monoamines are synthesized at the initial stages of embryogenesis. They are intracellular regulators at the initial unicellular stages. Later, they determine the intercellular relationships as local hormones and prenerve mediators. According to Buznikov (1971), acetylcholine participates in cellular division as an initiator and regulates the state of the cytoplasmic membranes of the intact cells. Mediator synthesis, which coincides with the membrane localization of the cholinoreceptor, becomes extremely important in phylogenesis and ontogenesis.

In a complex organism, most organs are under double neural control, i. e. adrenergic and cholinergic control. Many effects of these systems cause opposite functional shifts. However, this functional antagonism is only a separate instance of interaction. There is a single regulatory system between whose various links antagonistic and synergic relationships may be formed. These relationships serve to attain an adaptive shift in the whole system.

It has been shown in Nachmanson's (1959) classical works that acetylcholine biosynthesis is an enzymic process of many links, including the acetylation of coenzyme A (CoA) and the transfer of the residue of acetic acid with CoA to choline. Acetyl-CoA is formed differently. Various products of metabolism, such as acetate, pyruvate, citrate, succinate, acetaldehyde and fatty acids, may be the sources of acetyl. In the animal organism, the formation of acetyl-CoA prevails in the oxidative decarboxylation of pyrotartaric acid under the influence of pyruvate dehydrogenase.

The synthesis of acetylcholine consists of the transfer of acetate to choline with the formation of ester, namely, acetylcholine. This reaction is catalyzed by choline acetyltransferase:

$$\text{acetyl-CoA} + \text{choline} \xrightarrow{\text{choline acetyltransferase}} \text{acetylcholine} + \text{CoA}$$

In our laboratory, we studied the age specifics of acetylcholine metabolism for several years (Verkhratsky, 1970, 1971; Frolkis, 1970). The investigations involved frogs, rats, rabbits and cats, and the objects used were the heart, the skeletal muscle, the motor nerve, the intestine, the kidney, the liver, etc. Hence, it was possible to establish some common regularities of mediator metabolism. Recently, a great deal of attention has been devoted to the specifics of acetylcholine metabolism in the brain during aging. However, only a few works have been written on the shifts in mediator metabolism in neural pathways, where information is transmitted from the centres to the periphery, and on acetylcholine metabolism in the effector organs.

To understand the molecular mechanisms of a change in cholinergic regulation during aging, it is necessary to analyze the age shifts in mediator synthesis, its reaction to cholinoreceptors and the dynamics of acetylcholine breakdown.

In determing acetylcholine biosynthesis in the auricles (the intensity of mediator synthesis was determined by the increment of its content prior to and after incubation), Verkhratsky (1970) established that it decreases progressively in old age. For instance, the content of acetylcholine in the heart of one-month-old rats grows from 5.61 ± 0.83 to $11.8 \pm 1.37\,\mu g/g$ per hour. In the heart of rats aged 8–10 months, it grows from 4.69 ± 0.53 to $6.33 \pm 0.34\,\mu g/g$, and in that of rats aged 24–26 months, it grows from 2.65 ± 0.42 to $2.99 \pm 0.52\,\mu g/g$ per hour.

The intensity of acetylcholine synthesis differs in various sections of the heart. It is maximum in the right auricle and minimum in the left ventricle. Acetylcholine synthesis is very intensive in the right auricle because a large amount of parasympathetic nerve endings and the pacemaker of the heart are localized in it. Cardiac automatism is believed to be connected with endogenous synthesis and the breakdown of acetylcholine. The diminution of the intensity of mediator synthesis may be one of the reasons why sinus automatism is affected and becomes durable and rigid in old age.

Acetylcholine biosynthesis may become less intense in old age because the content of acetyl-CoA decreases. According to Nikitin and Martynenko (1963), the concentration of CoA in the heart of old rats decreases by 15 per cent and that in their liver by 22 per cent, while the intensity of acetylation diminishes by 10 per cent in them. Moreover, the shifts in the metabolism of ATP, which provides energy for acetylation, may influence mediator biosynthesis. According to Frolkis and Bogatskaya (1965), the amount of ATP and especially creatine phosphate decreases, and the synthesis of these macroergic substances greatly diminishes in the heart, the skeletal muscle, the brain and the liver in old age. An especially important fact is that choline acetyltransferase becomes less active in old age. Verkhratsky (1971) studied the age changes in the activity of choline acetyltransferase in the myocardium, *Musculus gastrocnemius* and the sciatic nerve of rats of different ages. The activity of choline acetyltransferase is the lowest in old animals; it diminishes to the greatest extent in the auricles and the sciatic nerve, but only slight changes occur in the skeletal muscles.

The content of the mediator in the tissue depends on the intensity of acetylcholine synthesis. According to our data, the content of acetylcholine is maximum in the heart and the opening of *Vena cava superior* and minimum in the left ventricle. Its content is much greater in the right ventricle of the heart than in the left one. This fact is in accord with the dynamics of the metabolism of some other physiologically active substances and shows that the right ventricle plays an important role in realizing the regulatory influences on the heart.

According to Verkhratsky (1970), noticeable changes in the content of acetylcholine in the sections of the heart do not occur with age. Our fellow

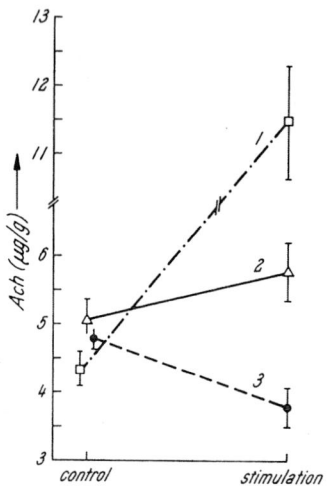

Fig. 46. Influence of the stimulation of the vagus nerve on the acetylcholine content in the orificium *V. cavae super.* in rats of different age. *1* rats 1 month old; *2* rats 8–10 months old; *3* rats 26–28 months old

workers' researches have shown that this unchangeability conceals a complex dynamics of shifts in the relationship between the mediator's synthesis and breakdown. These changes are revealed when the functional tests for the mediator system are reproduced. The synthesis of acetylcholine intensifies, it is released from the presynaptic terminals, and the mediator breaks down when the appropriate cholinergic nerves are stimulated. In our laboratory, we compared the shifts in the content of acetylcholine in the heart of white rats of different ages after stimulating the vagus nerve for one minute. To suppress the activity of choline esterase, proserine in a concentration of 25 μg per 100 g of weight was administered to the animals. Fig. 46 shows that the differences in the content of acetylcholine in the opening of *Vena cava inferior* of rats aged 8–10 months are clear-cut when the vagus nerve is stimulated. In this respect, the content of acetylcholine grows substantially (by 163 per cent) in one-month-old rats and decreases in old rats. A distinct negative chronotropic effect originates in the animals of all the three groups when the vagus nerve is stimulated. This effect is produced by the intensive extrusion of acetylcholine from the vesicles of the presynaptic fibres and its subsequent hydrolysis. As a result, the content of the mediator in the sphere if its action decreases. At the same time, mediator synthesis is greatly activated. The acetylcholine content in old animals decreases when the vagus nerve is stimulated apparently because the "power" of the mediator synthesis system diminishes. Such a direction of the shifts has been revealed in *Musculus gastrocnemius* of proserine-treated rats when the sciatic nerve was stimulated for 30 seconds in a continuous tetanus rhythm. In old rats, the acetylcholine content decreased noticeably (from $0.14 \pm 0.01 \, \mu g/g$ to $0.10 \pm 0.009 \, \mu g/g$ of wet weight) in 30 seconds, but it grew in 300 seconds. In adult rats, however, the acetylcholine content virtually did not change (it grew from $0.18 \pm 0.02 \, \mu g/g$ to $0.20 \pm 0.03 \, \mu g/g$ of wet weight).

These data show that the basal level and potentiality of the acetylcholine synthesis system decreases in old animals. This is a cause of the age changes in cholinergic neural influences on the tissue, i. e. their attenuation during prolonged cholinergic stimulation; for instance, the heart slips away more rapidly from the influence of the vagus nerve.

It is believed that the working ability of the synapses and the development of fatigue in the central and peripheral synapses are due to the "exhaustion" of the acetylcholine synthesis systems. The given age changes in acetylcholine biosynthesis probably promote the development of these states.

The level of cholinergic processes is determined by the intensity of not only the synthesis, but also the hydrolysis of the mediator. The cholinergic synapse can be highly labile only when the acetylcholine portions which act on the postsynaptic membrane are effectively inactivated. The effect of acetylcholine, which has been secreted into the synaptic cleft and has acted on the cholinoreceptor, stops mainly due to the action of the enzyme acetylcholinesterase (acetylcholine acetylhydrolase), which hydrolyzes acetylcholine into choline and acetic acid, both of which are scarcely active. Besides acetylcholine acetylhydrolase, the organism has a less specific enzyme, namely, pseudocholinesterase (acylcholines acylhydrolase), which hydrolyzes not only acetylcholine, but also some other choline ethers, apparently protecting the organism from death when the acetylcholine content grows sharply, and also splitting butyrylcholine that is synthesized in the liver. The localization of acetylcholinesterase on the postsynaptic membrane as well as the presynaptic membrane has already been described. Acetylcholine acetylhydrolase of the postsynaptic membrane plays the main role in conduction through the synapse. Cholinesterase is found not only in the synaptic region, but also in subcellular formations. Apparently, it participates in the intracellular "non-mediator" action of acetylcholine. Bertolini and others (1960) have thoroughly studied the age changes in the hydrolysis of acetylcholine and determined the activity of cholinesterase in rats 24, 180 and 840 days old. In comparison with rats 24 days old, the activity of cholinesterase in rats 180 days old was lower by 18.6 per cent in the brain, by 30.8 per cent in the liver, by 42.2 per cent in the lungs and by 0.72 per cent in the kidneys, but it was higher by 22.2 per cent in the heart and by 22.1 per cent in the striated muscles. In rats 840 days old, the activity of cholinesterase in all the tissues which were examined was reduced by 59.6, 12.9, 53.2, 47.1, 86.5 and 56.6 per cent, respectively. Verkhratsky (1970) observed that the activity of false cholinesterase in human blood serum was reduced and that the activity of true cholinesterase decreased less in erythrocytes than the activity of cholinesterase in blood serum. The activity of true and false cholinesterases changes differently in various organs and various sections of the same organ. Hence, there are differences in the nature of the age changes in the synthesis and hydrolysis of acetylcholine in various organs. This undoubtedly influences the dynamics of the cholinergic regulation of the organs.

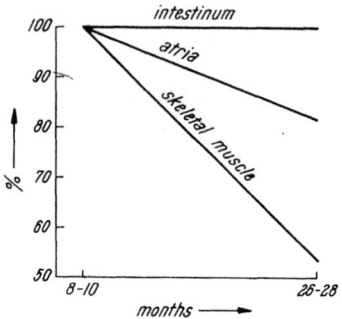

Fig. 47. Age changes in cholinesterase activity in muscular tissue with a different extent of subordination to neural control

The evolution of the cholinergic mediatory process is to a definite extent connected with a change in the intensity of neural influences on the tissue. Orbeli (1935) emphasized that the study of the physiological mechanisms which reflect various stages of the evolutionary process within the organism should be one of the approaches used in evolutionary physiology. He wrote that there were several transitional forms in evolution: the smooth muscle was at one end or near one end, while the skeletal muscles were at the other, more perfect end. Fig. 47 gives data on the age changes in the intensity of acetylcholine hydrolysis in the intestine, the auricles and the skeletal muscle, which are various levels of the evolutionary development of the muscle tissue and its neural control.

Neural control is known to play a differentiated role in regulating the function of these organs. The intestinal function is regulated mainly by the local humoral and mechanical factors. The vagus nerve diversely influences the heart, but even a denervated heart adapts itself to the organism's requirements. The skeletal muscles are included in the activity with impulses coming along the motor nerves, but denervation causes the death of the muscle fibres. The greater the neural control over the activity of an organ, the more substantial are the changes in the mechanisms of cholinergic regulation during aging. The evolutionary level determines the extent and type of neural control, but the type of neural control influences the extent of the age changes. Fig. 48 gives data on a change in the hydrolysis of acetylcholine in the skeletal muscles of adult rats after denervation and shows the shifts in this process in old rats. It can be seen that the shifts hardly coincide by their extent and direction. Hence, the age changes in the cholinergic processes in the effectors cannot be completely regarded as the attenuation of neural influences in old age.

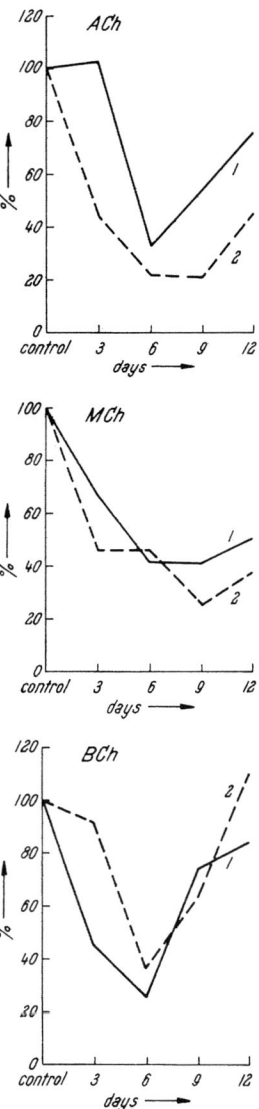

Fig. 48. Shifts in the hydrolysis (percentage of the initial level) of acetylcholine, acetyl-β-methyl-choline and butyrylcholine in the denervated *Musculus gastrocnemius* of mature rats *(1)* and old rats *(2)* at different times after the section of the sciatic nerve

As we have seen, there is a functional link between the synthesis of acetylcholine, its extrusion into the synaptic fissure and disintegration. These processes can be regarded as links of a single self-regulatory system. Choline, which is formed as a result of the hydrolysis of acetylcholine, is believed to influence its synthesis, while the acetylcholine being separated not only acts as a substrate of cholinesterase, but also influences its activity. Hence, a decrease in the activity of cholinesterase in some synapses in old age can be regarded as an

9 Frolkis, Aging

adaptive mechanism which preserves synaptic conduction. When the hydrolysis of the mediator becomes less intense as its synthesis diminishes, the amount of acetylcholine required for drawing cholinoreceptors into the reaction is preserved in the synaptic region.

Acetylcholine which has been released into the synaptic fissure interacts with the cholinoreceptor, causing a change in the conformation of the cholinoreceptive protein and shifts in membrane permeability, and also opening the appropriate ionic canals and changing the level of polarization of the cell membrane. Turpaev (1962) and his fellow workers have studied the protein nature of the cholinoreceptor. They learned that the substances which interact with the sulfhydryl groups can block cholinoreceptors. In Turpaev's laboratory, the ability of the mercury ions to interact with the cholinoreceptor is regarded as the basis of the separation of the cholinoreceptive protein. As acetylcholine interacted with the sulfhydryl groups of protein, it changed the nature of the interaction between the sulfhydryl groups and mercury. An "acetylcholine wave" appeared on the titration curve, indicating that a part of the sulfhydryl groups becomes less accessible for mercury in the presence of acetylcholine (Turpaev, 1962, and others). The chemicopharmaceutical method of studying cholinoreceptors is widely used. The cholinoreceptor is believed to have two active regions (Mikhelson, Zeimal, 1970). One of them is an anionic region which interacts with the cationic head of acetylcholine. The other is a dipole structure which binds the esterase part of the mediator molecule. Several patterns of the arrangement of active regions on the surface of the postsynaptic membrane were proposed as a result of using specific blockers of the cholinoreceptor (alpha-tubocurarine, diethylene, decamethonium).

The state of the cholinoreceptor link of cholinergic transmission during aging has been studied least of all. In our laboratory, we used several methods to characterize it. The data obtained suggest that the number of cholinoreceptors in several structures diminishes and their reaction to the action of the mediator changes with age. The changes themselves only in the cholinoreceptor link can be a cause of the age changes in cholinergic regulation in old age.

In our laboratory, Rogova and Khilko (1971) determined the influence of acetylcholine on the fraction of proteins, including the cholinoreceptive protein, that has been separated by Turpaev's method (1962). In their experiments, they used the extracts of the cerebral cortex and the cerebellum of rats of different age, determining the threshold concentrations of the mediator that cause the "acetylcholine wave," i. e. the concentrations of acetylcholine that inhibit the interaction between the cholinoreceptive protein and mercury. Fig. 19A, B shows the results of three types of experiments involving rats 1, 6 and 26 months old. The mediator concentration, which causes the "acetylcholine wave," in the extracts of the cerebral cortex was 1×10^{-13} g/ml in rats aged one month, 1×10^{-13} g/ml in rats aged 6 months, and 1×10^{-21} g/ml with variations ranging from 1×10^{-20} to 1×10^{-23} g/ml in rats aged 26 months. Thus, the concentrations of acetylcholine which interact with the cholinoreceptive protein of the cerebral cortex are smaller in old animals.

Such a direction of the changes has been revealed also on the cholinoreceptive protein which was separated from the cerebellum. For instance, the threshold concentration of acetylcholine was 1×10^{-5} g/ml in rats one month old, 1×10^{-5} to 1×10^{-6} g/ml in rats 6 months old, and 1×10^{-5} to 1×10^{-10} g/ml in old rats. These age specifics of the influence of acetylcholine on the receptive protein are apparently connected with the state of the sulfhydryl groups. According to Oeriu (1972), aging is characterized by a decrease in the number of sulfhydryl groups and an increase in the number of disulphide bonds. However, it should not be assumed that such a shift originates in all the proteins with age. According to Goldshtein and Khilko (1969) as well as Khilko and Rogova (1971), the number and reactivity of the sulfhydryl groups increase and the number of disulphide groups decreases in myogen A and myosin by old age. The content of the sulfhydryl groups (freely and inertly reacting ones, masked –SH groups, and –S–H groups which were obtained during the rupture of the S–S bonds) does not change with age. The comformation changes in the cholinoreceptive protein in old age probably demask the sulfhydryl groups, and they become more accessible for acetylcholine and react with smaller concentrations of the mediator.

Chemicopharmacological data indicate that the number and properties of the cholinoreceptors change in old age. Cholinoreceptors are known to play a definite role in the mechanism of neuromuscular transmission. There is a group of curare-like preparations (alpha-tubocurarine, Diplacin) which selectively block cholinoreceptors and thus disturb neuromuscular transmission. In our laboratory, we determined the doses of these substances (in the case of their application and administration into the femoral artery) that disturb synaptic conduction. Conduction was determined by lability and the threshold values of the current. In rats 26–28 months old, conduction was disturbed by smaller amounts of curare-like substances in comparison with younger animals. Changes in the lability of the neuromuscular synapse occurred when Diplacin was administered in a dose of 150–175 µg per 100 g of body weight to old animals and in a dose 220–250 µg per 100 g of weight to adult animals. When alpha-tubocurarine was administered, the figures were 1.0–1.5 and 3.0–4.0 µg per 100 g of weight, respectively. N-Cholinoreceptors are in the neuromuscular synapse. Such nicotine-sensitive receptors are localized also in autonomic ganglia. Duplenko (1965), our fellow worker, has shown that smaller doses of benzohexonium block ganglionic conduction in old animals in comparison with younger animals (Fig. 41).

M-Cholinoreceptors, which are localized in the heart, the vessels and the smooth muscles of the gastroenteric tract, can be blocked by atropine. Shevchuk (1971) studied the specifics of the change in the contractility of the myocardium and cardiac output under the action of acetylcholine prior to and after the administration of atropine. To assess the interaction of atropine and the cholinoreceptors, he used the calculation proposed by Clark (1926) and Turpaev (1962). An analysis of the curves of the effectiveness of the action of acetylcholine, being dependent on the concentration of atropine, has shown that the dissociation constant of the atropine-receptor complex is 0.053 µg per cent for adult animals and 0.018 µg per cent for old animals, i. e. the sensitivity of old animals to atropine is 3.2 times higher than that of adult animals.

9*

Calculations have shown that the amount of cholinoreceptors decreases in old age.

Most researchers now acknowledge that the cholinoreceptor and cholinesterase are different proteins. According to Verkhratsky (1970), the localization of cholinesterase in the cell does not change substantially in old age. Cholinoreceptors are localized mainly in the synaptic regions. The specifics of the reaction to acetylcholine suggest that, in old age, cholinoreceptors are disturbed over a larger area of the cell membrane.

Cyclic nucleotides are known to play a definite role in realizing the action of many hormones and mediators (catecholamines, glucagon, vasopressin, etc.) on the cell. Adenylate cyclase is believed to be a subunit of a receptor, while cyclic AMP, the second intracellular messenger. It has been shown that, besides adenylate cyclase, all the animal cells and bacteria have the enzyme guanylate cyclase, which causes the synthesis of cyclic guanosine monophosphate (cyclic GMP). The level of cyclic GMP in the cell is determined by the intensity of not only its synthesis, but also its breakdown under the action of specific phosphodiesterase. Cyclic GMP plays a big role in regulating some of the most important intracellular processes. According to many researchers, it is an antagonist of cyclic AMP.

The dynamic relationships between the cyclic AMP system and the cyclic GMP system greatly diversify the regulatory influences on the cell. The synthesis of cyclic GMP intensifies under the action of acetylcholine and cholinomimetics (Schwegler, Jacob, 1976; Keely, Lincoln, 1978). In this case, the amount of cyclic AMP either does not change or even diminishes. Hence, the effects produced through cholinoreceptors are realized through the guanylate cyclase-cyclic GMP system. Therefore, in order to assess the age specifics of the realization of cholinergic effects, it was important to establish the nature of the changes in the system of cyclic GMP synthesis during cholinergic stimulation.

Kulchitsky (1977) compared the shifts in the content of cyclic GMP in the homogenates of the hearts of mature and old rats caused by various concentrations of acetylcholine (0.5, 1.0 and 2.0 μM). He established that the basal level of cyclic GMP in the myocardium does not change with age (31.5 $\pm$ 2.9 and 28.5 $\pm$ 1.5 picomoles per gram of tissue of mature and old rats, respectively). Fig. 49 shows that the content of cyclic GMP increases more in the heart of old rats when the acetylcholine concentrations are small (0.5 and 1.0 μM), but the relationships change when the concentration increases (2.0 μM), i. e. the effect is more pronounced in mature rats. Acetylcholine hydrolysis becomes less intense in old age, as a result of which the effects of acetylcholine may change. Therefore, the influence of acetylcholine on the level of cyclic GMP was studied when cholinesterase was blocked by proserine (Fig. 49). However, the regularity did not change in this respect. Attention should be drawn to the similarity of the changes in the content of cyclic GMP and the functional responses under the action of acetylcholine, namely, the growth of sensitivity and the diminution of reactivity. This in itself suggests that the shifts in the synthesis of cyclic adenyl nucleotide largely determine the change in the function under the influence of the mediator.

Thus, the above-mentioned data show that, with age, substantial changes occur in all the three links of the realization of cholinergic effects, namely, the synthesis of acetylcholine, its hydrolysis and the state of cholinoreceptors. These changes occur at all the stages of cholinergic transmission to the periphery, i. e. autonomic ganglia and peripheral cholinergic synapses. The shifts in acetylcholine metabolism in the tissue and the brain attest to the fact that the whole system of cholinergic regulation changes with age.

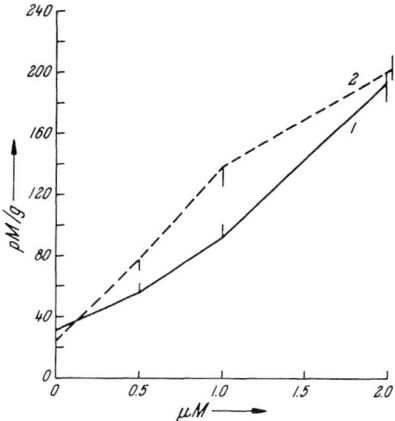

Fig. 49. Influence of acetylcholine on the content of cyclic GMP in the myocardium of mature rats (1) and old rats (2)

With age substantial disturbances occur in the parasympathetic ganglia inside the organs. For instance, the amount of large neurons increases in the heart of old rats; tigroid is distributed unevenly in them, the capsule of the neurons of the heart thickens, the impregnation of the neuroplasm of the ganglion cells by silver is heterogenous, i. e. hypo- and hyperimpregnation occurs, and contact between the nucleus and the neuroplasm decreases (Davydenko, 1972; Guseinov, 1972). Besides destructive shifts, adaptive changes have been observed in the synaptic apparatus. These changes include an increase in the number of the endings being revealed and the proliferation of simple and complex terminals. According to Davydenko (1972), the number of nerve fibrils, which are revealed by the histochemical test for cholinesterase and which cover the neuron, increases with age. This fact should be attributed to an increase, with age, in the number of synaptic endings.

Besides destruction and gross structural disturbances, adaptive reactions occur in the parasympathetic ganglia of not only the myocardium, but also the intestine in animals and man. These reactions include the hyperfunction of individual neurons, the redistribution of synapses on the body of the nerve cells, an increase in the number of synapses, the appearance of large mitochondria when their amount diminishes, rarely polyploidy, and the plication of the membrane of the cell and the nucleus.

The ganglia of the autonomic nervous system are characterized by the spatial summation of stimuli. On every postganglionic neuron, there are synapses formed by many preganglionic fibrils. When a group of preganglionic fibres is stimulated, a wide range of postganglionic fibres may be drawn into the reaction even if the force of stimulation of every fibre has a prethreshold value. The functioning of the neuron chains and the spatial summation of stimuli become limited when the structure and functions of the neurons are disturbed and they die. In this respect, an increase in the number of terminals on the body of the nerve cells is of adaptive significance.

Local peripheral reflexes, in which parasympathetic ganglia participate, are now believed to be of great significance in the regulation of the heart and the gastrointestinal tract. These reflexes allow important mechanisms of self-regulation to be realized at the level of an organ. Gross structural and functional changes in the bodies of the nerve cells and in their processes affect the realization of local reflexes.

In studying the structural and ultrastructural changes in neural ganglia, Davydenko (1972) concluded that the sensitivity of ganglia to adrenaline and reserpine increases. The changes in the Nissl substance, enzymic distribution and silver impregnation were more pronounced and prolonged when adrenaline and reserpine were administered to old animals. Parasympathetic ganglia become less labile in old age (Frolkis, 1970). As a result, the parasympathetic effects on the periphery become somewhat limited and the range of the reactions decreases.

Acetylcholine acted as a local hormone at the early stages of phylogenesis and ontogenesis. This mechanism was preserved also in higher animals. Among various sites of acetylcholine action in a cell, its possible influence on diverse enzymic processes is believed to be of great significance. There may be two sources of intracellular acetylcholine: its synthesis in the cell itself and the penetration of synaptic acetylcholine into the cell. The intracellular localization of cholinesterase is evident from the participation of intracellular acetylcholine in regulating metabolism.

The hydrolysis of ATP under the influence of myosin ATPase is an extremely important link in the realization of any contractile act. A group of proteins with cholinesterase activity is separated together with myosin. Acetylcholine can either activate or suppress ATPase activity, depending on the concentration of acetylcholine, but its effective concentration largely depends on the cholinesterase activity of myosin (Oganesyan, 1967). A metabolically self-regulating cycle then originates. Irregular changes occur in its various links with age. According to Grabina (1972), the ATPase activity of myosin grows (from $23.2 \pm 2.8\,\mu g$ P/protein in mature rats to $37.5 \pm 3.9\,\mu g$ P/protein in old rats), but the activity of cholinesterase diminishes with age (from 27.5 ± 3.3 to $7.3 \pm 1.2\,\mu g$ of acetylcholine per milligram of protein in mature and old rats, respectively). Such a sharp diminution of the cholinesterase activity of myosin promotes the manifestation of the action of intracellular acetylcholine on myosin and on the contractility of the muscle fibres. This direction of shifts intensifies the negative inotropic action of acetylcholine on the myocardium. The influence of acetylcholine on the ATPase activity of myosin is more pronounced in old animals. For instance, it has been shown in experiments *in vitro* that the ATPase activity of myosin decreases by 61.3 per cent in the muscles of old rats but virtually does not change in the muscles of mature rats under the influence of acetylcholine (40 μg/ml).

The mechanisms of the non-mediator action of acetylcholine are mobile and can change substantially in conformity with the conditions of activity. These regulatory relationships change with age.

We and Grabina have illustrated that fact by taking the example of the action of diverse anticholinergic substances. Various organophosphorus compounds, while suppressing cholinesterase by phosphorylating its esterase centre, penetrate differently into the cell. For instance, the molecule of phosphamide has tertiary nitrogen, which determines the possibility of its passage through the cell membrane. Dimehtyldichlorvinylphosphate (DDVP) which has quaternary nitrogen, penetrates into the cell and blocks only the membrane cholinesterase.

The administration of phosphamide in various doses suppressed the cholinesterase activity of myosin. However, the administration of DDVP (1.0 μg/100 g of weight) for three days activated myosin cholinesterase in mature rats, increasing its amount from 20.2 $\pm$ 1.44 to 30.3 $\pm$ 0.85 μg per milligram of protein in two hours, but it only slightly activated myosin cholinesterase in old rats (its amount increased from 6.0 $\pm$ 0.45 to 8.0 $\pm$ 0.67 μg per milligram of protein). A substantial shift in the cholinesterase activity of myosin occurred in old rats when DDVP was administered for seven days, but it was less than that in mature rats. Apparently, endogenous acetylcholine accumulated because the membrane cholinesterase was blocked by DDVP. Consequently, the enzyme is inductively synthesized, as can be seen from the fact that the activation of intracellular cholinesterase was precluded by simultaneously administering actinomycin D, which blocks the DNA-dependent synthesis of RNA. Hence, the inductive synthesis of the enzyme attenuates with age, being reflected in acetylcholine mebatolism. The attenuation of both cholinesterase synthesis and the intracellular hydrolysis of acetylcholine contributes to the revelation of the non-mediatory action of acetylcholine. For instance, the ATPase activity of myosin increased by 41 per cent in mature rats and by 68 per cent in old rats when DDVP was administered for seven days. Thus, the intracellular non-mediatory action of acetylcholine becomes more significant, and conditions for including acetylcholine in the regulation of enzymic reactions are created in old age.

Effects of Cholinergic Influences

The whole set of changes in acetylcholine metabolism and in the state of cholinoreceptors produces the age dynamics of the cholinergic regulation of the functions that was thoroughly described by us earlier (Frolkis, 1970). The experiments with rats, rabbits, cats and dogs have shown that, in old age, the thresholds of the influence of the vagus nerve on the heart (Fig. 28) grow, the heart slips away more rapidly from the influence of this nerve, and the thresholds of the influence of the motor nerves on the skeletal muscles increase. If the negative chronotropic influence of the vagus nerve on the heart attenuates, its influence on atrioventricular conduction intensifies (due to a change in the state of the atrioventricular node) in old age. Smaller intra-arterial acetylcholine doses cause muscle contraction, a change in cardiac activity, etc. New data on the shifts in the functional cholinergic effects in old age have recently been obtained in our laboratory. The acetylcholine doses which cause changes in hemodynamics and myocardial contractility are smaller in old rats than in mature ones (0.05 and 0.1 μg/kg) (Shevchuk, 1973). However, the effect is more pronounced in mature rats when large doses of the mediator (2.0–5.0 μg/kg) are administered. Cholinergic influences play a decisive role in regulating the functions of the salivary glands. Faizulin (1979) studied the specifics of the secretory potentials of the cells of the parotid gland of animals of different age with respect to the action of acetylcholine. In mature rats, the secretory potentials are two-phased with clearly defined hyperpolarization. In old rats, depolarizing effects are mainly observed and clearly defined dose-dependent effects are not produced. An important fact is that the sensitivity of various tissues to acetylcholine changes differently with age. For instance, we did not find any age differences in the threshold acetylcholine doses which cause a change in the contractility of the intestine of animals of different age. The sensitivity of the resistive vessels of various organs changes differently, i. e. the sensitivity of the vessels of the extremities and the kidneys grows, but that of the intestine vessels does not change. According to Faizulin (1979), the cells of the parotid gland are more sensitive in mature rats than in old ones.

Tonic parasympathetic influences attenuate with age. By blocking the M-cholinoreceptors of the myocardium, atropine attenuates the tonic effect of the vagus nerve on the heart. The higher the tonicity of the vagus nerve, the greater are the shifts after its effect is blocked. When 1.0 mg of atropine was administered, the heart rate increased by 36.5 ± 3.6 per cent in young persons and by 19.7 ± 1.9 per cent in elderly persons. After the orthostatic test and physical loads, the influence of atropine on the shifts in blood circulation was less pronounced in elderly persons (Dukhovichny, 1968).

The data obtained show not only the phenomenology of the age changes in cholinergic regulation, but also their mechanism. Cholinergic neural control attenuates at the level of parasympathetic ganglia and postganglionic fibres due to the destruction of the nerve endings, the diminution of mediator synthesis and a decrease in the mobility of the acetylcholine metabolic system. The manifestation of substantial parasympathetic effects further the diminution of the number of cholinoreceptors on the postsynaptic membrane. In this respect, an increase in the sensitivity of the cells of some tissues to the mediator and the stronger influence of its non-mediatory effect are of adaptive significance. This increase is due to the attenuation of acetylcholine hydrolysis when the reaction of the cholinoreceptor changes. The shifts in the synthesis of the most important intracellular mediator of the reaction, i. e. cyclic GMP, play a big role in the formation of those specifics. The age changes in the synthesis of cyclic GMP coincide with the shifts in the reaction of the tissues to acetylcholine.

A decrease in the activity of intracellular cholinesterase is especially important, since it furthers the manifestation of the non-mediatory metabolic effects of acetylcholine. All these shifts in various links of acetylcholine metabolism and the state of cholinoreceptors are expressed differently in various organs. They produce age changes in cholinergic regulation that range from substantial attenuation of neural control to its almost complete unchangeability. Cholinergic influences cause many functional as well as metabolic effects in the organism, including a decrease in oxygen consumption, a shift in the activity of some respiratory enzymes, an increase in the contents of glycogen, ATP and creatine phosphate, and a change in protein synthesis.

The "acetylcholine injection" concepts conceal the metabolic essence of the influence of acetylcholine from researchers. The changes in cholinergic regulation in old age can be a cause of not only the changes in the rhythmic and contractile functions of the heart, the motor and secretory functions of the gastrointestinal tract, neuromuscular conduction, and so forth, but also the shifts in their trophism and metabolism. According to our data, the accumulation of endogenous acetylcholine due to membrane cholinesterase blocking intensifies the ATPase activity of myosin in the skeletal muscles and increases the content of glycogen in the myocardium and the content of creatine phosphate more in old animals than in mature ones. These contents increase by 23 and 11 per cent and by 13 and 7 per cent in old and mature animals, respectively. According to Verkhratsky (1970), acetylcholine stimulates protein biosynthesis more in the auricles of old rats, but it suppresses this synthesis more in the liver of mature rats. The attenuation of cholinergic processes is one of the reasons why the organism becomes more sensitive to hypoxia in old age. Hence, the shifts in cholinergic regulation can greatly influence cell metabolism.

The mechanisms of adrenergic and cholinergic regulation are considered separately as a result of a thorough scientific analysis. They are really individual links of a single mechanism of self-regulation of metabolism and functions, links which determine a wide range of reactions. Substantial non-compensative deviations of the systems from the homeostatic level do not occur owing to the mechanisms of counter-regulation. The activation of a section of the autonomic nervous system stimulates many mechanisms of another section. Hence, adrenergic reactions of an isolated heart may originate when the concentration of acetylcholine gradually grows, while cholinergic effects may be produced by adrenaline.

We and Karpova studied the age specifics of the relationship between adrenergic and cholinergic mechanisms by taking the example of the regulation of cardiac activity. To this end, an investigation was made of the influence of adrenaline and noradrenaline on the synthesis and hydrolysis of acetylcholine in the heart as well as the influence of both the stimulation of the vagus nerve and acetylcholine on the content of catecholamines in the myocardium. Adrenaline caused greater changes in both the intensity of acetylcholine hydrolysis and the activity of cholinesterase in old animals in comparison with mature ones. The activity of acetylcholine transferase decreased inconsiderably in old animals.

Thus, adrenaline causes changes in various links of acetylcholine metabolism in the heart. These changes are greater in old animals than in mature ones. The shifts in acetylcholine metabolism are expressed in a change in the cholinergic regulation of the heart. According to Karpova (1974), the thresholds of the influence of the vagus nerve on the heart of old rats decreased from 0.84 ± 0.01 V before adrenaline injection to 0.41 ± 0.03 V after its administration, but it did not change in adult rats (0.28 ± 0.02 V in the control untreated animals and 0.26 ± 0.03 V in adrenaline-treated rats). This functional effect is probably due mainly to a decrease in the intensity of acetylcholine hydrolysis under the influence of catecholamines.

The content of noradrenaline diminishes in the myocardium when the vagus nerve is stimulated and acetylcholine is administered. For instance, the stimulation of the vagus nerve by a current of 3.5 V for 60 seconds reduces the content of noradrenaline in the heart of mature rats by 18 per cent, while the administration of acetylcholine (15 μg/100 g of weight) reduces the content of noradrenaline by 26.5 per cent ($p < 0.02$). In old rats, the noradrenaline content decreases inconsiderably when the vagus nerve is stimulated, but it decreases by 34.2 per cent when acetylcholine is administered. Thus, the relationships between the adrenergic and cholinergic regulations of the heart change with age.

Hence, changes occur with age in all the links of cholinergic regulation, namely, the brain, the ganglionic apparatus, the peripheral synapse, and the intracellular effects of acetylcholine.

6. Insulin Provision of the Organism During Aging

Robert Burns once said that there were a thousand illnesses, but only one health. Indeed, many predispositions to pathology originate during a single biological process of aging. These predispositions include the relationship between the age changes in the insulin provision of the organism during aging and diabetes.

Diabetes occurs more frequently in elderly and old subjects. According to Yefimov and others (1973), diabetes mellitus occurs eight times more frequently in persons above 60 than in persons under 40. Among those suffering from diabetes mellitus, 80 per cent are more than 40 years old and 50 per cent are more than 50 years old. In the U.S.A., the following number of cases of diabetes were recorded per 1,000 head of population: 1.1 case among men and 0.7 case among women under 25 years of age, 4.9 and 3.8 cases among men and women, respectively, 25–44 years old, 11.2 and 13.7 cases among men and women, respectively, 45–54 years old, 25.2 and 31.5 cases among men and women, respectively, 55–64 years old, 37.4 and 50,3 cases among men and women, respectively, 65–74 years old, and 31.5 and 38.8 cases among men and women, respectively, who were more than 75 years old. Therefore, it is quite natural to believe that the causes of the development of diabetes can be understood, an effective system of its prevention can be created, and new ways of treating it can be outlined when the mechanisms of the shifts which occur in old age are revealed.

However, there is another circumstance due to which ever growing interest is being taken in the problem of age and the insulin provision of the organism. Insulin is a hormone with a wide range of action. The metabolism of proteins, lipids and carbohydrates, the membrane processes, and so forth, change greatly under the influence of insulin. Hence, it was quite correct to assume that the age changes in the insulin provision of the organism played a certain role in the genesis of aging. The words "insulin provision" reflect a systemic approach to the analysis of the regulatory influences of insulin. They imply not only the amount of insulin in the blood, but also the specifics of its binding, the synthesis and breakdown of the hormone, the response of insulinocytes of the pancreas to neural and humoral stimuli, the response of the tissues to the action of the hormone, etc. In other words, they imply the whole system of the hormone's participation in metabolic processes. In our laboratory, we estimated the age changes in insulin provision by analyzing the shifts in its various links. These researches clearly show that even if we know about the changes in one link, we cannot understand how and why disturbances occur in insulin provision as the organism grows old, disturbances which create the predispositions to diabetes,

Content of Insulin and Carbohydrate Tolerance

It has long been known that the organism's tolerance for glucose decreases in old age. According to Balodimas (1967), the percentage of the cases in which tolerance for carbohydrates decreased was 0.5 among persons 24 years old, 23 among persons 45–54 years old, 36 among persons 55–64 years old, and 43 per cent among persons 65–74 years old. Smolyansky (1965) found that the tolerance for carbohydrates is reduced in 83.5 per cent of elderly persons.

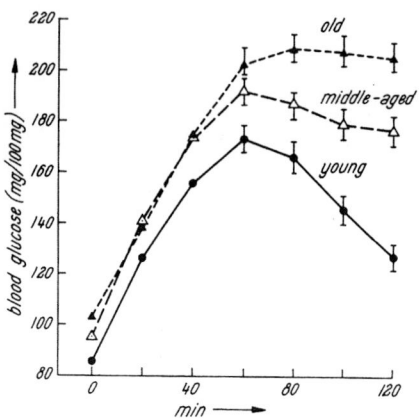

Fig. 50. Change in the blood sugar level during a glucose tolerance test against the background of hydrocortisone in three age groups which did not have diabetes in the family anamnesis. The standard error is given after 60 minutes. Before 60 minutes, the differences between the groups are not statistically great. The data have been obtained from 15 young persons (21–44 years old), 26 middle aged persons (45–64 years old), and 20 old persons (65–95 years old). See Shock, N., Andres jr., R. (1968): Adaptive Capacities of an Aging Organism. Kiev: Institute of Gerontology

According to Korkushko and Orlov (1974), the figure is 65 per cent, while Nonaka and Kono (1978) have found it to be 74 per cent. Kimmerling and others examined 100 men of normal weight with normoglycemia who were 22–60 years old. Their data show that tolerance for carbohydrates and sensitivity to insulin does not change with age. According to the researchers, this was because stout persons were not in the group of persons who were examined. Hosakawa and Kihara wrote about the possible relationship between the poor tolerance for glucose in elderly subjects and the conditions which are conducive to obesity. A higher level of hyperglycemia and the slower restoration of the initial level of blood sugar in elderly and old persons after a glucose load are an objective indicator of a decrease in tolerance for glucose.

The glucocorticoid test gives a definite idea about the state of the hormonal regulation of carbohydrate metabolism. According to Shock and Andrew (1968), the administration of cortisone after administering glucose causes longer and stable glycemic shifts in elderly persons (Fig. 50). We have obtained similar results in experiments with old rabbits after the administration of hydrocortisone. Hence, the sensitivity of the system which regulates carbohydrates metabolism to cortisone increases in old age. In old persons, insulin synthesis is activated more faintly in response to hyperglycemia which originates under the influence of cortisone. In any case, the results of the load of glucose and cortisone clearly show that tolerance for glucose decreases. There are two categories of elderly and old persons: tolerance is hardly changed in some of them, while it is substantially reduced in others.

In spite of the great differences in carbohydrate tolerance, the initial content of blood sugar virtually does not change with age (82 ± 5 mg per cent in young persons and 78 ± 4 mg per cent in elderly persons; 108 ± 4 mg per cent in young rats and 110 ± 6 mg per cent in old rats). Toshino and others have revealed a linear relationship between age and the content of glucose in the blood. The level of blood sugar is an extremely important homeostatic parameter. The homeostatic level of blood sugar is maintained even in very old age owing to the irregular changes which occur in different directions in various links of the regulation of insulin provision. However, the reliability of this system of regulation and its potentialities decrease with age, greatly reducing carbohydrate tolerance.

Various researchers offer different interpretations of the age decrease in carbohydrate tolerance. According to Kreteanu and Hurjui (1972), this decrease is a normal physiological manifestation of the adaptation of the regulatory mechanisms to the changed metabolic level. Rost and others (1967) as well as Heldmann and others (1970) are also of this opinion. Taking account of the physiological essence of a decrease in carbohydrate tolerance in old age, Kretsyanu and Khurzhui propose that age corrections should be made in the standard criteria of the diagnosis of diabetes mellitus. The researchers holding the opposite view interpret the decrease in carbohydrate tolerance in old age as latent diabetic disturbances, potential diabetes and latent diabetes (Schneider, 1971; Duncan, 1976). Dilman and Ostroumova (1973) regard the age changes in glucose tolerance as prediabetes. According to WHO experts, the term "prediabetes" should be used as a retrospective definition when the existing diseases are analyzed. Vasyukova and others (1979) believe that a decrease in carbohydrate tolerance in old age is an expression of pathology.

In their work, Nonaka and Kono (1978) draw the conclusion that a decrease in glucose tolerance in old persons is determined by mechanisms other than insulin insufficiency during diabetes. They refer to the fact that in the case of a glucose load, the relationship between the area of insulin and the area of glucose in persons 60–89 years old differs little from this relationship in persons 20–49 years old, that glucagon does not reduce glucose tolerance in old persons, that the activity of beta-H-acetylglucosamynidase of the serum of old persons is comparable with this activity in young persons but is 30 per cent lower than the given activity in diabetics, and that the activity of the glycolytic enzymes (hexokinase, pyruvate kinase) and the enzymes of gluconeogenesis (fructoso-1,6-diphosphatase, glucoso-6-phosphatase) is reduced in the liver of old rats, while the activity of the enzymes of gluconeogenesis increases in diabetes.

According to various authors, a decrease in carbohydrate tolerance is observed in persons above 50 in 40–85 per cent of the cases, while diabetes is observed in 7–9 per cent of the cases in them. Hence, certain conditions are needed for diabetes to develop in elderly persons with low carbohydrate tolerance. The age changes in insulin provision, while not being a form of diabetes, create prerequisites for its development. The limitation of the adaptive abilities of the system being regulated brings about its gross changes. For a long time, everything seemed to be clear; functional activity and the potentialities of the beta cells of the pancreas decrease with age. In this respect, the content of insulin in the blood decreases, and then carbohydrate tolerance diminishes. However, this concept was reviewed owing to the wide use of the radioimmunological methods of determining the content of insulin in the blood of a large number of people. It was reported that the content of insulin in the blood does not change in old age. Many researchers are even of the opinion that its content increases. According to our data (Frolkis *et al.*, 1971; Frolkis, 1977), the insulin activity of the blood decreases, but the content of the hormone increases with age. The rise of insulin content in the blood of old subjects and animals was shown both using the radioimmunological method and separating free and bound insulin on ion-exchange resins (Table 3). It is now being more frequently reported that the concentration of insulin in the blood increases in elderly and old persons.

Table 3. *Content of insulin in the blood of persons and rats of different ages*

Insulin	Persons		Rats	
	young	elderly	mature	old
Free, mg/g 3 hours	2.45 ± 0.18	4.85 ± 0.50*	3.80 ± 0.51	7.20 ± 0.73*
Bound, mg/g 3 hours	2.13 ± 0.15	4.20 ± 0.36*	2.81 ± 0.50	6.40 ± 0.41*
Immunoreactive, μ U/ml	9.5 ± 2.0	16.7 ± 2.1*	28.4 ± 1.2	53.0 ± 3.6*

* $p < 0.05$.

Livergant and others (1974) have shown that at the same level of glycemia, the content of immunoreactive insulin (IRI) in persons who are more than 40 years old is 73.6 per cent higher than in young persons. According to Lewis and Wexler (1974), the content of insulin is 60.8 ± 4.3 microunits per millilitre in the blood of rats 3 months old, 81.8 ± 4.0 microunits per millilitre in the blood of rats 6–8 months old, and 250.9 ± 26.2 microunits per millilitre in the blood of rats 18 months old. An increase in the content of insulin in the blood has been reported by Gatsko (1975) and by Feldman and Plank (1976). However, Wagner and others (1977) as well as Nonaka and Kono (1978) found that the basal level of the hormone in the blood remains unchanged in elderly persons. Goddling and others (1975) have reported that the insulin level decreases in old age. We believe that such diversity in the reports on insulinemia is due to the fact that, in most cases, persons with normal and reduced glucose tolerance were examined. Kulchitsky and Orlov (1977) have shown that the content of insulin increases in elderly persons with reduced glucose tolerance, but it decreases in elderly persons with normal glucose tolerance (Fig. 51).

Thus, an interesting situation exists: not a reduced (as was believed earlier), but an increased insulin content is coupled with a decrease in carbohydrate tolerance.

Insulin occurs in various forms in the blood (Staroseltseva, 1976). Free insulin reacts with antibodies and affects the absorption of glucose of adipose and muscular tissues. Bound insulin does not react with antibodies and is not determined radioimmunologically; it influences adipose tissue. According to our data, the content of free and bound insulin grows in old age (see Table 3).

The content of blood insulin is not a criterion of its physiological activity. It is necessary to determine not only its amount but also its true physiological activity, which is tested by the diaphragmatic synthesis of glycogen with respect to free insulin and by the intake of glucose by epididymal fat with respect to bound insulin. Table 3 shows that the insulin activity of the blood decreases in both persons and rats. The age decrease in glucose tolerance can be explained by the diminution of the effectiveness of endogenous insulin in spite of the growth of its content.

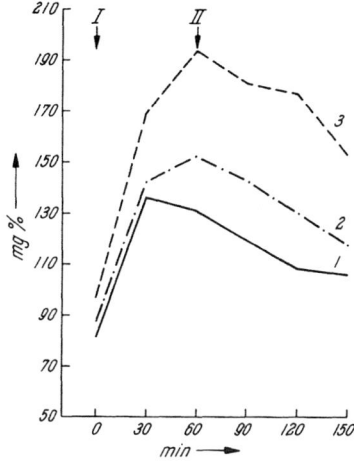

Fig. 51. Level of glycemia in persons of different ages with different glucose tolerance after a double glucose load. *I* first load; *II* second load. *1* young persons with normal glucose tolerance; *2* elderly persons with normal glucose tolerance; *3* elderly persons with impaired glucose tolerance

There may be various assumption of the nature of a decrease in the physiological activity of the hormone in old age. Firstly, the precursor of insulin, i. e. proinsulin, whose biological activity is low, may enter the blood from the beta cells. Indeed, Duckworth and Kitabachi (1976) have shown that the amount of proinsulin increases in elderly persons with normal carbohydrate tolerance when there is a peroral load of glucose. However, Mako and Starr (1977) have shown that the content of immunoreactive insulin increases more than the content of proinsulin when glucose tolerance is low.

Proinsulin is known to consist of one polypeptide chain, which begins with the B-chain and ends with the A-chain. C-Peptide, which contains 27–33 amino acid residues, is between them. Proinsulin is split into insulin and C-peptide in the granules of the Golgi apparatus. According to our data, the content of C-peptide is higher in the blood of persons 60–70 years old (3.06 ± 0.21 ng/ml) than in the blood of persons 20–29 years old (1.85 ± 0.27 ng/ml). An increase in the content of C-peptide in old age indicates that a greater amount of proinsulin is converted into insulin in old age. This phenomenon is the basis of a real increase in the concentration of the hormone in the blood. However, this fact does not rule out the possibility that a large amount of proinsulin can get into the blood. Secondly, changed insulin with low activity and low affinity for receptor may be produced in the genetic apparatus of the beta cells. Thirdly, the content and activity of the counterinsulin factors may grow with age. The antagonists of insulin can be divided into two groups: some of them produce effects which are opposite to those produced by insulin, while others influence the activity of the hormone itself. The hypoglycemic effects of insulin are "opposed" by a group of hormones which cause severe hyperglycemia. These hormones include adrenaline, glucagon, corticoids and the somatotropic hormone. Many persons are affected by diabetes apparently because of a "break" in one non-compensative link of neurohormonal regulation. Crepaldi (1978) drew the conclusion that a decrease in glucose tolerance in old age is not in accord with a change in the formation of the counterinsulin hormonal factors. He observed that the secretion of glucagon, the somatotropic hormone and cortisone does not change substantially in elderly persons with low tolerance after loads caused by the administration of glucose, arginine and insulin. Hence, glucagon, the somatotropic hormone and cortisone are not responsible for the prolonged hyperglycemic shifts. However, the change in the hormonal counterinsulin factors undoubtedly plays a definite role in reducing the insulin activity of the blood. According to some authors, the content of the somatotropic hormone somewhat grows with age (Vasyukova *et al.*, 1979), the content of adrenaline increases in elderly persons as that of noradrenaline decreases (Voronkov, 1975), the content of glucagon does not change with age, while glucocorticoids cause greater glycemic shifts in old persons and animals. However, not only the content of the counterinsulin hormones, but also the reaction of the tissues to them (sensitivity and reactivity) is important.

It was shown in our laboratory that the sensitivity of the system of glycemic regulation to several hormones increases, while its reactivity decreases in old age. It has been shown that glycemic shifts are more pronounced in old rabbits when a small dose of adrenaline is administered, but they are more pronounced in mature rabbits when a large dose of the hormone is administered. We obtained essentially similar data in our experiments with hydrocortisone: small doses of the hormone caused greater hyperglycemia in old rabbits, while large doses of the hormone made it more pronounced in mature rabbits.

The somatotropic hormone is of great importance. It produces a great counterinsulin effect and at the same time promotes the accumulation of the antagonists of insulin in the blood and enhances its ability to bind with proteins. In this respect, mention should be made of the data presented by Dilman and Ostroumova (1973), who believe that an excess of the growth hormone is a factor which causes hyperinsulinemia, disturbing metabolism and promoting diabetes, atherosclerosis and other diseases which affect elderly and old persons most frequently. Fourthly, antibodies with respect to insulin probably accumulate with age. Indirect evidence of this is the fact that several autoimmune affections are often found together with the main disease in diabetics. Many authors believe that resistance to insulin during long treatment with the hormone is due to the specific antibodies which circulate in the blood and inactivate endogenous and exogenous insulin. The most common type of anti-insulin bodies is IgG in persons, while IgA occurs rarely and IgM and IgE occur even more rarely in them. After studying the autoimmune reactions of the cellular and humoral types with respect to insulin and antigen from the pancreas of persons of different age, Zaichenko (1977) drew the conclusion that the number of autoimmune reactions to insulin does not increase in old age, suggesting that the autoimmune mechanism does not participate in inhibiting insulin activity. An interesting fact is that the autoimmune reactions of the humoral and cellular types to the antigens of the pancreas become more frequent with age. This mechanism probably plays a definite role in upsetting the insulin apparatus. However, it should be proved that these antibodies are specific for the beta cells. Fifthly, there are grounds to maintain that the inhibitors of insulin play an important role in reducing the biological activity of the hormone in old age. This is evident from the data obtained by our fellow workers (Potapenko, Paramonova, 1977). Insulin which is added to the blood serum of mature animals increases the absorption of glucose by the diaphragm by 15–25 per cent. The addition of such a dose of insulin to the blood serum of old rats does not change the intensity of glucose intake. The hypoglycemic effect of the same insulin dose which was administered to rabbits differed in conformity with the solvent in which the hormone was administered. The effect was maximum when insulin was added to a saline, but it was somewhat less when insulin was preincubated with the serum of adult rats. The effect was minimum when insulin was incubated with the serum of old rats. The influence of insulin on the cell membrane is considered to be of great importance in the mechanism of the hormone's biological action. Insulin hyperpolarizes many cells. If insulin diluted with the blood serum of an adult rat is administered in a dose of 1.6 unit per kilogram of body weight to test rats, the membrane potential of the fibres of *Musculus gastrocnemius* will increase from 75.1 ± 1.7 mV to 82.7 ± 1.0 mV in 90 minutes. Insulin diluted with the blood serum of old rats does not produce such an effect. Potapenko and Paramonova (1977) have shown that crystalline insulin diluted with the blood serum of young animals and administered in a dose of 1.6 unit per kilogram of body weight causes great hemodynamic effects (a decrease in the cardiac output, arterial pressure and the heart rate) as well as substantial electroencephalographic shifts, but insulin which is administered in the same dose after preincubation with the serum of old rats does not produce such an effect. Gatsko (1975) has shown that the serum of old rats which is added to insulin weakens its effect on glycogen formation in the diaphragm. Thus, the blood of old animals contains a substance (or substances) which inhibits the physiological effects of the hormone.

There is a definite bond between the inhibitor and the insulin molecule (Frolkis *et al.*, 1971). This is evident from the fact that blood was liberated from the inhibitors and antagonists of free insulin by means of ion-exchange resins (the sulphocationite SDV-3).

A comparison was made between the activity of free insulin in the blood and insulin which was purified with the ion-exchange resin. In mature animals, the activity of "pure" free insulin which was separated from the blood hardly differed from the activity of this fraction in the blood (2.64 ± 0.58 and 1.80 ± 0.1 mg/g, respectively, in three hours), but in old animals, the activity of the "pure" fraction was almost 6.5 times higher than that of free insulin in the blood (8.0 ± 0.8 and 1.3 ± 0.1 mg/g, respectively, in three hours). Hence, the biological activity of insulin sharply increases and the action of a high content of the blood hormone is revealed when the blood of old persons and animals is liberated from the inhibitors and antagonists of insulin.

Non-esterified fatty acids, beta lipoproteins, sinalbumin and other substances of a protein nature can act as the inhibitors of insulin. The substances which affect the bonds between protein molecules can also affect the bonds between insulin and the inhibitor, weakening the latter's influence on the hormone. Sodium dodecylsulphate (DDS) was used to ascertain this assumption. It dissociates protein molecules and enhances the sensitivity of the peptide links to proteases. The experiment was carried out in the following manner: the insulin activity of the blood was tested prior to and after the addition of DDS in a concentration of 100 mg per cent. DDS intensifies insulin activity by 110 per cent (from 0.70 ± 0.12 mg/g to 1.47 ± 0.20 mg/g) in the blood of old rats and by only 52 per cent in the blood of young rats. A special series of investigations has shown that DDS does not influence the activity of crystalline insulin. Hence, it can be assumed that firstly, DDS liberates the insulin molecule from its link with the inhibitor, and it becomes more active, and, secondly, DDS increases the permeability of the membranes of the myofibrils of the test object (diaphragm) and enhances the entry of insulin into the cell. The first assumption is apparently more real, since DDS intensifies the activity of insulin more in the blood of old animals. The influence of DDS on the activity if insulin in the blood of old animals confirms the link between the hormone and the protein inhibitor.

Thus, the biological activity of insulin decreases in old age as a result of the action of a set of factors. The accumulation of the hormone inhibitors, which reduce the effectiveness of the metabolic influences of the hormone, is especially important in this respect.

At present, various methods of diabetes treatment are used, including the administration of insulin and the activation of its secretion. The data on the inhibition of the hormone's action make another method of therapy promising, it activates endogenous insulin and ruptures its link with the inhibitor.

Hence, the growth of the concentration of blood insulin with age is an adaptive reaction which reduces the blood sugar level.

The content of blood insulin may increase as a result of its intensified synthesis, secretion and reduced breakdown. Insulin breaks down in several tissues. However, it breaks down especially intensively in the liver with the participation of insulinase. Glutathione insulintranshydrogenase, which ruptures the insulin molecule into A- and B-chains, is the main insulin dehydrating enzyme. According to our data, the activity of insulinase is almost halved in the liver of old rats: it is 89.7 ± 4.81 per cent in rats 8–10 months old and 48.3 ± 8.9 per cent in rats 24 months old. Hence, the attenuation of insulin breakdown due to a decrease in the activity of insulinase is probably one of the causes of the accumulation of insulin in the blood with age.

Structural and Functional Changes in the Insular Apparatus

An extremely important link in the whole system of providing the organism with insulin is associated with the influence of glucose on the beta cells of the pancreas. An adequate relationship between metabolic processes and hormone secretion is largely formed at this stage. It is believed that beta cells have specific glucose receptors which exert their influence through the cyclic AMP system. The receptors are acted on probably not by glucose itself, but by its metabolite, e. g. glucose-6-phosphate.

The age changes in the secretion of insulin have a definite structural basis. The ratio between alpha and beta cells changes with age. According to Avtandilov (1970), their ratio is 1 : 4.3 in mature age and 1 : 2.9 in old age. Shevchuk (1963) has shown that the number of Langerhans' islands averaged 207 in rats 2 weeks old, 130 in rats 2–4 months old, 80 in rats 7–12 months old, and 95 in rats 1.5–2.0 years old per hundred square millimetres of the pancreas. According to Reaven and others (1979), the number of beta cells grows with age. In every island, they total 2,330 in rats 2 months old, 2,760 in rats 6 months old, 3,410 in rats 12 months old, and 5,060 in rats 18 months old. The content of insulin in the pancreas of rats 18 months old is double that in the pancreas of rats 2 months old. Stupina and Shaposhnikov (1977) have shown that with age great ultrastructural disturbances occur in beta cells. The nuclei of these cells become scalloped at the edges. Consequently, the membrane surface increases and the nuclear cytoplasmic relationships are preserved. Moreover, perinuclear space substantially increases. An important fact is that the nucleus has a large number of condensed chromatin, indicating a change in the relationship between active and passive chromatin, which substantially influences hormone synthesis. The state of the protein-synthesizing apparatus of beta cells changes in old age: the endoplasmic reticulum becomes substantially enlarged and relatively ribosome-impoverished. An enlarged content of primary lysosomes and autophagosomes is characteristic of old cells. Mitochondria, which are the main energy-producing systems, also substantially change in beta cells. They swell in many cells, the matrix is clarified, cristae undergo discomplexation, and vacuolized and destroyed mitochondria are observed. The secretory granules in the beta cells of old rats substantially differ from one another in their size.

There is another population of beta cells whose structural changes indicate their hyperfunction. According to Gatsko (1975), the elements of the granular reticulum become hypertrophied, the number of free ribosomes increases, cisternae become larger, and the volume of the vesicles in the Golgi apparatus grows in many beta cells with age. This type of reorganization of beta cells becomes significant adaptively when the organism grows old.

The disturbance of the integrity of the membrane which limits the granules is the most typical of the electron microscopic pattern of beta cells in old rats. As a result of this disturbance, some granules with a destroyed membrane fuse with one another, forming conglomerates which look like bunches of grapes.

Thus, opposite tendencies in the dynamics of the structural changes in beta cells occur when the organism grows old. These tendencies are the degradation and atrophy of some cells and the compensatory, adaptive hyperfunction of others. The dynamics of the relationship between these tendencies and a change in the number of beta cells ultimately determine the potentialities of the insular apparatus. This functional direction of some cells is the cause of hyperinsulinemia, which develops in old age due to hyperfunction, being followed by the subsequent destruction of the active beta cells.

The specificity of the response of beta cells to the blood sugar stimulus is one of the most important functional indices of the state of these cells.

Some researchers indicate that the insulinemic reaction is maintained in elderly and old persons, although it occurs slowly in them. Others believe that it is reduced in them, and still others assert that hyperinsulinemia occurs in them. According to Nonaka and Kono (1978), the nature of insulinemia after a glucose load in persons 60–89 years old does not differ from that in persons 20–49 years old. In their opinion, reduced tolerance to glucose cannot be attributed to disturbed insulin secretion that is characteristic of diabetes at its initial stage. An interesting fact is that Nonaka and Kono did not observe any disturbances in the response of alpha cells and in the release of glucagon during a sugar load. D'Onfrio and others (1970) as well as Shimizu and others (1978) have noted that the beta-cell response to the administration of glucose is insufficient.

By producing a double glucose load, Ciaponi and others (1978) have shown that the response is reduced in some elderly persons who are not suffering from obesity or diabetes, but it is greater in others and hyperinsulinemia develops. According to Yoshino and others (1981), the content of insulin after the administration of glucose grows more in old age than at any other time. However, Soerjodibroto and others (1979) have shown that, after an alanine load, the level of plasma insulin grew less, while that of glucagon grew more in elderly animals than in young ones. Wagner and others (1977) have shown that when glucose is administered, the content of immunoreactive insulin in the serum of persons 18–29 years old increases about five times, but it increases about three times in the serum of persons 50–59 years old. Gatsko (1975) has observed a hyperinsulinemic type of response in old animals when a glucose load was produced. Some researchers believes that the sensitivity of beta cells to glucose sharply diminishes in old age, while others hold that it does not change, and still others maintain that it grows substantially. Interesting data have been obtained when the pancreas was perfused with glucose and when glucose acted on isolated beta cells. Tanaka and others (1978) have shown that the reaction of alpha and beta cells to the perfusion of the pancreas with hyperglycemic (300 mg/ml) and hypoglycemic (20 mg/ml) solutions decreases in old rats. Less insulin and glucagon are ejected into the blood in old age. The initial phase of insulin secretion especially changes. As a result of these experiments, it was concluded that the pancreatic cells become less sensitive to glucose in old age. According to Reaven and others (1979), the glucose-stimulated secretion of insulin by beta cells progressively diminishes with age. They have estimated that it is 1.3, 1.0, 0.4 and 0.3 nanounits per cell per minute, respectively, in rats which are 2, 6, 12 and 18 months old. The authors believe that the change in glucose tolerance with age is due to a decrease in the glucose-stimulated secretion of insulin and not to a change in the amount of beta cells. Comparing the responses of beta cells to stimulation by glycose and leucine, Reaven and others (1980) have concluded that insulin secretion decreases in response to the stimulating agents owing to the age-dependent change in the properties of beta cells, and not to the nature of the stimulating agent.

The data presented by Kulchitsky and Orlov (1977) somewhat explain the contradictions in the reaction of the insular apparatus to glucose. The nature of the hyperinsulinemic reaction differs in persons with different glucose tolerance (Fig. 51). Taking account of the glycemic responses, the persons being examined were divided into three groups: (a) virtually healthy young persons (20–29 years old) with normal glucose tolerance, (b) virtually healthy elderly and old persons (60–75 years old) with normal glucose tolerance, and (c) virtually healthy elderly and old persons with disturbed glucose tolerance.

There is a direct link between glucose tolerance, a patient's age and the nature of insulinemia. The first type of insulinemia, i. e. the rapid growth of the content of insulin in the blood and then its gradual diminution, has been observed in young persons and elderly persons with normal glucose tolerance. The second type of hyperinsulinemia, i. e. the rapid and prolonged growth of the content of insulin in the blood, has been observed in elderly persons with low glucose tolerance, and the third type of insulinemia, i. e. the diabetic type, has been observed in patients suffering from diabetes mellitus (although hyperglycemia is pronounced, insulinemia is reduced). Thus, many contradictions in the assessment of insulinemia disappear when it is taken into account that elderly persons are not a homogeneous population. In old age, the blood sugar level is not adequately reduced when a greater amount of insulin is ejected. Moreover, endogenous insulin becomes less effective in old age. Hence, more pronounced hyperinsulinemia caused by the administration of glucose is of adaptive regulatory significance.

In old age, the mechanisms of hyperinsulinemia during hyperglycemia may differ from one another: (a) hyperinsulinemia may originate because insulin does not adequately intensify both the passage of glucose into the cells and its further transformation (in this case, hyperinsulinemia is the inevitable outcome of prolonged hyperglycemia, which follows the sugar load; (b) hyperinsulinemia may be the outcome of the greater sensitivity of beta cells or the central mechanisms of their regulation of glucose. Experiments with isolated beta cells and the old animals' pancreas being perfused show that their sensitivity to insulin is normal, reduced or enhanced in old age. The results obtained by several researchers are contradictory largely because of the different experimental conditions. The data presented by Gatsko (1977) are interesting. In her *in vitro* experiments, she determined the insulin secretion of an isolated pancreas of adult and old rats, depending on the amount of glucose being added. She found that the reaction of the beta cells of the pancreas to small glucose doses occurs more intensively in old animals; age differences are levelled out when moderate doses are administered, and a greater amount of insulin is secreted in mature rats when the glucose doses are large. Hence, according to Gatsko's data, reactivity decreases, but the sensitivity of the insular apparatus to the action of glucose increases with age. Pronounced hyperinsulinemia may be due to the specifics of the reaction of the tissues to the action of insulin. Hyperglycemia is preserved for a longer time as a result of the attenuation of the influence of insulin on the transfer of glucose into the cell. Consequently, more portions of insulin are ejected. As we have already mentioned, such hyper-insulinemia is due to a decrease in the physiological effectiveness of the hormone in the blood and to a change in the reaction of the tissues to its action. The regulation of the secretion of not only insulin, but also glucagon changes in old age. Klung and others (1980) determined the content of immunoreactive glucagon in the blood of the portal vein after glucose was administered. The content of glucagon decreased by 50 per cent in rats 2 months old, but the content of insulin increased 2 or 3 times in old rats under the same conditions.

Specifics of the Tissue Reaction to the Action of Insulin in Old Age

The influence of insulin on the aging organism can be objectively characterized by using a large variety of hormone doses. According to our data, the possible range of the reaction of the tissues to the action of the hormone diminishes and tissue reactivity decreases with age. Hence, insulin causes shifts of a smaller amplitude in the organism of old animals. However, the sensitivity (which is determined by the threshold doses of the hormone) of several tissues grows in old age. According to Czech (1976), the sensitivity of the diaphragm and adipose tissue of rats to insulin decreases in old age. Gomers and others (1977) did not observe any age distinctions in the reaction of adipose tissue to insulin.

Fig. 38 A, B gives data on the hypoglycemic reactions in rabbits of different age after insulin was administered intravenously. When the hormone is administered in large doses, hypoglycemia and the passage of glucose into the cells are more pronounced in mature rabbits, and when it is administered in small doses, the given processes are more pronounced in old rabbits. This regularity, i. e. a decrease in reactivity and an increase in the sensitivity of the tissues to insulin, has been revealed by studying other aspects of the action of the hormone on metabolism and the functions, the membrane potentials of the cells, the bioelectric activity of the brain, and the cardiovascular system (Belonog, 1977; Martynenko, 1977; Shevchuk, 1977).

According to Martynenko, the membrane potential of the skeletal muscle fibres of mature rats does not noticeably increase (it increases from 79.5 ±1.1 mV to 82.9 ±1.5 mV) when insulin is administered in a dose of 0.04 unit per 100 g of weight, but it increases (from 78.8 ± 0.6 mV to 84.1 ± 0.2 mV) in old rats when the same dose is administered. As the hormone dose increases, the age changes are levelled out at first, and then the reaction becomes more pronounced in mature rats. The growth of the membrane potential entails a decrease in cellular excitability, which is determined by stimulating the cells with the microelectrode. The shifts in the transfer of ions through the membrane are more pronounced in mature rats when insulin is administered in doses which are higher than the threshold doses (0.16 unit per 100 g of weight). The concentration of total and intracellular potassium (per dry or wet weight) increases in 60 minutes in mature animals and in 120 minutes in old animals.

Belonog (1977) compared the shifts in the electric activity of the brain of young and old persons when insulin was administered in a dose of 0.05 unit per kilogram of weight. The shifts in the electroencephalogram occured more often in old persons (in 80 per cent of the cases) than in young persons (in 15 per cent of the cases) when the hormone was administered in that small dose. Shevchuk (1977) showed that the shifts in cardiac output, the stroke volume, the cardiac index, and so forth, are more pronounced in old rats when a small dose of insulin (0.025 unit per 100 g of weight) is administered, and that these shifts are more pronounced in mature rats when insulin is administered in a dose of 0.16 unit per 100 g of weight. These hemodynamic effects are associated with the action of insulin and not with hypoglycemia. Hemodynamic changes were not prevented even when insulin and glucose were simultaneously administered.

The influence of insulin on both the processes of protein biosynthesis and the genetic apparatus of the cells is an important link in the complex mechanism of the hormone's action. Goldstein and others (1977) have shown that qualitative changes occur in this influence with age. When insulin is administered to adult rats, only inactive chromatin participates in hormonal induction and the incorporation of the labelled precursor into it increases four times in two hours. In old rats, the label is incorporated into not only inactive, but also active chromatin. However, the label is incorporated into inactive chromatin later and less in old rats than in mature ones.

Gatsko (1977) determined the influence of various doses of insulin on the lipolytic activity of adipose tissue. In mature rats, lipolysis in adipose tissue was suppressed more as the amount of insulin grew in the medium. In old rats, the outflow of non-esterified fatty acids from adipose tissue was inhibited to the greatest extent when a minimum dose of the hormone was administered. This phenomenon was observed also when insulin acted on glycogen synthesis in the diaphragm of rats of different age. In old rats, glycogen is deposited to the greatest extent in the diaphragm when the concentration of insulin is 0.05 U/ml. An increase in the content of insulin is accompanied by a decrease in its effectiveness. In mature animals, the minimum effect was produced when the concentration of insulin was 0.05 U/ml and the maximum effect was produced when its concentration was 0.1 U/ml. Hence, the dose-effect ratio changes under the action of insulin and the reaction range diminishes in old age. When the physiological effectiveness of the hormone is reduced, the sensitivity of some tissues to the hormone increases for adaptive purposes. However, it is not enough to maintain adaptive reactions in a wide range of shifts which occur in the organism. In old age, a decrease in tissue reactivity is one of the main mechanisms of the development of insulin insufficiency. Insulin influences the cell through the highly sensitive specific receptors which are on its membrane. It has been established that insulin receptors are present on the membranes of the fat cells, the liver, muscular tissue, fibroblasts, lymphocytes and neurons. Direct experimental data show that the number of insulin receptors decreases in old age (Clark *et al.*, 1975; Olefsky, Reaven, 1975).

Thus, insulin binding by the adipocytes of rats is inversely proportional to their age. This fact is in accord with a decrease in the biological effects of insulin, particularly those produced by stimulating glucose oxidation in the adipocytes.

According to Muggeo and others (1979), the number of monocyte binding sites is almost halved in persons who are more than 50 years old. It should be noted that not only age, but also various physiological and pathological factors change the concentration of insulin receptors and their affinity for insulin. This affinity rapidly changes in accordance with the diet, physiological processes and the time of day. The number of receptors is subject to a smaller change. A decrease in the number of insulin-binding sites on the cell membrane is one of the main causes of both the diminution of cellular reactivity with respect to the action of insulin in old age and the disturbance of clear dose-dependent responses to the administration of the hormone. When there are a limited number of receptors, the sensitivity of some cells to insulin can grow because, in old age, they lose their equilibrium easier and a reaction occurs.

One of the main mechanisms of insulin action, i. e. the transfer of glucose through the membrane, is an active process. It is coupled with the transport of sodium ions from the cell and the activation of K^+, Na^+ and ATPase. Zierler (1960) and after him many other researchers attribute glucose transfer to the fact that insulin hyperpolarizes the membrane of the muscle and fat cells and increases the charge being fixed on their surface. This is believed to deform the membrane and produce conformation changes in its proteins. The laminar structures of lipoproteins assume a micellar or globular configuration. In this case, pores are probably formed, water-soluble substances occasionally pass through them into the cell, and glucose is transported inside the cell. We have shown that insulin hyperpolarizes the cell membrane. In small doses, it causes greater hyperpolarization in old rats, and in large doses, it causes greater hyperpolarization in mature rats. Several metabolic shifts which occur under the influence of insulin and which can be attributed to both a change in the membrane state and the development of hyperpolarization are in accord with those specifics. The age changes in the reaction of the cells to insulin are probably due to those membrane processes.

The hexokinase reaction, which leads to glucose phosphorylation, is an extremely important link in the transformation of glucose in the cell. Insulin intensifies the activity of hexokinase. Litoshenko (1977), our fellow worker, showed that the activity of the insulin-sensitive isoenzymes of hexokinase (II and IV types) in adipose tissue and the liver decreases in old animals. This may play an important role in limiting the reaction of the tissues to the action of the hormone. Parina and others (1976) have presented interesting data by showing that the administration of insulin does not change the activity of hexokinase in the liver of rats one month old, but it enhances substantially this activity in old rats.

Regulatory Mechanisms of Insulin Provision

Hypothalamic influences are of great importance in the mechanism which regulates insulin secretion. Insulin secretion is regulated hypothalamically by neural cholinergic mechanisms with the participation of somatotropine and somatostatin. Bezrukov and Epstein (1977) have shown that the regulatory hypothalamic influences on insulin secretion attenuate with age. The ventromedial nucleus of the hypothalamus is known to inhibit the lateral hypothalamus, while the stimulation of the latter intensifies (through the cholinergic mechanisms) insulin secretion by the beta cells of the pancreas (Stulnikov, 1973). Hence, cholinergic mechanisms are activated and the content of insulin in the blood increases when the ventromedial nucleus of the hypothalamus is destroyed and the structures of the lateral hypothalamus are "liberated" from the influence of this nucleus. Bezrukov and Epstein have shown that the level of blood insulin grows more in mature rats than in old ones when the ventromedial nucleus is destroyed. In mature animals, this level reaches 142.5 ± 23.5 μU/ml, while in old animals, it reaches 63.7 ± 7.8 μU/ml. This fact is due to a change in the relationship between individual hypothalamic structures which regulate the function of the insular apparatus. The attenuation of the inhibiting influence of the ventromedial nucleus on the lateral hypothalamus is manifested in the smaller growth of the insulin content when the ventromedial nucleus is destroyed in old animals.

The activity of the lateral hypothalamus under ordinary conditions intensifies when the inhibiting influence of the ventromedial nucleus attenuates. As a result, the stimulation of insulin secretion is more pronounced. Hence, the malfunction of the hypothalamus and the activation of the lateral hypothalamus play a definite role in the mechanism of a change in the content of blood insulin in old age. In other words, the range of the regulatory influences of the hypothalamus is narrower in old animals than in mature ones. Consequently, the changes in insulinemia are more pronounced and mobile in mature animals when glycemic shifts occur in them. Thus, the shifts in hypothalamic regulation bring about an increase in the content of insulin in the initial state, on the one hand, and limit the potentialities of the regulation of the insular apparatus during glycemic shifts, on the other.

There is every reason to believe that the age changes in the neural regulation of the insular apparatus and a diminution of the range of the regulatory influences are due to not only intracentral shifts, but also the disturbances which occur in the peripheral cholinergic synapses. According to our data (Frolkis, 1970), the activity of cholinesterase decreases much more (by 83.0 ± 5,2 per cent) in the pancreas than in any other organ (the heart, the skeletal muscle, the liver, and so forth) in old age. A decrease in cholinesterase activity somewhat indicates that substantial changes had occurred in synaptic conduction. Account should also be taken of our laboratory data on the great structural and functional changes in parasympathetic ganglia (Duplenko, 1965).

Thus, the organism is insufficiently provided with insulin in old age due to a decrease in the functional abilities of the insular apparatus, the structural changes in the beta cells, the attenuation of neural regulatory influences, and the inhibition of insulin. Consequently, the insulin activity of the blood decreases as the hormone content increases and the reactivity of the tissues diminishes with respect to the action of insulin. The necessary level of insulin regulation cannot be maintained for a long time when insulinase becomes less active, tissue sensitivity grows and the hormone content increases.

The insufficiency of the organism's insulin provision is due to a set of pancreatic and extrapancreatic factors. Insulin becomes less effective when the content of the inhibitors increases and the role of the counterinsulin factors grows. In this respect, glycemic shifts activate the function of beta cells and cause the intensified synthesis and secretion of insulin. Consequently, these cells hyperfunction, and then the insular apparatus is depleted. An important fact is that this activation occurs when a part of the cells undergoes age atrophy. The load then becomes greater on a smaller number of insulinocytes. The primary age changes in beta cells and their shifts caused by vascular sclerosis are extremely important. Proinsulin or synalbumin, which is the B-chain of insulin, may probably be secreted into the blood when gross age changes occur in the insular apparatus. The amount of inhibited insulin in the blood grows when that substance appears in the blood. This situation is aggravated by the fact that the changes which occur in both lipid metabolism and the content of fatty acids due to insulin insufficiency suppress insulin activity by themselves. All these pancreatic and extrapancreatic shifts are aggravated by the disturbances of the neural regulation of the pancreas and a decrease in its reactivity.

Inhibitors suppress the activity of free insulin and apparently do not influence bound insulin. Consequently, another vicious circle is created. When insulin activity is suppressed, hormone synthesis and the content of not only free, but also physiologically effective bound insulin simultaneously grow. As a result, the influence of the hormone on adipose tissue intensifies, lipogenesis is activated, and obesity may be promoted. The above-mentioned relationships between aging and vitauct in the insulin provision system greatly differ from one another. These relationships are the cause of the existence of two populations of elderly and old persons, namely, persons with normal carbohydrate tolerance and those with low carbohydrate tolerance.

Influence of the Change in Insulin Provision on Metabolism

A large number of applications of insulin action shows why the insufficiency of insulin provision plays a certain role in the formation of many disturbances in old age (Frolkis et al., 1977).

As the organism's insulin provision decreases with age, low carbohydrate tolerance is found in an increasing number of persons. When relative insulin insufficiency develops, glucose utilization is upset above all in muscular tissue and also in hepatic tissue.

Insulin insufficiency retards the rate of the membrane transfer of glucose into muscular tissue. This fact apparently plays a definite role in reducing the oxidative conversions of glucose with age and enhancing the significance of glycogenolysis in the energy generation processes. Glycogenolysis may be intensified through the cyclic monophosphate system. In the case of insulin insufficiency, the changes in this system may activate the kinase of phosphorylase b and cause the conversion of inactive phosphorylase b into active phosphorylase a. We have discovered such a direction of the given process in the heart of old rats. In their heart, unlike in the heart of adult rats, almost all phosphorylase b is converted into phosphorylase a. The changes in phosphorylase activity apparently intensify glycogenolysis during aging. Consequently, the glycogen content decreases in the cardiac and skeletal muscles and the liver in old age. This fact is especially clearly revealed when their activity changes. A decrease in the content of this reserve carbohydrate may also be due to a diminution of its synthesis with age as a result of the attenuation of the activity of UDPG-glycosyltransferase, which is the regulator enzyme of glycogen synthesis that is induced by insulin. When insulin becomes less effective biologically with age, the activity of the enzyme decreases as a result of either the disturbance of its conversion into an active form or the direct diminution of the concentration of glucosyltransferase due to the disturbance of its biosynthesis.

When the insulin-dependent hexokinase isoenzymes (types II and IV) become less active, the drop in the blood sugar level is no longer maintained and the synthesis of fatty acids and triglycerides is disturbed in adipose tissue. This synthesis may be disturbed when the rate of glucose phosphorylation, the activity of glucose-6-phosphate dehydrogenase and the NADPH pool diminish. Lipid metabolism is disturbed when insulin provision decreases in old age. Consequently, the glucose-fatty acid cycle is disturbed. This cycle is part of the homeostatic system which regulates the energy processes in the organism. Fatty acids then accumulate in the blood as less glucose is taken in by muscular tissue. Moreover, fatty acids are oxidized less intensively with age. As a result, free fatty acids accumulate in the blood in old age. When the amount of free fatty acids increases due to insulin insufficiency, the biological effect of insulin decreases as a result of the counterinsulin action of these acids. Consequently, prolonged glycemic shifts occur and hyperinsulinemia develops.

The disturbances in insulin provision may be the cause of the insufficient use of acetoacetic acid. Consequently, cholesterol synthesis may intensify. When insulin provision is reduced, the intensification of gluconeogenesis (which is one of the main causes of the excessive synthesis of cholesterol from aectyl-CoA) may promote the accumulation of cholesterol. This fact and the growth of the content of triglycerides promote the formation of lipoproteins of low and very low density in the liver. However, beta lipoproteins, just as free fatty acids, are the non-hormonal antagonists of insulin. Thus, shifts which aggravate insulin insufficiency occur during the changes in it.

This insulin activity of the blood decreases with age. It is tested by glycogen synthesis in the diaphragm and is connected mainly with free insulin. However, the content of bound insulin which is tested on adipose tissue and is connected with apparently non-inhibited insulin increases. Hence, a vicious circle originates, namely, the inhibition of free insulin intensifies hormone synthesis, as a result of which its bound form grows.

In old age, the intensity of lipogenesis may be on a sufficiently high level owing to the preservation of the effects of the influence of insulin on adipose tissue even when the organism's insulin provision is reduced. This occurrence is due to the great activity of hexokinase of type I, being connected with lipogenesis from glucose in the absence of insulin. In this respect, lipogenesis may decrease as a result of the disturbance in the conversion of acetyl-CoA (whose amount diminishes with age) into fatty acids and triglycerides (Nikitin, Martynenko, 1963). Pashkova and Popova (1970) indicate that the intensity of lipolysis and lipogenesis decreases with age.

In old age, the influence of relative insulin insufficiency on metabolism may be produced also through such an important mechanism as a change in the rate of ion transport through the cell membrane. This transport is realized with the participation of Na^+, K^+-dependent ATPase, whose activity is regulated by insulin. A decrease in insulin activity is somewhat responsible for the diminution of the activity of this extracellular transport mechanism of the cell in old age. In this respect, mention should be made of the data on a decrease in the general activity of ATPase in the kidneys, the liver, the brain and especially the muscles of animals with experimental diabetes and on the growth of this activity when insulin is administered.

The shifts in ion transfer can produce changes in the electric properties of the cells, in protein biosynthesis, and in the activity of the genetic apparatus. Thus, relative insulin insufficiency may influence the relationships between the state of the cell membrane and the activity of the genetic apparatus. According to the genoregulatory theory (Frolkis, 1969), these relationships are important mechanisms of aging.

When insulin provision decreases in old age, shifts occur in the processes of protein biosynthesis and, consequently, in the activity of several enzymes (hexokinase, lactate dehydrogenase, UDPG-glycosyltransferase, pyruvate kinase, lipoprotein lipase, etc.), for which the inductive influence of insulin is consequential. This fact undoubtedly determines several changes which are found in various metabolic cycles in old age.

Thus, the given data show that relative insulin insufficiency plays an important role in the age changes in various types of metabolism.

The insulin mechanism is only a link in the complex system of neurohumoral regulation, which changes substantially with age. Therefore, in all the metabolic shifts which were analyzed, insulin does not play an exceptional role in their formation; it simply participates to a different extent in changing the neurohumoral regulation of metabolism.

7. Thyroid Regulation in Old Age

Goethe once said that what is in the air and requires time can originate simultaneously in a hundred minds without being borrowed.

When the age changes in the functions of the endocrine glands are being studied, attention is usually given mainly to only one link in hormonal regulation, i. e. to the secretory function of the glands. This is a great shortcoming of the investigation of these changes.

To reveal the true direction of the shifts which occur as the organism ages, it is necessary to assess the whole pattern of hormonal self-regulation. A systematic approach is being taken now, when the study of the role of hormonal regulation in the mechanism of aging is at a new stage. Therefore, our topic is "thyroid regulation and aging" instead of the "thyroid gland and aging." In this respect, we will consider the hypothalamic regulation of the function of the thyroid gland, a change in its structure, metabolism, activity, shifts in the content of the thyroid hormones in the blood, the reaction of the tissues to the action of hormones, the metabolism of hormones in the tissues, and the effect of the thyroid hormones on the state of the hypothalamic centres. During the last decade, we have obtained data on the age changes in all the links of thyroid regulation. We have carried out many researches in this respect together with Verzhikovskaya and Valueva (Verzhikovskaya, 1971; Frolkis et al., 1973; Verzhikovskaya, Valueva, 1977; Frolkis et al., 1978; Verzhikovskaya et al., 1978).

Structural and Functional Changes in the Thyroid Gland

The thyroid gland changes structurally and functionally, and its relative mass diminishes, as the organism ages. In old animals, the follicles become polymorphous, their diameter decreases, and the follicular epithelium becomes smaller, flattened and atrophied. Histochemical investigations (Lasada, Roberts, 1975) have shown that the metabolic process in the thyroid gland diminish and the "growth" synthesis of protein as well as the mitotic activity of the cells decrease with age.

The structural changes in the thyroid gland are irregular, and adaptive shifts occur in it in old age. These shifts include the appearance of the hypertrophied cells with ultrastructural features of hyperfunction. A pale-coloured colloid is found in most follicles. This indicates that its reserves are being depleted. The interstitial tissue grows in the thyroid gland and its fibrosis and hyalinosis become distinct as the organism ages. The stroma of the organ is so sclerosed in old age that it squeezes the parenchymatous cells and causes their atrophy. The connective-tissue reaction, vascular sclerosis, capillary depletion, and a decrease in the number of anastomoses outside the organ worsen the trophicity of the thyroid gland. However, the sequence of the age changes in the thyroid gland shows that the disturbance of blood supply is an important, but not the primary cause of its aging.

An electron microscope investigation of the thyroid tissue of rats 28 to 32 months old has revealed the predominance of dark thyrocytes, a decrease in the number and a change in the shape of the microvilli of the apical part of the cytoplasm membrane, nuclear deformation, a diminution of the quantity of the endoplasmic reticulum, the loss of its correct orientation, the flattening of the cisternae, the disappearance of the distinctive outline of Golgi's apparatus, a decrease in the number of mitochondria and "colloidal" granules, a sharp thickening of the basilar membrane of the follicles, and the depletion of the capillary network (Fig. 52 A, B, C). It can be concluded from electron microscope investigations that the ultrastructure of the thyroid gland changes with age; these changes are associated with the processes of iodide oxidation, the synthesis and iodination of thyroglobulin, and the formation of iodotyrosines and iodothyronines as well as metabolic and oxidative processes in the gland.

Direct investigations have shown that functional changes occur in the thyroid gland as the organism ages. The iodine-accumulating function of the gland and the extent of isotope uptake decrease, while the time of isotope elimination increases. According to Valueva (1978), the diminution of the iodine-accumulating ability of the thyroid gland and a change in all the subsequent stages of iodine transformation in its cells are associated only with a decrease in metabolism and synthesis. Iodide which has been captured from circulating blood is included in the hormone-formation process, which is connected with the synthesis and iodination of specific protein and the formation of iodized amino acids. The thyroidal uptake of iodine is regarded as active transfer that is coupled with the simultaneous consumption of energy formed by aerobic cellular metabolism, which requires the presence of NADP and oxygen.

The initial stages of hormonogenesis as well as the subsequent conversion of iodine and the synthesis of the specific glycoprotein of thyroglobulin require energy which is formed as a result of cellular oxidation.

The tissue respiration of the thyroid gland is far less intense in old animals (3.78 ± 0.68 ml of oxygen per milligram of dry tissue per hour in 8–10 month-old rats and 2.52 ± 0.2 ml of oxygen per milligram of dry tissue per hour in 28–32 month-old rats). One of the causes of its diminution is the insufficiency of the oxidative substrates. The tissue respiration of the thyroid gland of old animals is activated when pyruvate, alpha ketoglutarate and succinate are added (Verzhikovskaya, 1971). Nevertheless, it is still less than that of adult animals under the same conditions. An interesting fact is that it is activated to the greatest extent when succinate is added. If the biosynthesis of the thyroid hormone decreases when succinate oxidation is more or less preserved and the oxidation of pyruvate and alpha ketoglutarate is reduced substantially, the energy supply of that synthesis is apparently connected with the processes which occur with the participation of NADH dehydrogenase. In

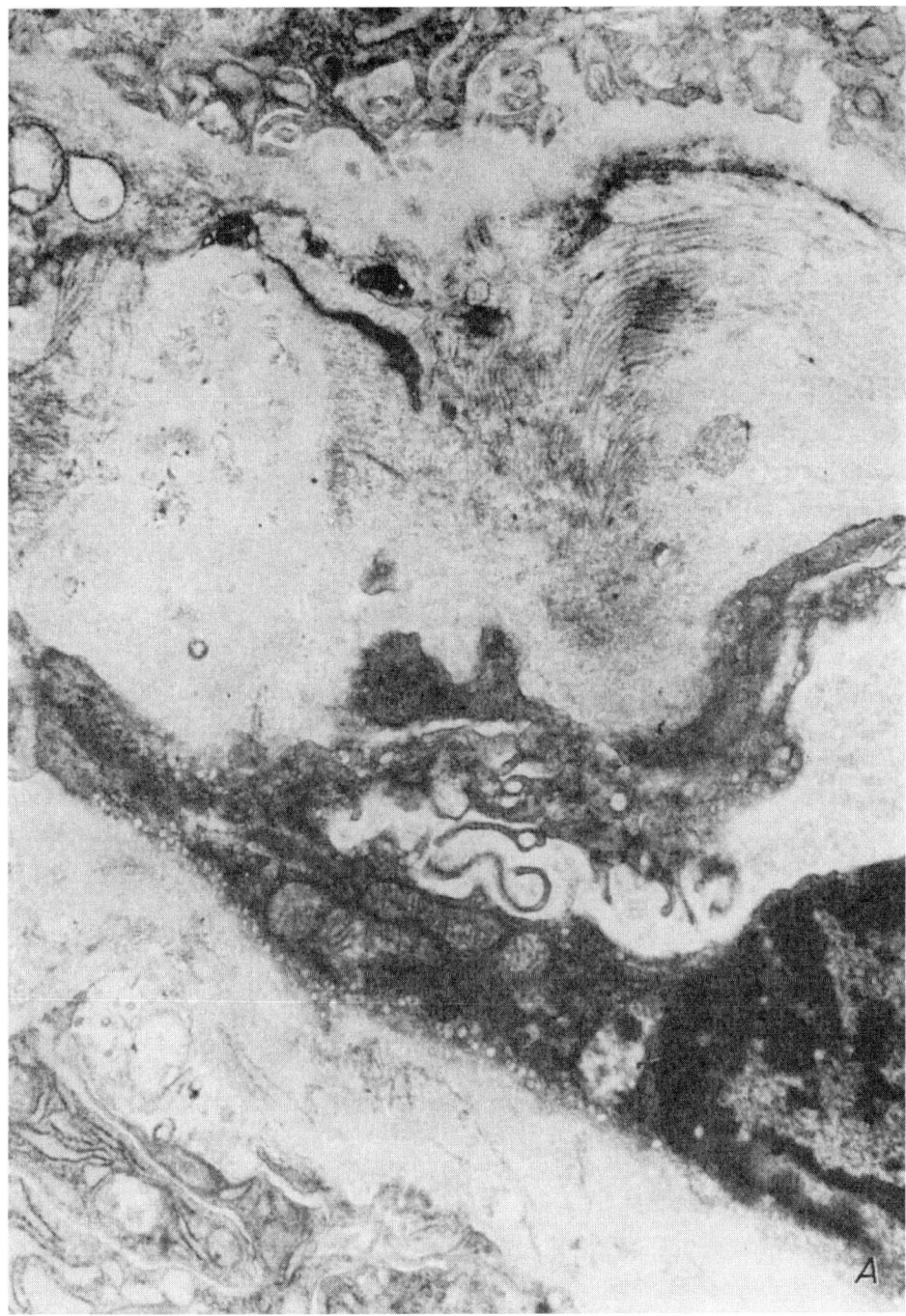

Fig. 52 A

Fig. 52. Ultrastructural changes in the thyroid gland in old rats; A region of the basal membrane;
B dark thyrocyte; C region of the thyrocyte

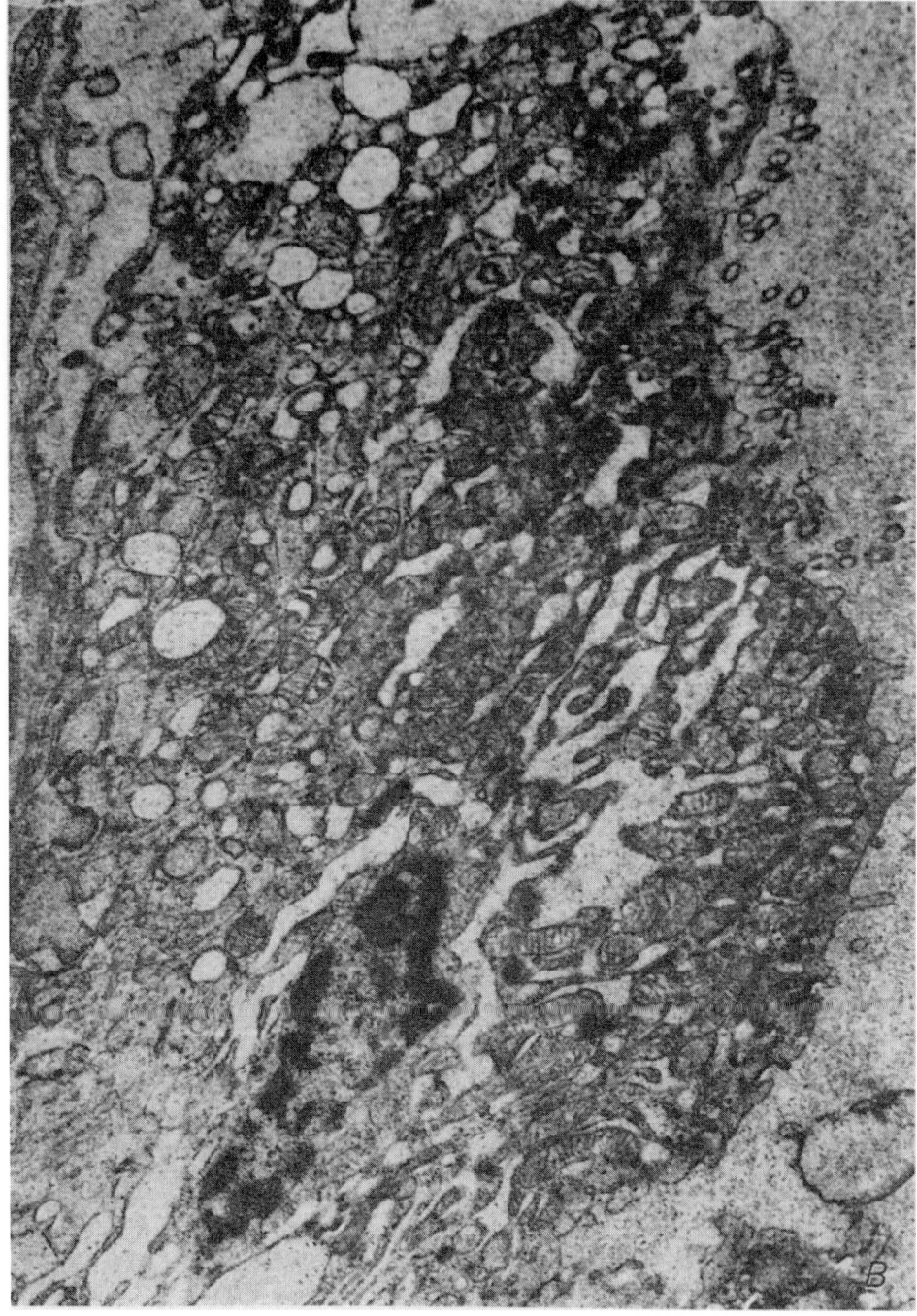

Fig. 52 B

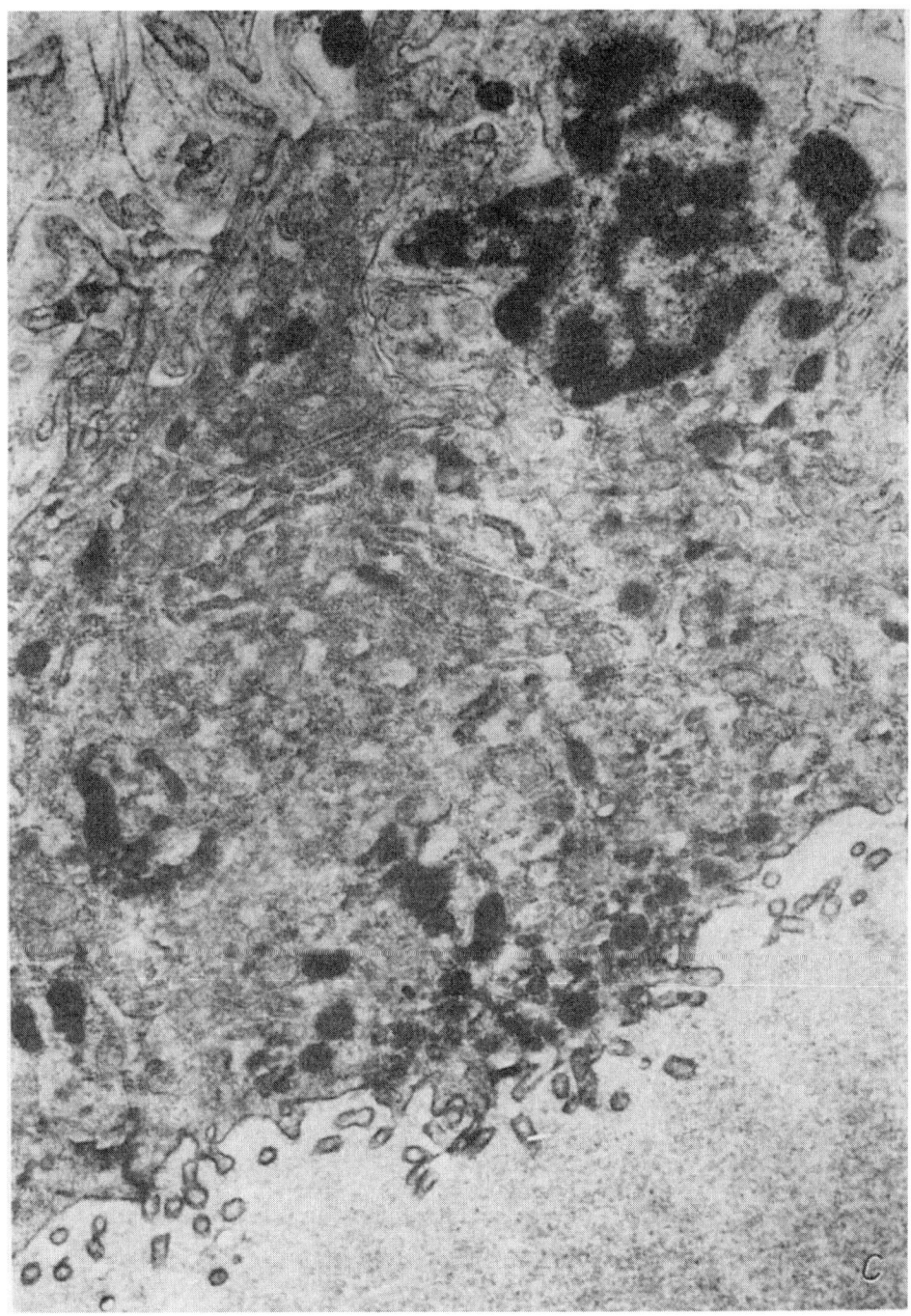

Fig. 52C

Table 4. *Content of iodinated amino acids and the quantitative ratios between them in the thyroid gland of rats of different ages*

Age (months)	Number rats	Monoiodotyrosine		Diiodotyrosine		T_4		T_3	
		μg/mg of tissue	percentage of total iodine	μg/mg of tissue	percentage of total iodine	μg/mg of tissue	percentage of total iodine	μg/mg of tissue	percentage of total iodine
1.5–2 (I)	10	0.15 ± 0.004	22.4 ± 1.3	0.36 ± 0.01	53.7 ± 2.4	0.14 ± 0.02	20.9 ± 1.5	0.02 ± 0.004	3.00 ± 0.7
8–12 (II)	10	0.25 ± 0.003	35.6 ± 2.7	0.27 ± 0.008	42.8 ± 1.5	0.09 ± 0.002	14.2 ± 1.1	0.02 ± 0.001	3.1 ± 0.5
P_{II-I}		< 0.001	< 0.001	< 0.001	< 0.001	< 0.02	< 0.01	> 0.5	> 0.5
28–32 (III)	10	0.43 ± 0.03	74.1 ± 5.2	0.1 ± 0.005	17.2 ± 2.3	0.05 ± 0.004	8.6 ± 1.5	0.005 ± 0.0003	0.86 ± 0.1
P_{III-II}		< 0.001	< 0.001	< 0.001	< 0.001	< 0.001	< 0.01	< 0.001	< 0.001

this respect, it should be taken into account that the thyroid gland can be activated non-specifically by succinates.

When the organism ages, changes occur at all the stages of the metabolism of hormones of the thyroid gland. Most of the iodine which enters the organism is in the form of iodide. In the thyroid gland, iodide is incorporated rapidly into thyroglobulin, whose hydrolysis engenders hormonally inactive monoiodotyrosine and di-iodotyrosine as well as the active derivatives of thyronine, i. e. thyroxine (T_4) and 3,5,3-tri-iodothyronine (T_3). The relationships between monoiodotyrosine and di-iodotyrosine as well as between iodotyrosine and iodothyronine are regarded as indicators of the intensity of hormone formation.

With age, the content of di-iodotyrosine, T_4 and T_3 decreases gradually, the monoiodotyrosine/di-iodotyrosine ratio and the iodotyrosine/iodothyronine ratio grow, and the amount of monoiodotyrosine increases substantially in the tissue of the thyroid gland. These changes are more pronounced in adult rats than in young animals, and are especially pronounced in old rats. The iodine-accumulating ability of the thyroid gland decreases and the activity of peroxidase diminishes in old age. Consequently, the content of oxidized iodine decreases and the synthesis of monoiodotyrosine increases (Table 4). This is evident from the fact that ^{131}I is eliminated from the thyroid tissue much slower in old rats than in rats aged 1.5–2 and 8–12 months. This has also been confirmed in the experiments with old dogs and hens, in which the iodine/iodine oxide ratio is increased (Book, 1976; Bobek, Krus, 1977).

The ascertained age changes at the initial stages of the biosynthesis of the thyroid hormones, i. e. iodotyrosines, apparently also determine the disturbances in the synthesis of iodothyronines, T_4 and T_3, which are formed as a result of the condensation of two molecules of di-iodotyrosine (T_4) or the molecules of di-iodotyrosine and monoiodotyrosine (T_3). According to Valueva (1978), the synthesis of di-iodotyrosine lessens substantially as the organism ages. This is mainly why the formation of T_4 and T_3 decreases. The content of di-iodotyrosine is somewhat higher in animals 8–12 months old than in old animals. This apparently determines the invariability of the content of T_3 in adult animals.

Thus, structural and functional changes develop gradually in the thyroid gland with age, limiting the hormone-formation processes.

Thyroid Hormones in the Blood

The larger part of the thyroid hormones in the blood is bound with serum proteins, while an inconsiderable part of them is in a free state. The amount of protein-bound iodine changes with age. Such iodine consists of thyroxine and other organic compounds of iodine. According to several authors, the amount of protein-bound iodine is increased in the blood of elderly and old persons (Cicinotta et al., 1974).

At the same time, much data indicate that the amount of protein-bound iodine in the blood decreases in old age. This is regarded as a manifestation of the hypofunction of the thyroid gland. According to Green (1974) as well as

Kaplan and associates (1975), the amount of protein-bound iodine is far less in elderly and old persons than in those between 20 and 30. Moreover, some researchers indicate that the amount of protein-bound iodine virtually does not change with age. The data obtained by the direct methods of determining T_4 and T_3 are of much greater value than all those indirect data. T_3 is synthesized in a far smaller amount than T_4. The extrathyroidal stock in the former is one-eighth of that of the latter. However, the former is three or four times more active metabolically than the latter (Gharib, 1974). T_4 has three-fourths of all the blood iodine. The levels of T_4 and T_3 and their free and bound forms in the blood are determined by the complex-formation of the thyroid hormones with definite proteins of blood serum. The binding of the thyroid hormones by specific blood proteins is an important factor that influences the rate at which the hormones disappear from the blood. This rate determines the turnover of hormones in the blood and the ratio of the free and bound forms of T_4 and T_3, which in turn determine the penetration of the hormones into the cells.

It has now been established that T_4 in human blood is associated with three serum proteins: thyroxine-binding globulin, albumin, and thyroxine-binding prealbumin.

T_3 also binds with the blood proteins, forming less stable complexes than T_4. T_3 is associated in human serum mainly with thyroxine-binding globulin and only then with albumin, but it does not bind with the thyroxin-binding prealbumin. The complex of T_3 and thyroxine-binding globulin are from three to five times more labile than T_4 in the same fraction (Pedersen, 1974). This explains the low content of T_3 in the blood in spite of its continuous secretion from the thyroid gland and its participation in the regulatory processes. Nouel and associates (1973) have shown that the concentration of T_3 in the blood diminishes with age. According to Herrmann et al. (1974), the content of T_4 decreases in old persons.

The content of the thyroid hormones and their complex formation with specific blood proteins change substantially with age (Frolkis et al., 1978; Valueva, 1978). The concentration of total T_4 in the blood of old animals decreases substantially in comparison with adults. However, the amount of free T_4 in rats 28–32 months old is virtually the same as in adult rats. This rise of proportion of free hormone against the background of decreased function of the thyroid gland is of adaptive importance in old age. It helps to maintain a definite level of thyroid regulation in old age. The thyroxine-binding ability of the blood is reduced as the level of total T_4 drops. Hence, the quantity of free T_4 remains invariable as the amount of total thyroxine diminishes. According to Valueva (1978), T_4 in old animals is bound only with thyroxine-binding globulin, and not with other proteins. The thyroxine-binding ability of the blood decreases due to a diminution of either the amount of protein molecules or the number of binding sites on every molecule.

It has been found that the amount of the specific thyroxine-binding alpha globulin in the blood progressively decreases in old age. However, in determining the thyroxine-binding capacity of the specific thyroxine-binding globulin that has been isolated from the blood of old rats, it has been established that the number of the protein-binding sites is the same as that in other groups

Table 5. *Content of total and free T₄, T₃ in the blood of rats of different ages*

Age, months	Number rats	Total T_4 μg/100 ml	Free T_4 %	Absolute content of free T_4 ng/100 ml	Total T_3 ng/100 ml	Free T_3 %	Absolute content of T_3 ng/100 ml
1.5–2 (I)	20	8.1±0.5	0.1 ±0.01	8.1±1.1	250±35	0.30±0.02	0.75 ±0.1
8–12 (II)	20	5.6±0.4	0.07±0.002	3.9±0.7	195±21	0.29±0.03	0.56 ±0.07
P_{II-I}		<0.001	<0.01	<0.001	>0.2	>0.5	>0.2
28–32 (III)	20	4.2±0.2	0.1 ±0.01	4.2±0.9	93±23	0.29±0.01	0.269±0.02
P_{III-II}		<0.001	<0.01	>0.5	<0.02	>0.5	<0.01

of animals 1.5–2 and 8–12 months old (81×10^{-10} M with 300 micrograms of protein).

Thus, the number of binding sites on the specific thyroxine-binding alpha globulin isolated from the serum of old rats does not change. However, the amount of this protein in animals 28–32 months old is far less than in mature and immature animals. Apparently, this ultimately determines the decrease in the thyroxine-binding capacity of the blood in old rats.

Along with a decrease in the contents of total T_3 and T_4, we see also a decrease in both total and free tri-iodothyronine (Table 5).

Thus, the content of free T_4 remains unchanged as the content of total T_3 and T_4 decreases with age. T_3 is known to be the most active form of the hormone. The transition of T_4 to T_3 is of great importance in the mechanism of the action of T_4 on tissue metabolism. Therefore, the preservation of a definite level of free T_4 cannot compensate completely for the shifts in thyroid regulation.

Hypothalamohypophysial Regulation of the Thyroid Gland Function

The thyroid gland is a link in the complex system of the thyroid regulation of metabolism and functions. The function of the thyroid gland is known to be hypothalamohypophysially controlled through thyrotropin (TSH). Thyrotropin regulates the release of iodized components from the intrafollicular epithelium into the blood, the absorption of iodine by the thyroid tissue, the oxidation of iodide to organic iodine, the formation of iodotyrosines and the condensation of their molecules, and the maintenance of the optimum level of the metabolism of substances in the tissue of the thyroid gland.

Separate links of the hypothalamus-hypophysis-thyroid gland system have been analyzed in a series of our works (Verzhikovskaya, 1971; Frolkis *et al.*, 1973; Frolkis *et al.*, 1978; Valueva, 1978; Verzhikovskaya *et al.*, 1978). In this respect, studies have been conducted with respect to the age changes in the TSH content, its release from the hypophysis under the effect of thyroliberin, and the age specifics of the reaction of the thyroid gland to thyrotropin. Some morphological changes also indicate a change in the thyrotropic function of the hypophysis. Monastryrskaya (1974) has reported that the number and size of basophils in the adenohypophysis of animals and man increase as the organism grows and develops. In old age, the number of these cells diminishes and degenerative changes occur, i. e. they reveal the vacuolization of the cytoplasm and the pycnotization of the nuclei. According to Voitkevich (1963), the amount of secreted basophilic cells diminishes and their structure is disturbed in old age.

Conflicting data on the content of TSH in the blood during aging were obtained by different methods (biological and radioimmunological) and by using incomparable analyzed groups. Dussault and Walker (1979) have reported a decrease in thyrotropin in the hypophysis and the blood of old rats, whereas Kirkham and others (1970) and Wenzel and others (1974) have observed a decrease in the TSH content in the blood of human subjects 20–60 years old. However, Weeke (1973) and Virkhunen and others (1974) showed that the basal

TSH level in the blood of subjects 16–70 years old does not change considerably with age.

Interesting research has been carried out by Sawin-Clark and others (1979). In their investigations of men and women 20–89, they discovered that the thyrotropin content increased with age, the increase being greater in women. An important fact is that the TSH level was relatively higher in elderly persons with increased T_3 and T_4 contents.

Table 6. *Content of the thyrotropin stimulating hormone (TSH) in adenohypophysis and the content of TSH, thyroxine (T_4) and triiodothyronine (T_3) in the blood of rats of different ages*

Age	Mass of adenohypo- physis, mg	TSH		T_4, µg per 100 ml	T_3, ng per 100 ml
		Adenohypophysis	Blood		
		I. U./mg	I. U. for the gland	ng/ml	
1.5–2 months (I)	3.0 ± 0.9	35.0 ± 1.3	105.0 ± 2.4	4.4 ± 0.3	8.1 ± 0.5	250.0 ± 35.0
8–10 months (II)	6.5 ± 1.6	57.0 ± 2.7	370.0 ± 3.7	6.1 ± 0.8	5.6 ± 0.8	195.0 ± 21.0
$P_{II–I}$	>0.05	<0.001	<0.001	<0.05	<0.001	>0.05
18–24 months (III)	7.0 ± 0.6	40.0 ± 3.1	280.0 ± 12.9	8.5 ± 0.8	4.0 ± 0.5	100.0 ± 15.0
$P_{III–I}$	>0.05	<0.001	<0.001	<0.05	<0.05	<0.001
28–32 months (IV)	7.2 ± 0.8	22.0 ± 1.7	158.0 ± 3.0	3.3 ± 0.5	4.2 ± 0.2	93.0 ± 4.3
$P_{IV–I}$	>0.05	<0.001	<0.001	<0.001	<0.001	<0.02

In our laboratory, studies were made of the TSH content in the blood and the hypophysis of four groups of rats (Table 6). The blood content of TSH was seen to increase until the animals were 24 months old, and then it decreased. The content of thyrotropin in the hypophysis is maximum in animals 8–10 months old. Apparently, the inconsistencies of the data on the content and secretion of the hormone can be explained by studying the fractional age groups. In any case, it should be noted that, firstly, the content of thyrotropin in the blood is maintained on a high level for a rather long time during aging, and that, secondly, the basal hormone level in the blood is maintained as a result of the great functional performance of the hypophysis. This is evident from the high TSH level in the blood and the low TSH level in the hypophysis of rats 18–24 months old.

In rats 18–24 months old, thyrotropin in the blood remains on a high level even when the functional activity of the thyroid gland decreases. Hence, the age changes in the thyrotropic function of the hypophysis are not the cause of alterations in the functions of the thyroid gland which occur with age (Valueva, 1978).

The thyrotropic function of the hypophysis is regulated hypothalamically by means of the thyrotropin-releasing factor (TRF). Winokur and Utiger (1974) have observed that the release of thyrotropin, especially in elderly men, is reduced when synthetic TRF is administered. The work carried out by Ohara and others (1974) is of great interest. They administered TRF in varying doses to persons 25–35 and 60–94. It turned out that the TSH level rises to a greater extent in old persons when the TRF dose is small (100 µg) and in young persons when the dose is large (300 μg). This level virtually does not change when TRF is administered in a large dose to old persons. Hence, according to Ohara and others (1974), the sensitivity of the thyrotropin-synthesizing system to the releasing factor grows, but its reactivity diminishes with age.

When various doses of TRF are administered, states which may originate under natural conditions in stress situations and during the activation of the hypothalamus are reproduced. In old age, the thyroliberin-thyrotropin link is activated much more when the hypothalamic structures are slightly stimulated. This link can become a limiting one in the whole system of thyroid regulation in situations in which the system must be activated substantially. Moreover, the link seems to break even when there is a large amount of activating thyroliberin.

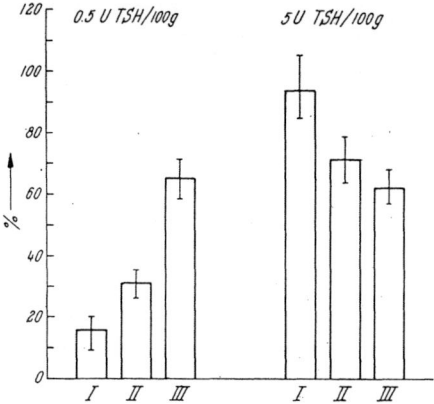

Fig. 53. Alterations of thyroxine in the blood (with respect to the basal level) 3 hours after the administration of thyrotropin in doses of 0.5 and 5.0 units/100 g. *I* rats 1.5–2 months old; *II* rats 8–10 months old; *III* rats 28–32 months old

The reaction of the thyroid gland to the effect of thyrotropin is another important link in thyroid regulation. Thyrotropin is known to influence the synthesis of the hormones of the thyroid gland through the adenylate cyclase system. The effect of thyrotropin on the thyroid gland is expressed at first in proteolysis, colloidal dissolution and the secretion of the thyroid hormones into the blood.

In our laboratory, Valueva studied the reaction of the thyroid gland of animals of different age to thyrotropin. For this purpose, thyrotropin in doses of 0.5, 1, 3 and 5 U/100 g of body weight was administered intraperitoneally to three groups of rats 1.5–2, 8–10 and 28–32 months old. The content of T_4 in the blood was determined after 1, 2 and 3 hours (Fig. 53). It was found that the sensitivity and reactivity of the thyroid tissue to the action of thyrotropin change as the organism ages. In old animals, the thyroid parenchyma becomes more sensitive to thyrotropin: when a minimum dose (0.5 U/100 g of body weight) is administered, the content of T_4 in the blood increases to the greatest extent in rats 28–32 months old. The thyroid gland does not react to this dose of the hormone in animals 8–10 months old. The reaction of the thyroid gland is marked most clearly in rats 1.5–2 and 8–10 months old when 1.0 and 3.5 U/100 g of thyrotropin are administered. In old rats, however, the rise of the T_4 level in the blood remains the same when these doses of thyrotropin are administered as when 0.5 U/100 g of the hormone is injected. Moreover, the response of the thyroid parenchyma to the administration of any dose of thyrotropin is retarded in old rats, i. e. the content of T_4 in their blood increases 3 hours after the administration of the thyrotropic hormone, while it increases in 1 hour in rats 1.5–2 and 8–10 months old. Hence, the sensitivity of the thyroid gland to thyrotropin increases, but the range of its reactions to the hormone decreases in old age. This is observed not only when the specific function of the gland is being studied, but also when the general metabolic shifts are being analyzed. For instance, the administration of 0.5 U/100 g of thyrotropin increased substantially oxygen consumption by the thyroid gland of old rats (by 34 per cent), while no changes were observed in mature rats. Inverse relationships originate when 1.0 U/100 g of the hormone is administered: oxygen consumption increases by 64 per cent in adult rats and only by 31 per cent in old rats (Verzhikovskaya, 1971). This has also been observed when the mass of the thyroid gland and the height of the thyroid epithelium change were studied. When 0.5 U/100 g of the hormone was administered for 3 days, the mass of the gland increased by 11 per cent, while the height of the thyroid epithelium, by 43 per cent in adult rats. However, they increased by 29.4 and 67.5 per cent, respectively, in old rats. These shifts were more pronounced in adult rats when the hormone was administered in a dose of 1.0 U/100 g. The range of the hypothalamohypophysial regulation of the thyroid gland decreases in old age in natural situations when stress occurs. It is still unknown at what stage of the metabolism in thyrocytes their reaction to thyrotropin changes.

According to some researchers (Scharrer, Scharrer, 1963), the neurosecretory elements of the hypothalamus are like translators. Knowing two "languages," i. e. the neural and the humoral ones, they translate everything into the "humoral" language, since the endocrine glands "do not understand" neural information. This widely held opinion turned out to be misleading. It has been proved for many glands that information is transmitted transhypophysially from the hypothalamus to the gland with the participation of sympathetic neural effects (Aleshin, 1971). Suffice it to recall that the hyperfunction of the thyroid gland can occur in many cases without an increase in the content of thyrotropin in the blood. In some patients, hypophysial extirpation did not lead to the disappearance to hyperthyroidism and some other disorders.

The hypothalamic influences on the thyroid gland involving the sympathetic nerve pathways become less effective with age. The impairment of sympathetic neural control with age has been demonstrated by the neural regulation of metabolism and the function of various tissues, i. e. those of the heart, the skeletal muscles, several vascular regions, the nictitating membrane, etc. The postganglionic nerve fibres of the thyroid gland originate in *Ganglion cervicale superius*. It has been shown in our laboratory that excitability, lability, and synthesis of acetylcholine in this ganglion decrease substantially with age (Duplenko, 1965; Frolkis, 1970). In old animals, smaller doses of the ganglion blocking agents disturb conduction in *Ganglion cervicale superius*. Moreover, the neural apparatus in the thyroid gland begins to be destroyed with age. Hence, parahypophysial hypothalamus neural control over the thyroid gland decreases with age.

Thus, the two ways (hypophysial and sympathetic) of regulating the function of the thyroid gland are redistributed with age. The impairment of neural control can change the reaction of the thyroid gland to thyrotropin, which plays a greater role in old age. Many adaptive reactions of the thyroid gland are limited when sympathetic neural control is impaired.

Specifics of the Influence of Thyroid Hormones on Tissue in Old Age

The influence of the thyroid hormones on the metabolism and function of the cells depends on the binding of iodothyronines by tissues and on hormone degradation. In old animals, the content of T_4 in the heart and the skeletal muscle sharply diminishes, but it hardly changes in the liver and the kidneys (Valueva, 1978). In the animal organism, deiodination is the main way in which the thyroid hormones undergo intracellular metabolism. At present, many investigations clearly show that the deiodination of the thyroid hormones is connected directly with the hormonal effect and is not a passive degradation of the hormones. It is believed that highly active iodide cations are formed when T_4 is deiodized, and that the hormonal effect is realized on the molecular and subcellular levels with the participation of these cations. According to Valueva (1978) as well as Macill and associates (1979), deiodination occurs only in one subcellular fraction: the microsomes (the smooth endoplasmic reticulum, which contains the deiodinase). Our data on the deiodinizing activity of the rat tissue in old age are given in Table 7. The deiodinase was isolated from the tissues and purified partially (by 90 times). Afterwards, its enzymic activity was studied by using T_4 and T_3 as substrates. The specific enzymic activity of deiodinase isolated from the liver, kidneys, heart and skeletal muscles of old animals was substantially higher than that of deiodinase isolated from those of adult animals. This activation of the processes of deiodination in the tissues and an increase in deiodinase activity are of adaptive significance. They are vitauct processes, because they compensate somewhat for the drop in the basal level of the blood hormone. An important fact is that the intracellular distribution of the hormone changes with age. According to Valueva (1978), more T_4 is incorporated into the microsomes and less of it is incorporated into the cytosol of the cells of the liver,

Table 7. *Thyroxine deiodizing activity of some tissues of rats of different ages* (nm of thyroxine which has disintegrated in 3 hours, 300 mg of tissue)

Age	Liver	Kidneys	Heart	Sceletal muscle	Adeno- hypophysis
1.5–2 months (I)	50.6 ± 1.3	57.6 ± 1.0	7.2 ± 0.7	16.0 ± 2.0	42.0 ± 3.0
8–12 months (II)	52.0 ± 1.1	58.4 ± 1.2	8.0 ± 0.9	14.0 ± 1.2	33.0 ± 4.0
$P_{II–I}$	> 0.5	> 0.5	> 0.5	> 0.5	< 0.05
28–32 months (III)	58.0 ± 1.0	69.1 ± 1.0	15.0 ± 1.0	21.0 ± 1.0	54.0 ± 5.0
$P_{III–II}$	< 0.001	< 0.001	< 0.001	< 0.001	< 0.001

kidneys, heart and muscles in old animals. The cells have specific thyroxine-binding cytosol proteins, which inhibit hormone deiodination. Using affine chromatography, the T_4-binding proteins with limited thyroxine-binding capacity and high specificity were isolated from the tissue cytosol of rats of different ages. The maximal binding ability of the proteins was measured by the graphs used by Scatchard (1949). With age, the content of thyroxine-binding proteins in the cytosol of the tissues being tested decreases and the maximal thyroxine-binding ability of the isolated proteins diminishes in comparison with adult animals. It is possible that the number of the T_4-binding sites on the protein cytosol receptors decreases or the sites lose their ability to bind the

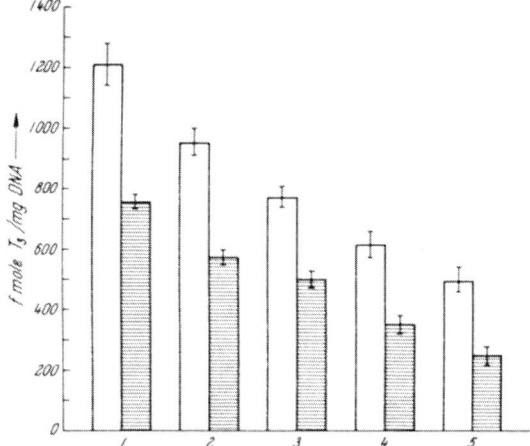

Fig. 54. Maximum T_3-binding ability of the nuclear receptors of the tissues of rats of different age. 1 hypophysis; 2 liver; 3 kidneys; 4 heart; 5 skeletal muscle. Light columns stand for adult rats, and black columns, for old rats

hormone. Thus, besides a diminution of the amount of T_4 in the cell, the enzymatic activity of deiodinase increases and the thyroxine-binding ability of the cytosol proteins of the tissues decreases in old animals. This shifts hormonal equilibrium in the cell towards the predominance of the free form of T_4, which can be subjected to deiodination in the microsomal fraction that contains deiodinase. Such changes should be regarded as an important compensatory mechanism in the thyroid control system.

A study of the indices of the T_3 kinetics in the entire organism and the T_3 content in separate tissues has shown that the concentration of the hormones in the tissues of old animals is maintained almost on the same level as in adult animals, although the synthesis of this hormone decreases in old ones. This is also evident from the half-life of T_3 in the blood of old rats, the space in which T_3 is distributed, and the clearance of the hormone with urine and feces. According to Frolkis et al. (1978), the content of T_3 in the organism remains unchanged as the hormone is synthesized less with age only because its extra-thyroidal formation from T_4 is less intense than in adult rats. The mechanism of the effect of T_3 on the protein synthesis processes is determined largely by the binding of the hormone with nuclear receptors. The maximal thyroxine-binding ability of the nuclear receptors isolated from the liver, kidneys, heart, skeletal muscle and hypophysis was substantially lower in old animals than in adult ones. An investigation of the binding of T_3 by the nuclear receptors from animal tissues revealed no age distinctions (Fig. 54). Thus, T_3 is bound less by the nuclear receptors of the tissues in old animals apparently because the number of receptors decreases.

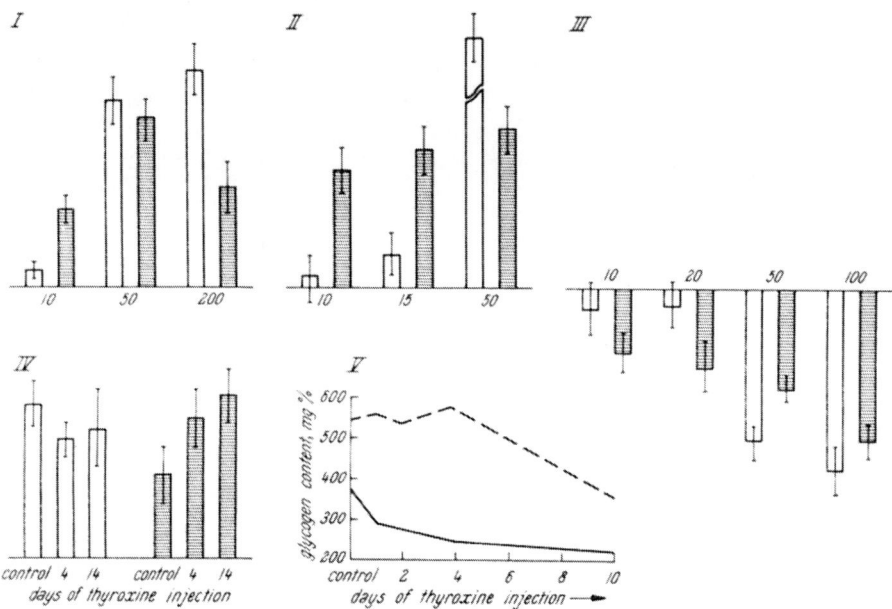

Fig. 55. Influence of thyroxine on various aspects of metabolism in mature and old rats. I–III changes after a single administration of various doses (μg) of the thyroxine on gas metabolism (I), urea nitrogen (II), and the cholesterol of blood serum (III). IV, V influence of the prolonged administration of the hormone on the intensity of tissue respiration (IV) and the glycogen level (V) in the heart. Light columns and the dashed line stand for mature rats, and the shaded columns and the continuous line, for old rats

According to Valueva (1978), that is due to a change in the capacity of the non-histone proteins. A decrease in the ability of nuclear receptors to bind T_3 can limit the regulatory effect of the hormone on the processes of protein biosynthesis in the tissue. When a set of changes occur in the metabolism of the thyroid hormones, the reaction of the tissues to their action change in old age. Indeed, we have shown in our work (Verzhikovskaya, 1971; Frolkis et al., 1973) that the sensitivity of the tissues to the action of the thyroid hormones grows with age, but the possible maximal effect decreases (Fig. 55). In other words, a smaller signal at the inlet to the system causes a change at its outlet. However, the possible amplitude of the outgoing signal decreases. For instance, gas exchange in old rats increases by 18.2 per cent after a single administration of T_4 (10 μg/100 g of weight), but it does not change in adult rats. The relationship changes when 50 μg of the hormone is administered: gas exchange grows by 22.1 per cent in old rats and by 38.8 per cent in adult animals. The serum content of cholesterol in old rats decreases after the administration of thyroxine in $5-20\,\mu g/100$ g, and in adult animals, after its administration in $30-40\,\mu g/100$ g.

Energy processes (tissue respiration, oxidative phosphorylation) are extremely important as regards the action of the thyroid hormones. These hormones influence apparently the order of the inner structure of mitochondria. The intensification of tissue respiration may be caused by the greater permeability of mitochondria and the entry of a large amount of oxidative substrates into them. Hyperthyroidism was reproduced by the daily administration of 0.2 mg of thyroidin per 100 g of body weight. The activation of tissue respiration and the dissociation of oxidative phosphorylation were observed at an earlier period in old animals.

In hyperthyroidism, another way of energy conversion, i. e. glycolysis, originates when oxidative phosphorylation is disturbed. According to our data, glycolysis intensifies sooner in the heart and the liver of old animals. These metabolic shifts correlate with the functional changes which occur due to the action of the thyroid hormones. We and Shevchuk have obtained data on the effect of the thyroid hormones on the hemodynamics and contractility of the myocardium. In this respect, the same regularity has been established, i. e. during hyperthyroidism shifts occur at an earlier period in old rats, while their maximal amplitude is greater in adult animals. Cardiac insufficiency occurs when the hormone is administered to old rats for a long time.

Hence, age differences are determined by the different hormone content: the smaller the amount of the hormone, the higher is the sensitivity to its action. Thyroidectomy was performed in mature and old animals, i. e. age differences of the hormone content were levelled out in them. The reactions of the tissues to the action of the thyroid hormones were determined against that background. It was found that the higher sensitivity of the tissues of old animals to the thyroid hormones is preserved after thyroidectomy. Thus, thyroidin feeding for 3 days causes an increase by 12.5 per cent in the gas exchange of adult thyroidectomied animals and by 35.5 per cent in old ones. The cholesterol level dropped by 17.5 and 37.6 per cent, respectively, while the intensity of the tissue respiration of the myocardium rose by 50.9 and 74.7 per cent, and that of the liver, by 14.1 and 49.1 per cent, respectively. Thus, an increase in tissue sensitivity to the thyroid hormones in old age cannot be connected with a decrease in their content in the tissues. It is connected with deiodination, during which the physiological effect of the hormones is produced. A decrease in both tissue reactivity and the reaction amplitude is apparently due to the diminution of the number of thyroreceptors. The period of hormone action is also of definite importance.

Feed-back Control of the Thyroid System

Thus, we have traced the changes in the system of the hypothalamus-hypophysis-thyroid gland tissues. The adaptive functioning of this system occurs via feed-backs, being realized mainly at the thyroid hormone-hypothalamic stage.

Table 8. *Effect of thyroxine (T_4) on the level of thyrotropin in the blood and adenohypophysis of adult and old rats*

Dose of T_4, g, per 100 g of the mass	8–10 months		28–32 months	
	blood, ng/ml	adenohypo- physis, I. U./mg	blood, ng/ml	adenohypo- physis, I. U./mg
Control (I)	6.1 ± 0.8	57.0 ± 2.7	3.3 ± 0.5	22.0 ± 1.7
2.0 (II)	5.0 ± 0.4	51.0 ± 3.7	1.5 ± 0.2	18.0 ± 0.5
P_{II-I}	> 0.05	> 0.05	< 0.001	< 0.05
4.0 (III)	3.2 ± 0.7	45.0 ± 1.5	1.3 ± 0.1	17.0 ± 0.7
P_{III-I}	< 0.001	< 0.001	> 0.5	> 1.2

We have reported age changes at the stage of the realization of feed-backs in the hypothalamus-hypophysis-thyroid gland system, which occur due to the effect of T_4 and T_3 on the synthesis and secretion of TSH (Frolkis *et al.*, 1978). In a series of experiments, T_4 solution was administered intraperitoneally in doses of 2 and 4 μg/100 g to rats 8–10 and 28–32 months old for seven days. The content of thyrotropin in the blood and adenohypophysis was determined 24 hours after the last injection. Table 8 shows that the administration of T_4 in a dose of 2 μg reduces substantially the synthesis and secretion of thyrotropin in old rats. These changes are statistically insignificant in adult animals. However, thyrotropin synthesis was not suppressed further when the dose of T_4 was increased to 4 μg in animals 28–32 months old. The content of thyrotropin in the blood and adenohypophysis of adult animals decreases substantially when that dose of the hormone was administered.

Intracellular deiodination processes are decisive in the mechanism of the hormonal effect of iodothyronines on various tissues, including the adenohypophysial tissue (Silva *et al.*, 1978). Therefore, the thyroxine-deiodizing ability of the hypophysis during different age periods should be measured so as to analyze the causes of the changes in feed-back.

The deiodinizing ability of the adenohypophysial tissue is greatly enhanced as the animals age. Experiments involving the use of a blocking agent of peripheral deiodination, i. e. 6-methylthiouracil, have revealed the significance of the deiodination processes in the age changes of the reaction of the hypophysial tissue to T_4. It has been established that the single administration of 6-methylthiouracil (10 mg/100 g) reduces substantially in 2 hours the amount of the T_4 being deiodized in the hypophysis of animals of all age groups and sharply enhances the synthesis and secretion of thyrotropin. This is evident from the shifts in the content of the hormone in the hypophysis and blood. Data on the effect of 6-methylthiouracil in old animals are interesting especially. In intact rats 28–32 months old, the content of thyrotropin in the blood and adenohypophysis is low, while T_4 is intensely deiodized in the latter. When 6-methylthiouracil is administered to old animals, the content of thyrotropin in their organism becomes larger, i. e. it reaches the level in adult rats after 6-methylthiouracil is administered to them (Frolkis *et al.*, 1978). Thus, the suppression of deiodination by administering 6-methylthiouracil had somewhat levelled out the age differences in the initial level of TSH in the hypophysis and the blood. In this case, the level of the thyroid hormones in the 6-methylthio-uracil-treated animals had remained the same as in intact animals.

Thus, the hypothalamohypophysial area becomes more sensitive to the hormone, but its reactivity, i. e. its ability to react to substantial changes in the content of the thyroid hormones in the blood, diminishes with age. The mechanism which enhances sensitivity to thyroid hormones is connected with the activation of the deiodination processes. What is important is that this mechanism determines "hypothalamic misinformation" on the state of the hormones in the blood. The levels of T_3 and T_4 drop in the blood of old animals. However, this does not activate thyrotropin synthesis because the deiodination processes intensify in the hypothalamohypophysial region. In other words, higher sensitivity may be the cause of misinformation of centres on the occurrences at the periphery.

Specifics of the Reactions of the Thyroid Control System

Substantial changes occur in all the links of the thyroid control system with age. On the whole, it becomes less active. Nagorny and Golubitskaya (1947) as well as Nikitin (1972) have observed that the shifts in the organism of old animals are less pronounced than in adult ones after thyroidectomy. This has been confirmed by our data, too. For instance, two weeks after thyroidectomy, gas exchange decreases by 41.7 per cent in adult rats and by 16.6 per cent in old ones, while the intensity of the tissue respiration of the myocardium diminished by 42.6 per cent in the former and by 6.5 per cent in the latter. An important fact is that the initial age differences in the intensity of gas exchange, tissue respiration, oxidative phosphorylation and the cholesterol content are levelled out after thyroidectomy. According to Pashkova (1975), the lipolytic activity of various tissues decreases much more in young animals than in old ones after thyroidectomy. Two important conclusions can be drawn from the results of her experiments. Firstly, thyroid control over tissue metabolism decreases with age. Hence, thyroidectomy causes less pronounced metabolic shifts in old rats. Secondly, many metabolic changes which occur with age are apparently caused by the impairment of thyroid control. This is evident from the fact that several age differences of metabolism and the functions are eliminated after thyroid-ectomy.

A study of the age dynamics of thyroid regulation has produced more evidence which corroborates the adaptive regulatory theory of aging. Manifestations of aging and vitauct occur in thyroid regulation during individual development. Substantial structural and functional changes in the thyroid gland, a decrease in the content of total T_4 and T_3 as well as in tissue reactivity, a diminution of the number of receptors, and so forth, are important manifestations of aging. At the same time, manifestations of vitauct and adaptive regulatory shifts occur in other links of the system. They include the greater sensitivity of the hypophysis to the releasing factor, the thyroid gland to thyro-tropin, the tissues to the thyroid hormones, and the hypothalamus to the thyroid hormones, the maintenance of the content of free T_4 in the blood, and the activation of the processes of deiodination, which is the basis of the greater sensitivity of the cells to the hormone. These shifts help to maintain a definite level of the whole system in spite of the pronounced age changes in the thyroid gland.

A comparison of the age changes in the thyroid function of the hypothalamohypophysial area and in the function of the thyroid gland shows that the gland becomes less active sooner and that the diminution of its activity is one of the primary mechanisms of the changes in the whole system. The content of thyrotropin in the blood of rats increases until they reach the age of 18–20 months. This adaptive reaction occurs due to the functional tension of the hypothalamohypophysial area because the concentration of thyrotropin in the hypophysis diminishes as its content in blood grows in the animals of that age. The content of thyrotropin decreases in the blood of rats 28–32 months old. This changes substantially the state of the whole thyroid control system.

Earlier, we have given data on the age changes in individual links of thyroid regulation. It was necessary to assess the state of the whole system under the conditions of functional tension. Many researchers have shown that the thyroid gland participates in many stress reactions. In our experiments, which were carried out together with Verzhikovskaya, we studied the shifts as the state of stress was imitated by the generally accepted methods (cold stress, hypo-dynamia, immobilization, administration of adrenaline). The iodine-accumulating function of the thyroid gland, the thyroxine-binding ability of the blood, the functional activity of the gland, the deiodizing ability of the tissues and the morphological changes in the thyroid gland were studied in adult and old animals.

The function of the thyroid gland is activated when the gland is exposed to the cold. Sympathetic neural effects play a big role in the mechanism of this activation. The thyroid hormones which entered the blood dissociate oxidation and phosphorylation and activate thermogenesis. In our experiments, we kept the animals in the cold chamber, where the temperature ranged from $+2\,°C$ to $+4\,°C$, for 24 hours or for 4 days (for 4 hours daily). The exposure to the cold activates the iodine-accumulating function of the gland. However, this shift is less pronounced in old animals. Substantial age changes occur in the transport forms of the thyroid hormones. In rats 8–10 months old, the ability of the serum proteins to bind the thyroid hormones increases, the total content of T_4 and fraction of free hormone in the blood grow, and the index of free T_4 rises. In old rats, the thyroxine-binding ability of the serum proteins also increases, but the content of total and free thyroxine decreases. Age differences of the functional changes in the thyroid gland are maintained even when the animals are exposed to the cold for 4 days. The thyroxine-binding ability of the serum proteins increases in adult as well as old rats. However, the content of total T_4 grows in rats 8–10 months old, while it does not change in old rats. In old animals, the concentration of free T_4 tends to diminish.

Hence, the thyroid control system of old animals reacts less actively to cold stress. In this stress, the function of the thyroid gland is activated largely under the effect of sympathoadrenal stimulation. Apparently, this mechanism becomes less active in old age. According to Verzhikovskaya, the release of catecholamines from the adrenal glands is less pronounced in old animals during stress. The catecholamines which entered the blood activate the function of the thyroid gland through the hypothalamic control mechanisms.

The functional activity of the gland decreases in stress caused by the immobilization (for 2 and 17 hours) or by hypodynamia in a special cage (for 4 days). The iodine-accumulating function of the thyroid gland decreases and the binding coefficient of T_3 diminishes somewhat during fixation. These shifts are less pronounced in old animals.

Thus, the thyroid control system participates less in the organism's most important adaptive reactions with age. This is expressed in the reactions involving both the activation and the suppression of the thyroid function.

A long time ago, Horsley (1884) indicated the parallelism between the aging symptoms and hypothyroidism. Gley (1922) and Shershevsky (1940) attached great importance to the age changes in the thyroid gland, regarding them as a significant prerequisite of the organism's aging. Obviously, the extremely complicated biological process of the organism's aging cannot be regarded as merely a change in the function of one of the glands. However, the growing hypofunction of the thyroid gland plays a substantial role in the mechanism of many age changes (in the diminution of the intensity of tissue respiration, a change in the correlation between oxidation and phosphorylation, the attenuation of the synthesis of several proteins, the growth of the cholesterol content, a change in the mobility of neural processes, and so forth). The change in the given metabolic parameters is expressed differently in various tissues. However, the peripheral mechanisms of hormone action in various tissues, e. g. transport through the membrane, the tissue contents, deiodination, the number of nuclear receptors, also change differently in old age.

The role that the age changes in the function of the thyroid gland play in aging should not be assessed unequivocally. It seems that substitution therapy (the administration of thyroid hormones) should retard aging, or at least it should prolong life. However, according to available data, thyroid hormones used in various doses do not change life span, or they may even shorten it (Everitt, 1970). A decrease in basal metabolism due to the hypofunction of the thyroid control system can apparently prevent exhaustive tensions as well as gross disturbances of metabolism and can prolong life. This is corroborated by data on the change in the thyroid function during experimental life prolongation, especially in the case of a growth-restraining diet (Nikitin, 1979). Such a diet is known to be one of the most effective ways of prolonging life. It prolongs life by 50–80 per cent. It was discovered that the thyrotropic function of the hypophysis is greatly inhibited in the 3 month-old test animals. However, this function is gradually restored as the animals reaches old age.

The researches carried out by Denckla (1974) as well as Mollerach and associates (1978) are very interesting. They have shown that a factor (hormone), which suppresses the thyroid function, begins to be synthesized in the hypophysis with age. Its action is the opposite of that of thyrotropin, and it probably blocks the thyrotropin-sensitive receptors in the thyrocytes. It reduces the intensity of basal and tissue metabolism by suppressing the thyroid function. According to Denckla, this factor can be regarded as the "hormone of aging." However, it has not been separated, while its action is described on the basis of the effects on the brain homogenate. Of course, if the gene regulation hypothesis is taken into account, there may be genes which did not act earlier, and new proteins, including those with regulatory effects, may appear in old age.

Thus, irregular changes originate in the thyroid control system with age, i. e. adaptive regulatory shifts are observed together with the phenomena of extinction. For instance, the structural and functional changes in the thyroid gland, which reduce its activity, are coupled with the greater sensitivity of the thyroid parenchyma to thyrotropin, while the low level of the thyroid hormones in the tissues is due to the intensification of deiodination, a change in the tissue reaction to the effect of iodothyronines, and so forth.

8. Neural Regulation of Tissue Trophism in Aging

George Bernard Shaw once wrote that a researchers who takes a phenomenon to pieces in quest of truth risks learning about nothing. Today, a researcher should take account to the general biological essence of a natural phenomenon when he thoroughly studies it. This applies also to the concept of the neural regulation of trophicity.

Even as early as 1784, Procháska asked the sacramental question: "Are nerves needed to feed the tissues?" As physiology rapidly developed, many discoveries were made with respect to neural influences on various aspects of tissue activity. The regulatory influences of the nervous system are wide-ranging. As early as in the 1920's, Pavlov emphasized that every organ was under triple neural control, i. e. it was controlled by functional nerves, which start or stop an organ's activity, by vascular nerves, which regulate vascular tone, and by trophic nerves, which directly influence the metabolic processes in the tissues. The existence of special trophic influences on the tissue is now recognized (Orbeli, 1935), and it may be that all these influences represent a natural control mechanism.

Another aspect of Pavlov's investigations of tissue trophicity should be mentioned. It is the ideas which he evolved in his works *Nitrogen Balance in the Salivary and Submaxillary Glands during Work* (1890) and *Laboratory Observations of the Pathological Reflexes of the Abdominal Cavity* (1898). These ideas are about the neural influences on the restoration of the working organ's structure and the effects which maintain its integrity. According to Pavlov, such complicated aspects of the trophic process as hypertrophy, atrophy and aging can be understood when the essence of these influences is revealed.

In 1938, Koshtoyants clearly defined the ontogenetic aspects of the problem of trophic control in his work *Trophic Influence of the Nervous System in Animal Ontogenesis.* According to him, they are (1) the investigation of the changes in the trophic influences of the nervous system in ontogenesis, and (2) the ascertainment of the trophic influences of the nervous system on the ontogenetic process proper. Using the denervation method, he showed the role of the trophic neural influences in the formation of the functional properties of the muscles at different stages of ontogenesis. These influences play a certain role in lability and excitability, and they determine the complexity of the reactions of the neuromuscular apparatus. In ontogenesis, just as in phylogenesis, there is a tendency towards an increase of the neural control over biochemical processes (Koshtoyants, 1951).

The study of trophism is very useful, because it obliges us to combine the available data on the relationship between metabolism, structure and functions of the cell, although they are usually treated separately. Neural control of tissue trophicity enables the tissues to become adapted to the future and current activity and ensures the most important adaptive regulatory processes. Orbeli (1935) reasonably defined the influence of the sympathetic neural system on tissues as an adaptive trophic influence. The neural control of trophicity is an extremely important manifestation of vitauct, which maintains a high level of tissue viability.

There are apparently two groups of facts whose comparison should naturally give rise to the following conclusion: age changes in the regulation of the trophism of cells and tissues play an essential role in the mechanism of their aging. One group of facts relates to clinical data on numerous trophic disturbances which occur with age (loss of hair and teeth, senile gangrenes, trophic ulcers, etc.). The other group relates to experimental data on the origin of the structural, metabolic and functional changes which occur in the disturbance of trophic innervation and which largely resemble shifts that develop as the organism ages. However, a comparison of these data does not help to establish the cause-and-effect relationships between them. Therefore, it is important to directly study the age changes in trophic regulation and to assess the role of these shifts in the primary and secondary mechanisms of the organism's aging.

Only a few works describe the trophic changes during aging. According to the adaptive regulatory theory of aging, age changes in the neural regulation of tissue trophicity determine the most important mechanisms of vitauct and aging.

We are convinced that the high level of the neural regulation of tissue trophicity helps to maintain the organism's adaptive possibilities for a long time and to greatly prolong life. When the age changes develop in the structures which control tissue trophism, they inevitably become one of the principal mechanisms of the organism's aging. The impairment of the neural influences on the tissues in old age has been dealt with at great length in the preceding chapters.

It should be emphasized that trophism is neurally controlled in various ways. However, as is usually the case, neural and hormonal influences should not be opposed to one another in this case. The hormonal regulation of trophism, which undergoes a great change with age, is determined largely by the neural influences that are realized through hypothalamus, which changes substantially with age.

Great importance is now being attached to the axoplasmic flow of substances in the regulation of tissue trophicity. Investigations in this field have been reviewed by Mezentsev and Messinova (1971) as well as Glebov and Kryzhanovsky (1978).

Back in 1944, Weiss found the presence of the axoplasmic flow from the perikaryon of the nerve cell along the axon. It is believed that the axoplasmic flow is realized along the neurotubules, which contain both the contractile protein, i.e. neurotubulin, and neurofilaments, which are twisted globular structures. The axoplasmic flow is an energy-dependent process, and the ATP-

ATPase-contractile protein system plays a big role in it. Proteins, RNA, amino acids, vesicles with transmitters, mitochondria, and so forth, move with the axoplasmic flow along the axon. In other words, this is a universal and "lively" transport system. The axoplasmic flow has two main components: the fast component (10–500 mm/day) and the slow component (0.5–5 mm/day) (Ochs, 1973; Jefrey, Austin, 1973). Synaptic vesicles, mitochondria, nucleotides, amino acids, structural proteins, etc., move with the fast axoplasmic flow, while neurofibrils, neurotubules, high molecular weight proteins (the molecular weight being of the order of 480,000), and RNA move with the slow one. The axoplasmic flow goes in two directions and, consequently, carries plastic information from the centre to the periphery and vice versa. An important fact is that the axoplasmic flow of substances is observed in the brain, where it maintains trophic processes. The application of colchicine on a nerve is known to stop the axoplasmic flow. Serious trophic disturbances occur in the tissues when a nerve is treated with colchicine for a long time. They occur apparently because the extremely important trophic support is switched off.

There are only a few works on the investigation of the axoplasmic flow during aging. This extremely important problem is only beginning to be worked out. Changes in the axoplasmic flow during aging are an important mechanism of the disturbance of tissue trophicity. These changes are very significant, as they can cause destructive atrophic changes (Gutmann, Hanzlikova, 1973; McMartin, O'Connor, 1979, etc.). Gutmann and Hanzlikova (1973) ligated the sciatic nerve of mature and old rats and found a smaller acetylcholinesterase accumulation above the ligature in old rats as compared with mature animals. Hence, it was concluded that the axoplasmic flow slows down in old age. McMartin and O'Connor (1979) have observed that the transport of proteins along the axons slows down substantially in old age. They used a set of methods to characterize the accumulation of acetylcholinesterase above the ligature. The experiments involving ligation only indirectly indicated the rate and intensity of the axoplasmic flow. Account should also be taken of the data given by Ranish and Dettbarn (1976), who have shown that only 10 per cent of acetylcholinesterase moves with the fast component of the axoplasmic flow. Ochs (1973) did not find any noticeable changes in the rate at which labelled protein moved along the sciatic nerve in old cats and dogs. In some old dogs, this rate even increased by 16 per cent.

Clear-cut data on the attenuation of the axoplasmic flow in old age have been obtained by us together with Tanin, Grabina, Novozhilov and Martsinko. Various approaches and objects were used to assess the state of this flow. The experiments involved nerve ligation, the investigation of the accumulation of substances above the ligature after a certain length of time, and the determination of the flow rate along the intact axons of various nerves.

In the first series of experiments, the change of the RNA content in various sections of the sciatic nerve was determined prior to and 2, 4, 8 and 12 days after its ligation. It was found that the content increases above the ligation site and that this increase is smaller in old rats than in mature ones. For instance, the RNA content in rats 8–10 months old increased by 32 per cent in 48 hours and by 51 per cent in 96 hours after the nerve was ligated; it increased by 12 and

39 per cent, respectively, in old rats. These data only indirectly indicate the deceleration of the axoplasmic flow in old animals. A clear-cut conclusion can be drawn only when the movement of substances along the intact nerve is studied.

A special series of experiments were carried out to study the distribution of proteins and labelled substances in the ventral roots of the spinal cord in the proximal-distal direction. Five microcuries of leucine marked with carbon 14 were injected into the anterior horn area through a special chemotrode.

The method proposed by Tikhonov and his associates (1973) was used to determine the axoplasmic flow rate, while the overall axoplasmic flow of substances was determined by Chihara's method (1979). A clearly defined peak of the activity of the labelled substances in the ventral roots was recorded at a distance of 18 mm in mature rats one hour after the administration of the label. It corresponded to the axoplasmic flow rate of 390 ±16 mm per day. The posterior roots were used as control; no such radioactivity peak was observed in them. In old animals, the label moved more slowly along the roots, i. e. it moved at a rate of 224 ± 32 mm per day (p < 0.01). The flow rate of the labelled proteins was determined separately. It was 320 ± 22 mm per day in mature rats and only 200 ± 40 mm per day in old ones (p < 0.01). Thus, the velocity of the axoplasmic flow of both the label and the newly synthesized substances diminishes with age.

We drew the conclusion that the axoplasmic flow slows down in old age when we studied the motion of the label along the optic nerve. In experiments involving rats 8–10 and 26–28 months old, ten microcuries of leucine marked with carbone 14 were injected into the eye. Then, the appearance of labelled protein was determined at various lengths of time. Having in mind that the label transferred by blood could also be incorporated, the area of the sciatic nerve where the concentration of the label was dozens of times lower than that of the optic nerve were used for control. The specific activity of the protein was determined in four areas of the optic nerve, beginning with the ocular end. As is seen in Fig. 56, the axoplasmic flow slows down in old age. This is evident from the fact that the rise of specific activity of protein is observed in respective nerve sections of old rats at later terms than in mature animals. In this case, the age changes in the axoplasmic flow may be associated with two factors: the attenuation of protein synthesis in the perikaryon of the nerve cells and the deceleration of the axoplasmic flow. This deceleration is evident from the fact that the specific activity grows just as intensively in the first section of the optic nerve of mature and old rats, while it grows several times more intensively in the second area of the optic nerve of mature rats than that of old rats. Moreover, the change in the axoplasmic flow is evident from the fact that the age differences have been established with respect to not only protein, but also amino acid, whose transfer along the optic nerve is retarded, too.

All these investigations show that the axoplasmic flow slows down in old age. The axonal transport of substances in the brain also changes with age. Geinisman and co-workers (1977) injected a tracer into the medial area of the septum of rats 3 and 25 months old, and then the radioactivity of the extract in the hippocampal sections was determined. The acid-soluble extract was transported axoplasmically at virtually the same rate in both age groups, while unsoluble glycoproteins moved at a much slower rate in old animals. The authors believe that the reduction of the number of synapses in the hippocampus may possibly play a certain role in the mechanism of the change in the axoplasmic flow in old age. The deceleration of the flow from the neuroglia to the nerve cells is also of definite significance. The deceleration of the axoplasmic flow of substances in the brain tissues has been observed in old age (Barondes, 1968).

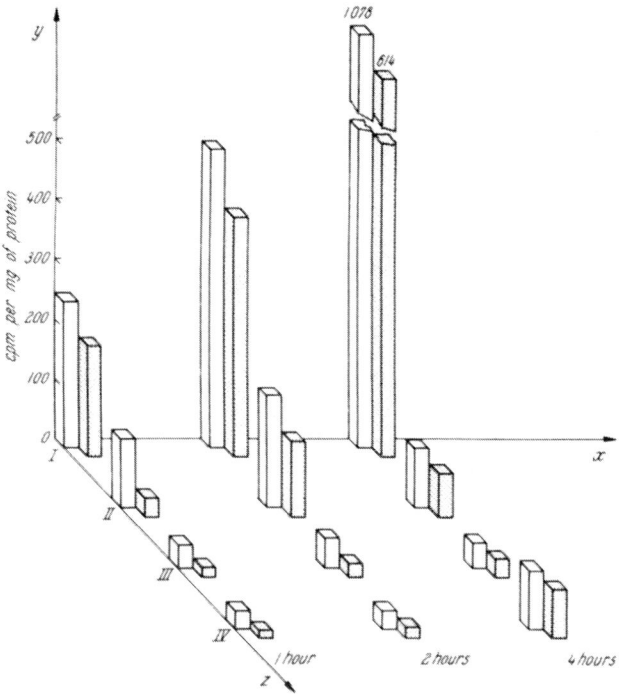

Fig. 56. The specific activity of labelled proteins in various areas of the optic nerve of mature rats (light columns) and old rats (dark columns) 1, 2 and 4 hours after the administration of glycine, 1–^{14}C (10 microcuries), into the eye. The y axis stands for the specific activity of protein, x stands for time (hours), and z stands for the areas of the optic nerve which are 3 mm long and which are in the proximodistal direction

The mechanisms of age changes in the axoplasmic flow remain unknown. It is known that several structural changes occur in the axon and the number of various inclusions increases with age. McMartin and O'Connor (1979) believe that the deceleration of the axoplasmic flow in old age is connected with the more frequent occurrence of permanent and temporary stoppages of the axoplasmic flow in the axons of old animals. Since not all the canals can be blocked, a part of the particles can move at a normal rate or, what is interesting, even faster than usual (Ochs, 1973). This acceleration of the axoplasmic flow along individual canals is of great adaptive significance, as it helps to maintain the optimum level of the flow. The observations made by Gutmann and

Hanzlikova (1973) are interesting in this respect. They have shown that the number of neurotubules and neurofibrils increases in the axon of old animals. This phenomenon is an important manifestation of vitauct, which preserves the viability of the neuron and its axon as well as trophic regulation.

There may be another mechanism of a change in the axoplasmic flow in old age. It is connected with the changes in the energy provision of the axoplasmic flow. Such an assumption is underpinned by the experiments carried out by

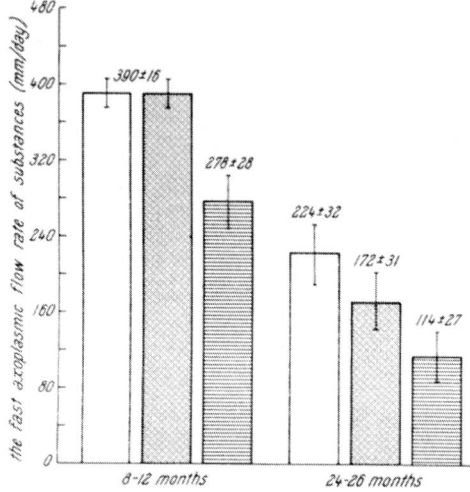

Fig. 57. The effect of hypoxia on the fast axoplasmic flow of substances in the male rats of different age. Light columns stand for control. Dotted colums are Patm = 349 Hg mm (6,000), and shaded columns are Patm = 270 Hg mm (8,000)

Martsinko. Hypoxia is known to ultimately disturb the oxidative processes in the tissues as well as the energy-dependent processes and cause an energy shortage. Experiments were carried out with rats 8–10 and 24–26 months old to study the effect of hypoxemia on the axoplasmic flow in the ventral roots. For this purpose the rats were placed at an altitude of 8,000 meters immediately after the label was administered into the anterior horns of the spinal cord, and then the axoplasmic flow rate was determined. It was found that hypoxia retarded the axoplasmic flow both in mature and old rats, but it was more retarded in old rats. Under these conditions, the axoplasmic flow rate is 278 ± 28 mm per day in mature rats, i. e. it drops by 25 per cent, while it is 114 ± 24 mm per day in old rats, i. e. it drops by 50 per cent. At an altitude of 6,000 meters, the axoplasmic flow rate does not change in mature rats, but it drops by 23 per cent in old animals. Hence, the axoplasmic flow is not sufficiently supplied with energy even in the initial state in old age. This as well as other causes decelerate the flow (Fig. 57). The fact that the age changes in the axoplasmic flow are connected with the shifts in the energy processes is evident from the data on its changes in the selective blocking of oxidative phosphorylation (the administration of 2.0 µg of 2,4-DNF/100 g of body weight). The axoplasmic flow is retarded more in mature animals when oxidation and phosphorylation are dissociated by the administration of 2,4-DNF.

A change in the axoplasmic flow in old age can affect both the trophicity of the neuron and the innervated tissues. Glebov and Kryzhanovsky (1978) have distinguished the following functions of the axoplasmic flow of macromolecules and organelles from the neuronal body into the area of nerve endings: (1) the effective and reliable transmission of nervous impulses; (2) the replenishment of the reserves of enzymes, metabolites and organelles that are needed for the synapses to function; (3) the growth of the processes of the neuroblast and the neurons of the growing organism, and the regeneration of the nerves and the presynaptic part of the synapses; (4) the realization of the trans-synaptic transmission of the trophogens (substances which induce metabolism in the effector cells) and trophic material (proteins, polypeptides), which make the effector structures highly plastic, and (5) the feed-back control of information from the synapses to the neuronal body. Hence, the disturbance of the axoplasmic flow can have serious consequences in the aging organism. Shifts may occur not only in the neuron, but also in the effector tissues, because (1) the disturbance of the axoplasmic flow causes changes in the presynaptic endings and the mechanisms of transmitter transmission, and (2) the transfer of trophogens through the synapse into the effector cell may be affected. This is one of the most important functions of the axoplasmic flow. Although it has been poorly studied, it explains the metabolic and regulatory link between the neuron and the innervated tissue. The exchange of plastic information (RNA, regulatory proteins) between the neuron and the innervated cell helps to combine them into a definite system. The breakdown of this link in old age can cause metabolic and functional disturbances.

Another function of the axoplasmic flow is of great significance in vitauct and the preservation of the neuron's viability. Hartmann (1931) amputated a piece of cytoplasm in the amoeba. As a result, the amoeba ceased to divide and, according to him, virtually did not age. Zhinkin (1966) believes that the nerve cell, like the amoeba in Hartmann's experiments, does not divide and does not age for a long time because a part of its protoplasm always flows out through the axon. Consequently, the neuron structures are renewed due to biosynthetic processes. Apparently, there is a definite link between the capacity of the axoplasmic flow and the neuron's life span.

Neural influences on the tissues are realized through the appropriate transmitter systems. Therefore, it is especially important to study the effect of the transmitters on tissue metabolism, particularly on protein biosynthesis as the basis of trophic processes, in order to ascertain the mechanisms of the age changes in trophic regulation. To understand this question, Verkhratsky (1977, 1978) studied the effect of catecholamines and acetylcholine on protein biosynthesis in the tissues of animals of various age. However, there is not much data on the effect of catecholamines on protein biosynthesis. Reshef and Hanson (1972) have shown that catecholamines cause the inductive synthesis of several enzymes. Rona and co-workers (1959) as well as Stanton and others (1969) have observed that the biosynthesis of total proteins is activated in the myocardium, while Wool (1960) noted that protein synthesis decreases in the liver and the

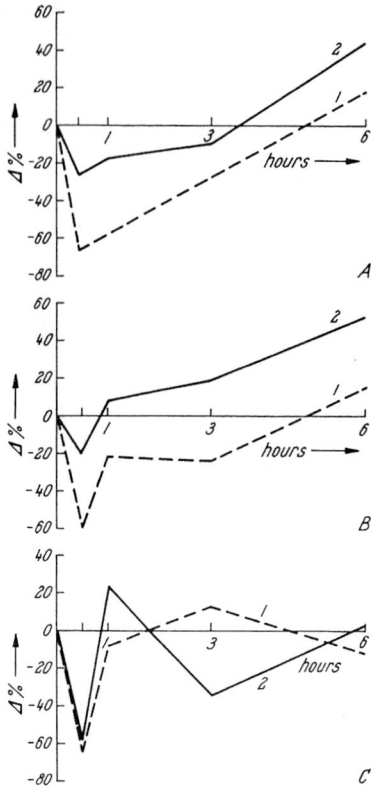

Fig. 58. Influence of the intraperitoneal administration of noradrenaline (300 μg/kg) on the intensity of protein biosynthesis in the auricles (A), the right ventricle (B) and the left ventricle (C) of the heart of mature rats (1) and old rats (2) with respect to the initial level

diaphragm. Verkhratsky (1977) studied the effect of noradrenaline on the incorporation of glycine into the total proteins of various organs. In the experiments which were carried out *in situ*, noradrenaline was administered intraperitoneally in a dose of 30 μg/100 g of body weight, and then the specific radioactivity of the amino acids, the specific radioactivity of protein and the relative specific radioactivity of protein were determined. Substantial changes occur in the biosynthetic processes under the effect of noradrenaline. These changes occur non-uniformly in animals of different age and have definite organ specificity. Moreover, the specificity of the reaction is so great that it can be expressed differently in various parts of the same organ. It can be seen from Fig. 58 A, B, C that noradrenaline strongly activates protein biosynthesis in the right ventricle of old animals, while it suppresses this biosynthesis in mature animals. These changes in protein biosynthesis are two-phased in myocardium of the left ventricle of both mature and old rats. In old animals, this difference in the direction of the effect of noradrenaline on the right and left ventricles may be the cause of the non-uniform trophic adrenergic influences on various parts of the myocardium. In this respect, the age differences of the structural changes

on the right and left ventricles should also be mentioned. The stimulating effect
of noradrenaline on protein biosynthesis in the skeletal muscle is more marked
in mature animals than in old ones. In his experiments with the liver sections,
Verkhratsky (1977) showed that noradrenaline has a non-uniform effect on the
synthesis of the total proteins of the liver: it activates this synthesis in old
animals and inhibits it in mature.

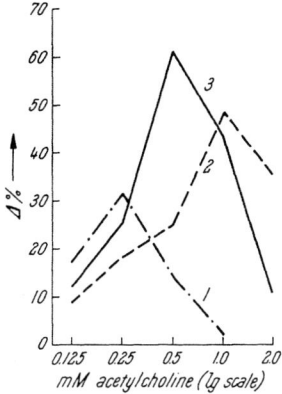

Fig. 59. Influence of the growing concentration of acetylcholine in the incubation medium on the
intensity of protein biosynthesis (relative specific radioactivity) in the sections of the auricles of rats
of different age: *1* young rats; *2* mature rats; *3* old rats

Thus, in the experiments carried out *in vivo,* noradrenaline causes a
two-phase change in the intensity of protein synthesis and occasionally its
pronounced stimulation. Protein biosynthesis was suppressed in the experiments
with the liver sections. Consequently, it was assumed that two components,
i. e. direct and indirect effects, are present in the mechanism of noradrenaline
action on protein biosynthesis. Catecholamines are known to activate the hypothalamohypophysial system, and probably they affect protein biosynthesis
through its regulatory mechanisms. Indeed, Verkhratsky has shown that
noradrenaline suppresses protein biosynthesis in the heart, liver, skeletal muscles
and the salivary gland after hypophysectomy.
    Neural trophic influences can involve the cholinergic mechanisms, which are
realized through the system of acetylcholine metabolism. It should be taken into
account that, besides producing the synaptic effect, acetylcholine can influence
the intracellular processes and produce the so-called non-mediatory action,
which is very important in the regulation of trophicity. In his experiments *in
vitro,* Verkhratsky (1978) studied the changes in protein biosynthesis in the
sections of several organs when various amounts of acetylcholine were added to
the incubation medium. Prozerine (neostigmine) was added beforehand to the
medium to prevent acetylcholine from being rapidly hydrolyzed. It can be seen
from Fig. 59 that acetylcholine causes a dose-dependent shift in the relative
specific activity of protein. In the auricles and ventricles of the heart, definite
concentrations of acetylcholine stimulate protein biosynthesis: this stimulation is
greater in old animals than in mature ones. That activation of protein

biosynthesis is an important link in the mechanism of the chronotropic influences of the vagus nerve on the heart (Frolkis *et al.*, 1977).

In the liver, acetylcholine suppresses protein biosynthesis in mature animals, but it does not change substantially this synthesis in old ones. It is known that the effect of acetylcholine is blocked by atropine, which forms a more stable complex with cholinoreceptors. Verkhratsky studied the effect of acetylcholine on protein biosynthesis in various organs after pretreatment with atropine. It was found that atropine did not change the inhibiting effect of acetylcholine on the incorporation of labelled amino acids into hepatic proteins, but blocked the stimulating effect of acetylcholine on protein biosynthesis in the auricles. Cholinoreceptors of the heart and the liver are known to belong to the group of M-cholinoreceptors, which are blocked by atropine. The inhibition of protein synthesis in the liver by acetylcholine is probably connected largely with its non-mediatory action, while stimulation in the heart, with its mediatory effects. Interestingly these two types of effects are marked non-uniformly in old age. Shifts of greater intensity in the protein biosynthesis of the heart caused by acetylcholine correlates with the more marked changes in myocardial contractility due to transmitter action.

Thus, the above data show that the cholinergic and adrenergic effects on protein biosynthesis change with age. Tissue trophicity is determined by a set of metabolic processes, which determine the cellular function. In the previous chapters, data were given on the substantial changes which occur in the adrenergic and cholinergic influences on the energy processes as the organism ages.

The altered effect of transmitters on many key enzymes of cellular metabolism plays a big role in the mechanism of age shifts in neural regulation. We have obtained data demonstrating that catecholamines in old rats cause qualitatively different shifts in the activity of several respiratory and glycolytic enzymes as well as the enzymes of acetylcholine synthesis. In old animals, acetylcholine inhibits more markedly the ATPase activity of myosin. The activity of the key enzymes of energy exchange is influenced to a different extent. Thus, transmitters change substantially the neural regulation of tissue trophicity.

Many works of Orbeli's school were on the adaptive-trophic effects of the sympathetic nervous system. The Orbeli-Ginetsinsky phenomenon (i. e. the greater contraction of the fatigued muscle when the sympathetic nerve is stimulated) is believed to be a classic example of the trophic influence of the sympathetic nervous system. The sympathetic effects on the skeletal muscle are realized because the transmitter going to the working muscle fibres is released into the blood (Govyrin, 1967).

It was important to see how the Orbeli-Ginetsinsky phenomenon occurred when the sympathetic nerve was stimulated and when catecholamines were administered with due regard to our data on both the weakening of neural influences on the tissues and greater sensitivity to humoral effects in old age. In our laboratory, Zamostyan (1964, 1971) showed that the influences of the sympathetic neurvous system on the skeletal muscles weaken and their sensitivity to catecholamines increases with age. In mature rats, for instance, the influence of the sympathetic nerve on the muscle is seen when the sympathetic trunk is stimulated by a current of 0.59 ± 0.06 V, while in old rats, by a current of 1.48 ± 0.16 V. In the case of sympathetic stimulation, the latent period of the influence is prolonged, coming to 5.23 ± 0.35 sec in mature rats and 9.8 ± 0.47 sec in old animals. After the stimulation of the sympathetic nerve, the restoration of the initial contraction values is greatly delayed in old rats. It takes, on the average, 45.20 ± 5.47 sec in mature rats and 79.88 ± 5.54 sec in old animals. The sympathetic effect is less in old rats (15.99 ±1.5 per cent against 23.12 ±1.91 per cent in mature rats).

At the same time, shifts in the contractility of the skeletal muscles are more pronounced in old animals when adrenaline is administered (33 μg/100 g of body weight). In mature rats, the value of muscle contractions rises by 12.56 ± 0.93 per cent due to adrenaline action, while in old animals, it rises by 22 ± 1.09 per cent.

The age differences of the shifts in energy exchanges during the Orbeli-Ginetsinsky phenomenon are related directly to these functional changes. According to Frolkis (1963), Zamostyan (1964), and Frolkis and Epstein (1966), the amounts of ATP, creatine phosphate and inorganic phosphorus do not change substantially in mature and old rats due to the above-mentioned dose of adrenaline. In old rats, however, adrenaline causes greater shifts in the turnover of these compounds. The specific activity and relative specific activity of ATP and creatine phosphate show slight changes in mature rats, but they increase considerably in old animals.

Thus, the influences of the neural and humoral links are redistributed during the sympathetic regulation of muscle trophism in old age. Changes in contractility are delayed in old animals during sympathetic stimulation apparently because of the differences in the reactions to noradrenaline which is released in the nerve endings.

In our experiments, the negative Orbeli-Ginetsinsky phenomenon (a drop in the contraction values) was reproduced more frequently when the sympathetic trunk was stimulated. The positive Orbeli-Ginetsinsky phenomenon originated when the functional state of the neuromuscular apparatus worsened, its blood supply became limited, and so forth.

Ever since the Orbeli-Ginetsinsky phenomenon was discovered, the participation of the vascular factor and direct trophic effects in its mechanism has been debated.

The regulation of the vascular component of the Orbeli-Ginetsinsky phenomenon changes with age. Using the resistographic method, Zamostyan registered the reactions of the extremity muscle vessels when the sympathetic nerve was stimulated and adrenaline was administered as the skeletal muscles were either at rest or working (Fig. 60). Vascular reactions to the adrenergic influences change in the working muscles. These shifts in vascular sensitivity are more pronounced in old animals than in mature rats. In the former, vascular reactions are "rejuvenated," i. e. the increased sensitivity to adrenaline and the thresholds of the sympathetic neural influences are reduced. This "rejuvenation" probably explains somewhat the mechanisms of the favourable effect of a physical load in aging. Thus, the neural and humoral components of the adrenergic regulation of tissue trophism change with age.

Denervation is one of the most favourite approaches in the experimental analysis of the trophic influences of the nervous system. When tissues are denervated, it is possible to ascertain the shifts in the metabolism and the function which occur as the trophic influences of the nervous system are switched off. The reaction of tissues to denervation changes considerably in old age. For instance, Danielson (1952) showed that nerves are regenerated more rapidly in young rabbits than in adult animals. According to Gutmann (1976), the skeletal muscle function is restored more rapidly in young animals after reinnervation.

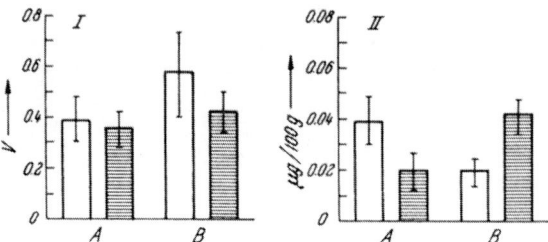

Fig. 60. Influence of the stimulation of the sympathetic nerve *(A)* and the administration of the threshold doses of adrenaline *(B)* on the vascular tonicity of the resting and working muscles of rats of different age: *I* rats 8–12 months old; *II* rats 26–30 months old. Light columns stand for threshold values at rest, and shaded columns, for threshold values during work

Age differences in metabolism are non-uniform in various tissues during denervation. This is apparently due to the substantial shifts in the level of trophic neural regulation and in the mechanisms of its interference in the metabolic processes of various tissues. The specifics of the tissue reactions of animals of different age to denervation have been clearly shown by Nikitin and his associates (1956). Changes in the mass and metabolism of the striated muscles and liver were registered after denervation. In the denervation of the liver, the changes in its mass and biochemism appeared to be more pronounced in old animals, whereas in the denervation of the skeletal muscles, they were more marked in adult rats. Apparently, the metabolism and the function of the skeletal muscles are more dependent on age changes in the nervous system when the level of regulation of these muscles is more perfect. Besides, account should be taken of the strong influences which immobilization has on the metabolism of the denervated skeletal muscle. Parkhotik (1964) showed that changes in tissue respiration, excitability, extracellular and intracellular fluid, and potassium and sodium concentrations in the skeletal muscles were less pronounced after denervation in old rats as compared with young animals. Moreover, the metabolism and function are subsequently restored more slowly after reinnervation in old age. Data have been obtained in our laboratory on the less pronounced rise of the membrane potential and the changes in the cholinesterase activity of the skeletal muscles after denervation in old animals.

All this indicates that the neural trophic influences are impaired in old age. Noting the similarity of the changes in protein metabolism in the muscles during denervation and aging, Gutmann (1976) believes that a decrease in the neuronal function is an important factor of aging.

Osseus tissue is a good object for studying the neural regulation of trophism. It is known to be innervated greatly by the somatic and sympathetic nerves (Kapustina, 1965). Osteoporosis, i. e. substantial structural and metabolic changes in osseus tissue, naturally and almost inevitably occurs with age. It is characterized by the porosity of osseus tissue, an increase in the osteon canal opening, a decrease in the number of cells, in the transverse bone bars and in the content of acid mucopolysaccharides, and by a change in the qualitative composition of these mucopolysaccharides. Substantial osteoporotic changes can cause several pathologic states, such as frequent fractures and pain syndromes.

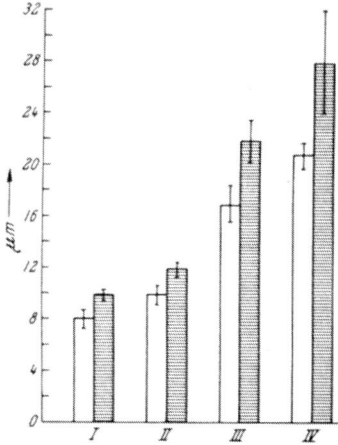

Fig. 61. Diameter of the canal openings of the osteons of the femur in mature rabbits (light columns) and old rabbits (shaded columns) 1–4 months after the ligation of the sympathetic nerve

In our institute, Orlova (1973) compared the structural, roentgenologic and metabolic changes when the osseus tissue of animals of different ages was denervated. The femoral and obturator nerves were cut in one group of mature and old rabbits, while the sympathetic trunk was cut at the level of the third lumbar vertebra in another group. Severe osteoporosis developed when the motor and sympathetic nerves were cut in the rabbits. Osteoporosis was more pronounced in old animals than in mature ones (Fig. 61). It was manifested in the thinning of the cortical layer of the femur, an increase in the osteon canal opening, and a decrease in the amount of mucopolysaccharides in the bone. Interestingly osteoporotic disturbances were more pronounced in the desympathization activity than when the motor nerves were cut. These disturbances were also quite well manifested on the intact side. These data confirm Orbeli's conception of the adaptive and trophic influence of the sympathetic nervous system. Trophic reflexes occur when the motor and sympathetic nerves are cut. These reflexes disturb the tissue trophism of the intact extremity. Prerequisites for reflex trophic disturbances originate in old age due to the changed metabolic background. Greater trophic disturbances of the intact extremity are connected with that fact. Reflex trophic disturbances can originate in different internal organs that are away from the damage site in various situations in old age, and pathology can occur in their basis.

Thus, both motor and sympathetic denervations cause great disturbances in osseus tissue. These disturbances are more pronounced in old age.

Age changes in the efferent pathway of regulating trophism were analyzed in all the above-mentioned investigations. However, the regulation of tissue trophism can be perfect only when the efferent trophic influences are adequate for the organism's adaptive reactions and for the current state of the trophic process in the tissues. Such integration can occur only when the central mechanisms of regulation constantly receive an information on the occurrences at the periphery. In other words, the tissue trophism regulation system can only be self-regulatory. Hence, information on a change in tissue trophism does not come from one type of receptors, but covers the whole complex range of the systems which receive it. This applies to vascular mechanoreceptors, vascular chemoreceptors, tissue receptors, muscular proprioreceptors, humoral effects and, in general, the most diverse information on the changes in the metabolism and function at the periphery. The centripetal as well as the centrifugal pathways of information are cut usually in denervation. However, clinicians and experimenters knew even in the nineteenth century that gross changes occurred in trophism (skin dryness, trophic ulcers, etc.) when only the sensory nerves were cut.

A physiologist can fix the limits of the trophic changes in the muscles when the efferent and afferent pathways are switched off, i. e. he can do this by cutting the posterior and anterior roots in which the excitation flows from the centre are separated from those going towards it. It was found that muscle trophism was disturbed to the greatest extent when the motor roots were cut, and that it was disturbed less in the case of deafferentation and desympathization. In our laboratory, we tried to ascertain some age specifics of a change in the trophism of the skeletal muscles in deafferentation (i. e. when feed-backs are switched off by cutting the posterior roots) in connection with our concepts of the irregularity of the changes which occur in various links of functional regulation (regulation centre, direct control, feed-back, object of regulation) as the organism ages.

According to Zamostyan (1971), the deafferentation of the posterior extremity did not affect the ability of the skeletal muscles to perform prolonged and stable work in mature and old animals. A study of other functional and structural indices has shown that the denticulate tetanus becomes a "continuous" one at lower stimulation frequencies, the lability of the neuromuscular apparatus decreases, and the structural trophic changes (edemas, ulcers, gangrene) become more pronounced in old rats after deafferentation. It follows from these and other data that the switching off of sensitive innervation affects the functional and structural properties of the skeletal muscles to a greater extent in old animals than in mature ones.

Thus, irregular changes develop in various links of the regulation of tissue trophism as the organism ages.

Why does denervation cause greater disturbances in mature animals in some cases, while in other cases, it does so in old ones? Apparently, two mechanisms play a significant role in the development of post-denervation disturbances. These mechanisms are: (a) the degree of neural control over the tissues (the greater it is, the more pronounced are the consequences of denervation), and (b) the ability of the local intracellular mechanisms of self-regulation to maintain the optimal level of the vital activity of the cell when neural control is absent. Consequently, denervation often causes greater gross changes in the activity of cells and tissues when neurotrophic control is impaired in old age.

Trophic regulation is realized in different ways. We will recall only one of them, which has been described in our works (Frolkis, 1970–1979). The activation of the genetic apparatus and protein biosynthesis in the cell results in the hyperpolarization of a cell. The rise of the membrane potential causes a change in cell excitability and in the transport of substances inside the cell, and also engenders shifts in the reaction of the cell to physiologically active substances. We believe that this mechanism is one of the concrete substrates of the neurotrophic influences. The rise of hyperpolarization is of adaptive and regulatory significance when the genetic apparatus is activated. The activation of protein biosynthesis requires considerable energy expenditure. Under these conditions, the development of hyperpolarization, a change in membrane resistance and a decrease in excitability protect the cell from great losses and promote the transport of glucose and amino acids. Thus, neurohormonal influences change all properties of a cell via this trophic mechanism.

9. Local Mechanisms of Humoral Regulation During Aging

The self-regulation of the organism's metabolism and functions is realized due to a complex hierarchy, i. e. to the subordination of its various levels to one another. The objects of regulation, namely, the organs and the tissues, are under the complicated neurohumoral control of the central nervous system. These higher forms of regulation were created on the basis of intracellular and inter-cellular regulatory factors during historic and individual development. However, the local regulatory mechanisms, which are of great adaptive importance in ensuring the adequate reactions of the cells, organs and tissues, did not lose any of their biological significance even though those forms were created. The interaction between the general and the local, and between the centralized and the local, is what determines the specific mechanisms of regulation.

Our data show that the central neurohormonal control of the local mechanisms of humoral regulation changes, the local humoral factors in the realization of the regulatory effects become more significant, and the peripheral reflex reactions become less intense with age.

Cyclic Nucleotides

Heinrich Heine once wrote that nature, like a great poet, attains great diversity with a small amount of means. Indeed, the diversity of the organism's energy requirements is ensured ultimately by a universal donator of the high-energy bonds, namely, by adenosine triphosphate (ATP). Moreover, the most important factors of intercellular and intracellular regulation originate on the basis of ATP exchange. They include cyclic adenyl nucleotides and the system of adenosine metabolism.

The system of the synthesis and breakdown of cyclic nucleotides is known to play a certain role in the realization of neurohormonal effects on the cell. They are synthesized under the action of a specific enzyme of adenylate cyclase, which is a part of a tricomponental structure: (1) the receptor which is on the outer surface of the cell membrane; (2) the conjugating subunit (the communicator or the transductor), which is deep in the membrane and which transmits the signal from the regulatory to the catalytic part of the enzyme, and (3) the catalytic subunit, which is on the inner side of the membrane and which realizes the conversion of ATP $= Mg^{2+}$ in cyclic AMP. Cyclic nucleotides act as a "secondary messenger" because they activate several enzymic systems which determine the metabolic and functional response of the cell. Their influence on protein kinases is the key link in the mechanism of the action of cyclic AMP. Various proteins, including those which participate in the regulation of the activity of the genetic apparatus, are phosphorylated with the participation of protein kinases.

According to Kulchitsky (1981), the content of cyclic AMP and cyclic GMP in the heart, the liver and the skeletal muscle does not change with age. I. V. Frolkis (1978) did not find any changes in the content of cyclic AMP in the wall of the portal vein. The basal level of cyclic AMP and cyclic GMP in the cerebral cortex, basal nuclei and brain stem does not change with age (Govoni et al., 1977; Schmidt, Thornberry, 1978). However, the reaction of adenylate cyclase of the cerebral cortex of rabbits and rats to the action of catecholamines and histamine either decreases (Makman et al., 1979) or does not change at all (Schmidt, Thornberry, 1978) with age. Some authors note that the reaction of adenylate cyclase of certain structures of the limbic system decreases under the action of catecholamines in old age (Govoni et al., 1977; Makman et al., 1979, etc.).

Kalish and associates (1975) have shown that the basal activity of adenylate cyclase in the rat liver increases and that this activity, stimulated by adrenaline and glucagon, grows substantially with age (from 6 to 24 months). Kranz and others (1976) have discovered that the activity of adenylate cyclase stimulated by adrenaline and histamine in the wall of the femoral artery is higher in old rats than in mature ones. Data on the invariability of the basal and adrenaline-stimulated activity of adenylate cyclase were obtained by means of erythrocytes, while the systems of the synthesis of cyclic AMP and cyclic GMP were unchanged in adipose tissue (Bylund et al., 1977; Giudiulli, Pecquery, 1978). According to Gatsko and others (1977) as well as Surikov and associates (1976), the activity of phosphodiesterase does not change in the liver and the heart, while according to Puri and Volicer (1977), it decreases in the *Corpus striatum* of the brain.

We have already seen that greater shifts in the content of cyclic AMP in the liver, the heart, the portal vein and the skeletal muscle occur in old animals under the effect of catecholamines. The shifts in the content of cyclic GMP in the heart are also more pronounced in these animals under the action of small doses of acetylcholine (see Fig. 49). The correlation between the functional effects and the nature of the changes in the content of cyclic adenyl nucleotides is interesting. For instance, the shifts in both the contractility of the myocardium and the content of cyclic GMP are more pronounced in old rats under the action of small doses of acetylcholine, but they are more pronounced in mature rats under the action of large doses of acetylcholine. Medved (1980) has shown that greater shifts occur in the content of cyclic AMP in the heart of old rats when vasopressin is administered. In every experiment, the shifts correlated with the severity of the functional changes in the heart.

Sodium fluoride activates adenylate cyclase when it is administered in definite doses. Kulchitsky (1981) has shown that the increment of the content of cyclic AMP is higher in the homogenates of the liver, the skeletal muscles and especially the heart of old animals when sodium fluoride is administered.

13*

Thus, the growth of sensitivity to regulatory factors, which has been described in several cases, can be associated with a change in the properties of adenylate cyclase. The irregular changes in the reaction of different tissues to the action of physiologically active substances are connected with the differently expressed shifts in the activity of adenylate cyclase and phosphodiesterase. The activity of adenylate cyclase cannot be used (as many do) to determine, for instance, the adrenoreception of the cell. The amount of the receptors of the cell and the activity of adenylate cyclase of the brain change differently as the organism ages. The enzymatic activity which is being determined depends not only on the amount of molecules of the enzyme, but also on the conformation properties of these molecules. The more clearly expressed stimulation of adenylate cyclase can be an important adaptive mechanism when the number of cellular receptors decreases in old age.

Adenosine Metabolic System

Great interest is being taken in adenosine, since it is believed that this compound plays a certain role in regulating the blood flow, especially the coronary blood flow, and in regulating the contractility of the myocardium.

It has been established that adenosine is a product of the degradation of adenine nucleotides: ATP, ADP and AMP. The total amount of adenosine, cyclic AMP, inosine and hypoxanthine (ATP conversion products) constitutes 0.1 per cent of the overall content of adenine nucleotides (Schrader, Gerlach, 1976). Adenosine is formed on the outer membrane of the myocardial cell as a result of the dephosphorylation of AMP, which is catalyzed by the enzyme 5'-nucleotidase. It has been shown that this enzyme is closely connected with the membranes. Thus, the adenosine formed on the outer cell membrane is secreted into the extracellular medium (Rubio *et al.*, 1973).

The metabolism of adenosine and the rate of its outflow from the myocardium are closely connected with the oxygen balance in the myocardium. This fact confirms the role of adenosine as a mediator of the metabolic regulation of the coronary blood flow. Any factor which upsets the balance between oxygen supply and the tissue's oxygen requirement causes adenosine to be formed more rapidly in amounts which are enough for vasodilation. The elimination of hypoxia blocks the further formation of adenosine.

Recent investigations have shown that adenosine plays an extremely important metabolic role which is independent of its coronarodilatory effect. It has been proved that adenosine has a stimulating effect on glucose metabolism and its transfer into the cell.

In our work carried out together with R. A. Frolkis, we studied the activity of the basic enzymes which participate in the synthesis and breakdown of adenosine, namely, 5'-nucleotidase, which catalyzes the conversion of AMP into adenosine, and adenosine desaminase, which desaminates adenosine. Fig. 62A, B shows that the activity of 5'-nucleotidase grows in the blood and especially the myocardial tissue of old rabbits. Enzymic activity in the myocardium is 51 per cent higher in old animals than in mature ones. The activity of adenosine desaminase is also higher, though to a smaller extent, in old animals. Such correlations between the activities of the enzymes, which synthesize and break down adenosine, suggest that the adenosine formation system is activated in old age. This reaction of the system of adenosine metabolism in the myocardium is of great adaptive regulatory importance when its blood supply is changed. It helps to improve blood supply and microcirculation in the organs, optimize their oxygen supply as the vessels are sclerosed with age, and change the permeability of the hematoparenchymatous barrier.

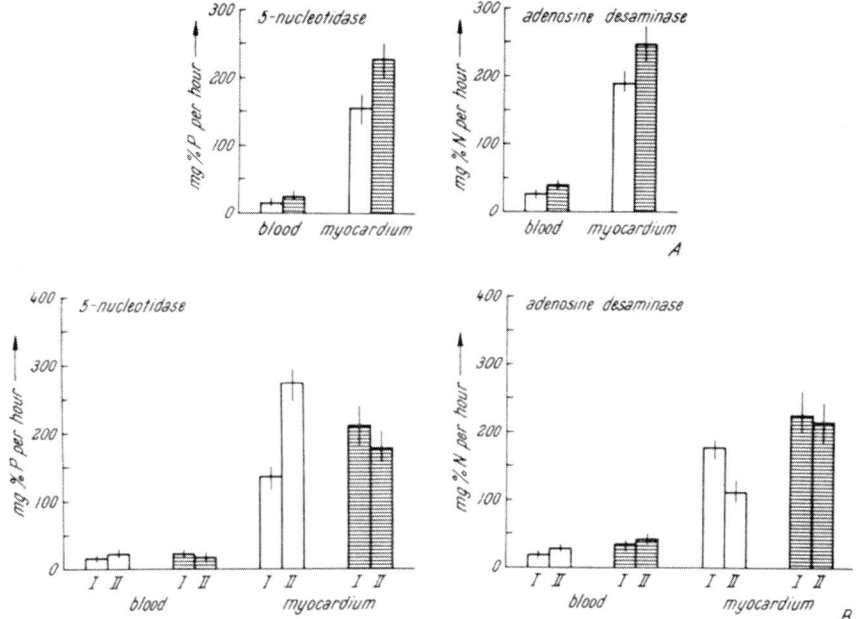

Fig. 62. Enzymes of adenosine metabolism in the blood and myocardium of animals of different age (A), and their change when vasopressin is administered for a long time (B). Light columns stand for mature rabbits, and shaded columns, for old rabbits. I before the administration of vasopressin; II after the prolonged administration of vasopressin

The activity of the adenosine metabolism system is known to change within a wide range. Its potentialities are revealed as the oxygen deficiency of the tissue grows. In our experiments with rabbits, we simulated the chronic hypoxia of the myocardium by administering vasopressin daily. Coronary insufficiency was indicated by ECG changes: the S-T segment sharply rose, the T-wave increased, arrhythmia developed, and so forth. These shifts were more pronounced in old animals. It can be seen from Fig. 62 A, B that adenosine is formed more rapidly in mature rabbits after vasopressin is administered, i. e. the activity of 5'-nucleotidase increases and that of adenosine desaminase decreases in them. These shifts in adenosine metabolism are very important when the coronary vessels undergo a spasm, which causes myocardial ischemia. Such changes do not occur in adenosine metabolism in old animals under the effect of the prolonged administration of vasopressin. Thus, the adenosine metabolic enzymes are activated in old age. However, their potentialities are reduced, thus limiting the participation of adenosine in adaptive reactions.

Kallikrein-Kinin System

Kinins are biologically active substances which act like local or tissue hormones. The concept of the kallikrein-kinin system has now been formed. The system has many components which are structurally and functionally interconnected in a complex manner. The biologically active nonapeptide bradykinin is the main operating unit of the system. In man and animals, kinins are formed from inactive protein precursors, i. e. kininogens, under the action of kallikreins, which are specific enzymes of blood plasma and tissues, and also plasmin, trypsin, and the enzymes of snake venoms (Habal, Movat, 1976). Kininogen is synthesized in the liver (Lukjan et al., 1975), while it is eliminated mainly by the kidneys. Kallikreins of blood plasma belong to the family of tripsin-like proteases, which hydrolyze strictly definite peptide bonds in the blood kininogen with the formation of bradykinin. A large part of kallikreins is found in plasma in the form of proenzymes, i. e. kallikreinogens (Yarovaya et al., 1979).

Human blood plasma contains few kinin-forming enzymes which belong to alpha and gamma globulins. The cascade of the reactions which lead to the formation of blood kinins ends with their destruction under the effect of kininases. Thus, the processes of the formation and breakdown of kinins are physiologically balanced. Tissues and especially the lungs play a substantial role in inactivating kinins; in the lungs, 80–90 per cent of circulating bradykinin is destroyed during one passage of blood (Overturf et al., 1975).

The kallikrein-kinin system of blood is one of the most important humoral systems of regulating the organism's homeostasis. Extremely small concentrations of kinins may influence the tonicity of the smooth muscle, reduce systemic arterial pressure, participate in microcirculatory processes, and stimulate leukocyte diapedesis. The action of kinins on the cardiovascular system is especially clearly expressed. In this respect, numerous investigations have shown that the tonicity of the coronary vessels decreases, while the coronary blood flow, venous return and cardiac output increase under the effect of bradykinin (Gomazkov et al., 1977).

The kinin system is closely connected with the blood clotting system. According to Chernukh and his associates (1975) as well as Gomazkov (1979), the kinin system's function is to maintain a balance between the tonicity of vessels and the rheologic state of blood. The systems of clotting, fibrinolysis and kinin formation are connected with a single activating agent: the Hageman factor.

We have shown together with R. A. Frolkis, Gunina, Pugach and Rushkevich that the kallikrein-kinin system of blood is activated to a certain extent with age. Fig. 63 shows that the content of kallikreinogen, i. e. the inactive precursor of kallikrein, decreases in the blood of old animals, while the antitryptic activity of the blood is suppressed. A moderate increase in the BAEE-esterase activity of the blood of old animals is apparently due to not only kallikrein, but also other blood enzymes which possess the properties of esterase activity, such as plasmin, trombin, and the activated Hageman factor.

Noteworthy is the fact that the activity of kininase diminishes substantially with age. This decrease in the enzymic breakdown of kinins can prolong the circulation of the biologically active peptides in the blood. We have shown that small doses of bradykinin (0.25 μg/kg) cause greater hemodynamic changes in old animals than in mature ones (Frolkis *et al.*, 1979a). This functional effect is probably connected with the suppression of kinin breakdown by kininase.

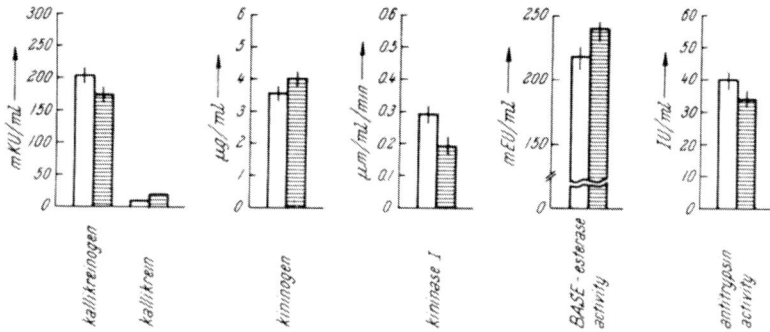

Fig. 63. Parameters of the kallikrein-kinin system of mature rabbits (light columns) and old rabbits (shaded columns)

Substantial changes in microcirculation occur with age: the number of capillaries decreases, the diffusion radius grows, capillary fibrosis becomes pronounced, the basal membrane becomes thicker and more densely packed, the precapillary connective tissue is collagenized, the capillaries become narrower, and so forth. Under these conditions, the action of blood kinins can be potentiated and microcirculation can be maintained on a definite level when kinin breakdown becomes less intense. These changes in the synthesis and breakdown of kinins are promoted by shifts which are connected with the development of tissue hypoxia in old age. Apparently, this explains the lower level of the kinin precursor, i. e. kininogen, in the myocardial tissue of old animals. Shifts in pH and a decrease in the level of ATP in the myocardium are believed to be important factors which help to convert kininogen into free kinins.

The kallikrein-kinin system is under neurohormonal control. According to our data, the stimulation of the hypothalamus activates substantially the kinin system (Fig. 64). In this case, the content of kallikreinogen as well as kininogen and the activity of kininase decrease, while the activity of kallikrein increases. This set of shifts in the system apparently causes the accumulation of kinins, whose biological activity is clearly expressed. The stimulation of the hypothalamus is known to cause substantial hemodynamic changes as well as the engagement of the depressor and pressor mechanisms in the realization of which the activation of the kallikrein-kinin system plays an important role. In old animals, the stimulation of the hypothalamus causes less pronounced shifts in the kinin system. There are various ways of realizing the effect of the hypothalamus on the kinin system. According to our data, the way involving the secretion of the hormones of the posterior lobe of the hypophysis, i. e. vasopressin, is important among them (see Fig. 64). The stimulation of the hypothalamus and the single administration of vasopressin cause the same type of shifts in the kallikrein-kinin system: a reduction of the content of

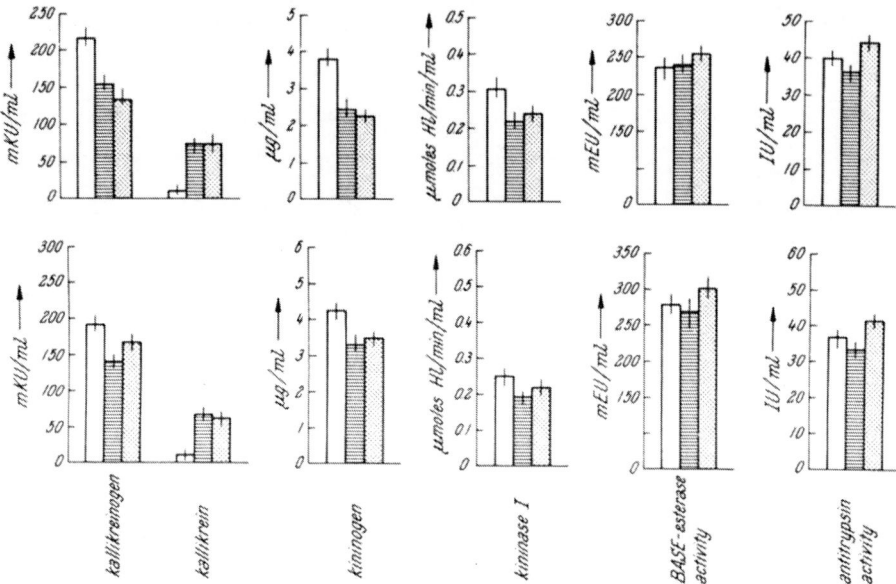

Fig. 64. Kallikrein-kinin system of blood in its normal state and when vasopressin is administered once and the hypothalamus is stimulated in animals of different age. Light columns stand for the initial indices of the kallikrein-kinin system, shaded columns, for the indices of the kallikrein-kinin system when vasopressin is administered once, and dotted columns, for the indices of the kallikrein-kinin system when the hypothalamus is stimulated. The graphs on top are for mature rabbits, and those below are for old rabbits

kallikreinogen, an increase in the activity of kallikrein and a decrease in that of kininase. Vasopressin is known to cause the spasm of many vessels, including coronary ones, and this leads to severe myocardial hypoxia. In this respect, the activation of the kinin system may apparently be of definite adaptive significance. The set of metabolic shifts, which develop under the effect of vasopressin, may probably become an important mechanism of the activation of the kinin system.

The changes caused by vasopressin in individual links of the kinin system are more pronounced in mature animals. The activity of kallikrein increases and that of kininase decreases to a greater extent in them. This suggests that the potentialities of the changes in the components of the kallikrein-kinin system diminish with age. We have already seen that the single administration of vasopressin causes greater myocardial hypoxia in old animals. This is expressed in the fact that the T-wave changes more persistently and more sharply, the S-T segment increases, while the content of ATP and creatine phosphate as well as myocardial contractility decreases. One of the causes of the more clearly expressed electrocardiographic and metabolic changes during the vasopressin-simulated coronary insufficiency in old animals is apparently connected with a smaller shift in the kallikrein-kinin system.

The age distinctions of the kallikrein-kinin system are more clearly expressed when the hypothalamus is stimulated than when vasopressin is administered. For instance, the activity of kallikrein is 1.5 time higher in mature animals than in old ones when vasopressin is administered once, while it is six times higher in the former than in the latter when the hypothalamus is stimulated. The activity of kininase decreases to a greater extent in mature animals when the hypothalamus is stimulated. All this shows that the hypothalamic control of the kallikrein-kinin system is impaired in old age.

Thus, the kallikrein-kinin system is activated with age. This can be regarded as an adaptive mechanism. The given activation of the local mechanisms of self-regulation occurs as central neural control diminishes. However, the system's potentialities, which are revealed when the hypothalamus is stimulated and vasopressin is administered, decrease with age.

Serotonin

Serotonin is widely distributed in the animal and plant kingdoms. In the organism, 90 per cent of it is formed in the enterochromaffin cells of the mucous membrane of the gastroenteric tract. A high content of serotonin has been observed in several regions of the cerebral cortex, the limbic system, the thalamus, the reticular formation, and so forth. Serotonin causes many metabolic and functional effects, reflexes from the vascular chemoreceptors, central nervous effects, a change in vascular tonicity, in cardiac output, in the tonicity of the smooth muscle, in the gastrointestinal tract, in the secretion of the digestive glands, in the kidney function, and so forth.

According to Kuznetsova (1970), the concentration of blood serotonin and that of the main metabolite of serotonin, i. e. 5-hydroxyindole acetic acid, decrease in the urine of elderly and old persons. For instance, the plasma concentration of serotonin is $0.15 \pm 0.018\,\mu g/ml$ in persons 20–25 years old, while it is $0.09 \pm 0.006\,\mu g/ml$ in persons 70–75 years old. Tryptophan is the source of serotonin in the organism. Substantial changes do not occur in the serotonin synthesis system in old age, i. e. the load of tryptophan causes approximately the same increase in the content of 5-hydroxyindole acetic acid in young and elderly persons. However, serotonin is deaminized more intensively in old age. The load of transamine blocks monoamine oxidase and levels out the content of serotonin in the blood of young and elderly persons. In old age, the activity of monoamine oxidase increases (Verkhratsky, 1971). The disturbance of the mechanisms of binding serotonin with thrombocytes plays, together with the growth of deamination, an important role in the genesis of the age changes in the content of serotonin in the blood.

In old animals, the content of serotonin decreases only in the brain tissues ($0.39 \pm 0.02\,\mu g/g$ in mature rats and $0.26 \pm 0.01\,\mu g/g$ in old ones), while it does not change in the liver, the heart and the small intestine. It follows that the concentration of serotonin decreases in the brain either because its synthesis becomes less intense or because the deamination processes intensify. After tryptophan loads, the increment of serotonin is the same in the brain of mature and old rats. Hence, its synthesis virtually does not change. However, Ipraside loads, which block monoamine oxidase, have shown that the serotonin breakdown becomes more intense in old age (Kuznetsova, 1970).

Besides a change in the serotonin metabolism, the sensitivity of the cardiovascular system and the brain to its action also changes in old age. For instance, the threshold dose which causes an increase in cardiac output and a decrease in peripheral vascular resistance is $0.01 \mu g/kg$ in old rabbits and $0.15 \mu g/kg$ in mature ones. When the doses are larger ($10.0 \mu g/g$), the hemodynamic response in old animals is less than in mature ones. In old animals, quantitative as well as qualitative distinctions are observed in the reactions to the administration of serotonin. For instance, cardiac output diminishes in old animals, while it continues to grow in mature ones when a dose of $50 \mu g/g$ of serotonin is administered. Apparently, the Bezold-Jarisch reflex originates earlier in old animals due to the growth of the chemoreceptors' sensitivity.

Kuznetsova (1970) has shown that the sensitivity of the brain structures to serotonin grows in old persons. The concentration of endogenous serotonin in the brain tissues was increased by means of transamine, which is an inhibitor of monoamine oxidase. Under these conditions, the EEG changes were more pronounced in elderly persons.

Thus, serotonin exchange in various organs changes differently, sensitivity grows, and tissue reactivity to the action of serotonin diminishes with age.

Prostaglandins

Prostaglandins play an important role in the mechanisms of the local regulation of both the metabolism and the function. Although this group of substances has long been known, the specifics of their metabolism and the mechanisms of their action have been intensively studied only in the last two decades. At present, 14 natural prostaglandins are known. They differ from one another in the number of the keto- and oxy-groups, the arrangement of these groups in the ring part of the molecule, and the amount of unsaturated bonds in the side chain. Prostaglandins are active within a wide range: they reduce the level of arterial pressure, enhance cardiac output, dilate the coronary vessels, change the excitability of the nerve centres, participate in the regulation of the secretion of several hypophysial hormones, stimulate the formation of thyroxine, etc. (Horton, 1972; Shkhvatsabaya, Nekrasova, 1977; Flower, 1978). According to Zerkal and Nikitin (1979), the content of individual groups of prostaglandins changes differently in various organs and tissues, while it remains unchanged in certain organs (including the testes) as the organism ages.

Our experiments with mature and old rats have shown that the content of prostaglandins of the E and A groups virtually does not change in the myocardium and the skeletal muscle, while it increases in the kidneys

(21.2 ±1.4 ng/g and 26.4 ±1.8 ng/g, respectively) and decreases in the blood (1.97 ± 0.02 ng/g and 0.71 ± 0.01 ng/g, respectively).

Many central neurohumoral effects on tissues are realized through the prostaglandin system. In some cases, prostaglandins participate in the realization of the hormone effect, while in others, the activation of that system is a counter-regulatory factor. For instance, the content of prostaglandins grows substantially in the kidney under the action of vasopressin; they suppress adenylate cyclase and curtail ultimately the vasopressin effect which is produced through cyclic AMP.

According to Medved (1980), the intravenous administration of vasopressin in a dose of 0.5 unit per kilogram of weight does not cause a change in the content of prostaglandins in the myocardium of mature animals, but it increases substantially this content in the cardiac muscle of old rats (from 14.8 ±1.5 to 29.3 ± 3.1 nanogram per gram of tissue). This increase is apparently an adaptive reaction that is aimed at levelling out the effects of vasopressin, which is known to cause severe myocardial ischemia. Medved showed that the electrocardiographic manifestations of coronary insufficiency, which is caused by vasopressin in old animals, are enhanced substantially when prostaglandin synthesis is blocked preliminarily by indomethacin.

Great interest is now being taken in the effect of catecholamines on the prostaglandin content. It is believed that prostaglandins can change the sensitivity of the adrenoreceptors, i. e. they can participate in the regulation of the adrenergic effects. For instance, adrenaline stimulates lipolysis and intensifies simultaneously the synthesis of prostaglandins in adipose tissue. The latter limits the action of adrenaline by inhibiting adenylate cyclase. Prostaglandin E weakens the pressor effect of noradrenaline, etc. When adrenaline was administered intraperitoneally (30 μg per 100 g of weight), the growth of the prostaglandin content differed in various organs. In most cases, the increment of this content was greater in old rats. For instance, the prostaglandin content virtually did not change in the myocardium of mature rats, but it increased from 16.6 ±1.4 to 30.5 ± 4.2 ng/g in that of old ones, from 16.7 ±1.2 to 35.5 ± 3.8 ng/g in the skeletal muscle of mature rats and from 13.0 ± 2.1 to 48.2 ± 4.3 ng/g in that of old ones, from 21.1 ± 6.5 to 39.0 ± 5.6 ng/g in the kidneys of mature rats, and from 25.2 ± 4.2 to 55.5 ± 2.4 ng/g in those of old ones. It virtually did not change in the blood of mature rats, but increased from 0.71 ± 0.01 to 2.93 ± 0.03 ng/g in that of old ones. This more clearly expressed activation of prostaglandin synthesis can be a mechanism which limits adrenergic reactions.

The content of prostaglandins as well as the sensitivity of the cells to it changes in old age. According to Goodwin and Messner (1979), the sensitivity of the lymphocytes to prostaglandin E is higher in old persons than in young ones.

Thus, the state of the local mechanisms of humoral regulation changes differently with age. In this respect, several systems of local humoral regulation are activated. This activation occurs as central neurohormonal control weakens, i. e. the correlation between the general and the local in the organism's general self-regulation changes and the role of the local humoral factors in the regulation of the organ's activity grows with age. An important fact is that substantial structural and metabolic disturbances occur with age in all the links of local reflex regulation, namely, in the autonomic ganglia, the postganglionic neurons and the receptor apparatus. This weakens the local and peripheral reflexes. In other words, the humoral component of regulation prevails over the reflex one also at the organ level as the organism ages. All this makes it possible for prolonged organotissue reactions with long latent and restorative periods to originate.

Local humoral factors determine the interaction of the cells at the organ level. Irregular shifts in the local humoral regulation systems is a cause of the change in the intercellular relationships in old age.

10. Neurohumoral Mechanisms of the Regulation of the Genetic Apparatus

Genoregulatory Hypothesis of the Processes of Vitauct and Aging

"The beauty presented by Nature to man becomes less visible, and his acquired beauty, engendered by spiritual wealth, becomes more visible with age. Therefore, we answer for ourselves in the second half of our life." – André Maurois.

The programmed age changes and the manifestations of vitauct largely appear during the genetically informative period. The disturbances of the genetic apparatus are accumulated by the time the organism reaches the concluding, genetically non-informative period (Frolkis, 1978).

Most researchers now acknowledge that the molecular and genetic changes are cardinal in the mechanism of aging. However, this does not make the debate on both their role and place in the genesis of aging meaningless. On the contrary, the debate becomes even more heated. The existing hypotheses of the whole organism's aging can be divided into two groups: (1) the organism ages as a complex biological regulatory system and (2) the organism's aging is a function of the aging of its individual cells. In the first case, it is maintained that the primary molecular age changes, which occur in certain groups of cells and are connected, for instance, with the neurohumoral regulation mechanisms, promote the secondary disturbances in the genetic apparatus in other cells. In the second case, the relatively independent shifts in the genetic apparatus, which cause every cell to age, are analyzed.

In 1965–69, we proposed the genoregulatory hypothesis of aging. According to this hypothesis, the primary mechanisms of aging are connected with a change in genome regulation and probably with the shifts in the regulatory genes. This hypothesis explains (1) the mechanisms of a change in the correlation of the syntheses of individual proteins, (2) the decrease in the potentialities of activation of the biosynthesis of definite proteins, (3) certain changes in the protein structure that are connected with the shifts in the polypeptide composition of proteins, (4) the change in the mechanisms of neurohumoral regulation of protein biosynthesis, (5) the mechanisms of the effect of the damaging exogenous and endogenous factors on the realization of genetic information, and (6) the fundamental possibility of activating the genetic loci, which determine the synthesis of proteins that were not characteristic of a given cell earlier. In other words, the direction of age changes in protein biosynthesis can be understood on the basis of the genoregulatory hypothesis. Of course, the molecular mechanisms of aging of various types of cells differ from one another. In some of them, the changes in genome regulation are of paramount importance. In others, the genoregulatory shifts are the outcome of the primary changes in other links of cell metabolism.

A fundamentally important fact is that the basic mechanisms of not only aging, but also vitauct can be understood by studying the specifics of the regulation of the genome and its structurally consolidated properties. The basic mechanisms of the organism's viability, i. e. the mechanisms whose purpose is to prolong life, are connected with the specifics of the genetic apparatus' regulation. Cutler (1978) has indicated that the processes of aging and antiaging can be traced throughout the storage and flow of genetic information. According to him, these processes are the same in various species of mammals, but the processes of antiaging are expressed to a greater extent in the longer-living species.

According to King and Wilson (1975), most differences between the mammalian species, which greatly differ from one another on their life span, are due to the specifics of genome regulation. Man and the chimpanzee, for instance, hardly differ from one another on the composition of their structural genes, although they began to follow different evolutionary routes 8–20 million years ago. Man's life span, which has changed in the course of several million years, is connected with the shifts in genome regulation. Thus, there is a relationship between the species specificity of genome regulation, on the one hand, and the life span, vitauct and aging, on the other.

In recent years, Vanyushin and Berdyshev (1977), Cutler (1978), Tereshchenko (1978) and others have indicated that the changes in genome regulation play a certain role in the mechanism of aging.

All the cells in the organism originated from a single precursor: the fertilized oocyte. Although there are many various cells in the complex organism, they all have the same genome, i. e. DNA, with the same set of information. Hence, cell differentiation depends above all on the specifics of the realization of genetic information and genome regulation.

Our concepts of the essence of the genetic apparatus regulation will change as science develops. Our concept of the relationship between the gene regulators, the gene operators, and so forth, may also change. New links will be discovered in the system of the genetic apparatus regulation, and old concepts will be discarded. However, the concept of the fundamental role of the processes of regulation in the realization of genetic information will remain undisputed.

The one-sided nature of molecular gerontology was expressed for a long time in a search for only the mechanisms which disturb and damage the genome. However, adaptive shifts and vitauct processes should be studied in order to understand the specifics of the development and formation of the life span of a species and an individual. Today, we can clearly single out a set of structural and functional changes in the genome that determine the course of vitauct and influence not only the reliability, preservation and transfer of genetic information, but also the viability of the cell and the organism.

DNA is a stable polymer. If its structure were very mobile, there would be chaos in protein biosynthesis, the genetic transfer mechanisms, and in the metabolism and the functions of the cells. The relative stability of the DNA structure has become the material basis of the unity of both changeability and heredity, unity which ensures evolution on Earth. At the same time, this reliability of the DNA structure is connected with the existence of the most important vitauct systems, whose purpose is to renew, or repair, DNA. As the cell actively functions, the DNA-protein set is constantly attacked by numerous damaging agents which are either exogenous or endogenous and have the most diverse "sites of action." For instance, the interaction between an electrophilic agent and DNA can cause 20 types of damages, including hydration, chain ruptures, and formation of crosslinks, dimers, phosphotriesters and adducts (Hart et al., 1979).

There are several reparative mechanisms. Among those in the mammalian cells, the greatest importance is attached to excisional and postreplicative (only for the dividing cells) reparation as well as the mechanisms which are responsible for restoring the DNA chain ruptures. These systems produce a restorative effect during the complex multistage process which occurs with the participation of various enzymes. For instance, excisional reparation has five stages, i. e. base ruptures, incision, excision, polymerization and ligation, in which DNAases, DNA polymerases and ligases participate.

The reparative mechanisms became more and more effective in the course of evolution. According to Cutler (1978), the mammalian species' life span grew in the last 50–60 million years mainly because the reparative potential increased (the correlation between the species' life span and the intensity of the reparation processes has already been discussed). However, the extremely great diversity of the damaging factors and the possible DNA modifications as well as the multistage nature and, consequently, the inertial nature of reparation hardly suggest the existence of a system which completely and rather rapidly eliminates absolutely all possible damages to the genetic apparatus. The limited nature of the functional abilities of the reparative mechanisms is especially manifested clearly when the damaging effects become more intense. This has often been proved experimentally in model experiments with mutagens, cancerogens and other damaging agents of a physical, chemical and biological nature. In the case of ionizing irradiation, for instance, the number of the non-repairing damages turned out to be a function of the fourth power of the exposure dose (Sacher, 1977).

The DNA-reparation system is a regulatory one. This is what creates the adequate relationships between the extent of damage to DNA and the activation of its reparation processes. Moreover, there are regulatory genome loci which are responsible for the synthesis of the DNA-reparation enzymes. Therefore, the age changes in genome regulation can either activate or suppress the DNA-reparation system and promote the processes of vitauct or aging.

It has been found that the reparative potential decreases substantially when the tissue culture ages (Hart, Setlow, 1976) and when the cells of the muscles, epithelium, lens and erythrocytes differentiate. In all the mammalian species which have been studied, the reparative potential was especially high in early embryogenesis, but it reached the level characteristic of a given species by the end of neonatal life (Peleg, Raz, 1977).

The age changes in the mechanisms responsible for the restoration of individual DNA ruptures have been studied well. The data obtained show that the reparative potential becomes insufficient in old age, and then DNA damages begin to accumulate. Using the slices of the brain, the liver and the myocardium fixed in ethanol as a matrix for DNA polymerase from the thymus, Price and others (1971) have shown autoradiographically that the number of single breaks decreases in the nuclei of the neurons and astrocytes of the brain, myocytes and cardiocytes as well as in the Kupffer cells of the liver of old mice. Gerasimova (1980) has shown that the number of breaks in single strands increases in the DNA of the cells of the liver and the mucous membrane of the small intestine. An increase due to age in the activity of DNA polymerase in such postmitotic tissues as the neurons of the brain and myocardiocytes suggested that the number of breaks and loops of the DNA of the brain and the myocardium grows with age.

The exchange of sister chomatids (ESC), being found in the dividing cells of various origin, is an interesting type of reparation. Kato and Stich (1976) have observed a decrease in the background level of ESC in the aging culture of the human fibroblasts. According to Schneider and others (1979), the background level of ESC did not change substantially as the culture of the IM-90 and I-38 cells aged. However, they found that the functional abilities of this reparative mechanism decreased with age when ESC was stimulated by various mutagens. It was observed that the background and mutagen-stimulated ESC decreased with age also during the early passages of the human skin fibroblasts taken from patients of various age.

All these age changes do not mean that the reparative potential is completely and irreversibly exhausted as the organism ages. There are data which show that the reparative processes can be stimulated at least in rather simple biological objects with a subsequent increase in the life span. The frequency of mutations and sensitivity to ultraviolet radiation increase substantially in the culture of paramecium, which is known to die after 150–200 divisions when conjugation is absent. However, the life span of paramecia increases to 194.3 ± 12.8 divisions (instead of the control $153.0 + 8.5$ divisions after ultraviolet exposure) when the old cultures are subjected to photoreactivation, during which the thimidine dimers are renewed (Smith-Sonneborn, 1979).

Thus, the reparation of DNA determines largely the extent of vitauct, while its disturbance determines aging. However, reparation is not absolutely reliable. It is believed that several damages to the genome are not repaired. They include the displacement of the strands with respect to one another, DNA depurinization, the built-in of molecules and double breaks. Hence, definite disturbances of DNA may originate during vital activity in spite of its reparation.

There are very important regulatory links between the genetic apparatus of the cell nucleus and the metabolism of the whole cytoplasm. These links enable the mechanisms of protein biosynthesis to become adapted to the changing conditions of cellular activity. It has been shown a long time ago that the disturbance of the nuclear cytoplasmic relations is an extremely important mechanism of cellular aging (Nikitin, 1978). This mechanism of genome regulation changes with age. According to Devi and others (1966), RNA synthesis on the DNA in the liver becomes less intense in old rats. However, the level of RNA synthesis remains just as high as in young rats when cytosol from the liver of old rats is added to the DNA of young ones. The level of RNA synthesis remains low when the cytosol of the hepatocytes of young animals is added to the DNA of old ones. It was found that the feed-back signals from the cytoplasm of the hepatic cells of old rats do not cause changes in the genetic apparatus. According to Hellthaler and others (1976), another nuclear cytoplasmic relationships exist in old age. The protein synthesizing ability of the microsomes of rats 3–5 months old was reduced to the level of old rats when cytosol from the liver of old rats was added to them. However, protein synthesis became just as intense when cytosol from the liver of rats 3–5 months old was added to the microsomes of old rats. Junghahn and Bielka (1974) have observed that the cytosol fraction from the liver of old rats stimulated protein synthesis to the greatest extent in polysomes.

Hence, the regulatory effects of the cytoplasm which changed with age can influence substantially the activity of the genetic apparatus of the cell. It follows that many shifts in protein biosynthesis in old age can be of a secondary regulatory nature. This is evident also from our experiments, which have been carried out together with Verkhratsky. The synthesis of mRNA and rRNA in the nuclei of young rats was suppressed when the cytosol of the liver tissue of old rats was added. The cytoplasm of young animals activated this synthesis in the nuclei of old ones, but it remained lower than in the other age groups. Thus, the regulatory effects of the cytoplasm as well as the state of nuclear RNA synthesis changed with age. The relationship between these factors differs in the primarily and secondarily aging cells.

Wright and Hayflick (1975) removed nuclei from the human cells and connected the nuclei-free cytoplasm with the undisturbed cells of different age. This was how *heteroplasmones* had originated. In their experiments, the cytoplasm of the young cells did not rejuvenate the old cells. However, heteroplasmones, which were reconstructed from the old cytoplasm and the young cells, possessed rapid growth properties.

The genic regulatory mechanisms are structurally consolidated. Chromatin, the structure which consolidates them, makes it possible to preserve and read genetic information and to regulate the genome.

Experiments involving the treatment of chromatin preparations with various nucleases show that DNA in chromatin is in the form of nucleosomes, i. e. particles which repeat themselves many times and are interconnected by short spacer regions. Nucleosomes are not fixed structures. The histone octomer, which consists of two molecules of the histone H2a, H2 b, H3 and H4, can slide along DNA and liberate loci for transcription or replication. Nucleosomes are believed to contain two symmetric subunits, each of which consists of 100 pairs of DNA bases, and one molecule each of the above-mentioned histones. These subunits can temporarily separate from one another and unwind the DNA spiral so as to free the regions being transcribed.

DNA is surrounded by two types of proteins. Histones are connected with definite DNA regions, which are not transcribed by RNA polymerase. The non-histone (acid) proteins hinder the inhibition of RNA synthesis by histones. An important fact is that histones can be phosphorylated with the participation of protein kinase. In this case, they lose their ability to inhibit DNA synthesis. Protein kinase is activated by cyclic adenyl nucleotides, which are synthesized with the participation of adenylate cyclase. Adenylate cyclase is a catalytic subunit of the receptors which are sensitive to many hormones and messengers. This is how the intracellular and extracellular mechanisms of genome regulation are interconnected.

After comparing his data and literature data on the molecular genetic changes during aging, Nikitin (1978) drew the conclusion that the "imprint of age" is manifested more when the genome of the cell is on a higher organizational level. He observed that the greatest shifts in aging occur at the chromatin level, i. e. at the level of the integral, structurally consolidated regulatory system. This is an important fact which substantiates the gene-regulatory hypothesis of aging.

Nikitin (1952) was probably the first to ascertain the role of a change in the link between nucleic acids and proteins in the mechanism of aging. Numerous investigations have recently shown that the DNA-protein link in the chromatin of the liver and of the cardiac muscle of dogs becomes stronger with age. This consolidation is a feature of aging which is so stable that even polyploidization does not prevent these changes from originating. It has been shown that the DNA-protein link in the diploid and tetraploid cells of the rat liver also becomes stronger.

Important information on the mechanisms of the change in genome regulation is obtained when the DNA-protein links are studied. According to Hahn (1970) and Verzar (1972), the mass of the DNA of the thymus gland of calves 1–2 months old has, on the average, 0.48 per cent of the histones, while that of old animals (9 years) has 0.88 per cent of the histones. The correlation between the non-histone proteins and DNA in the liver of old rats is almost one-half of that in the liver of rats which are 1 month old. The ratio between the non-histone proteins and histones gives a definite idea of the state of proteins in chromatin. It is 0.62 ± 0.01 in the liver of rats 3 months old, 0.53 ± 0.01 in that of rats 12 months old, and 0.43 ± 0.01 in that of rats 24 months old.

The formation of chromatin adducts, being based on the origination of crosslinks in them, is believed to be one of the main causes of aging. One crosslink can inactivate two large macromolecules. In such cases, the mechanisms of the realization of genetic information are switched off.

Important mechanisms of genome regulation, which change as the organism ages, are connected with the shifts in the correlation between active and repressed chromatins. The shift in the correlation between these chromatins is an important regulatory phenomenon which determines the adaptive abilities of protein biosynthesis. Active chromatin is known to be greatly enriched with protein due to the enzymes which participate in the transcription of RNA, whose synthesis continuously occurs on chromatin. The researches carried out by Khilobok and others (1977) have shown that the given parameters are to a certain extent specific to age: the portion of repressed chromatin increases and that of active chromatin decreases in the nuclei of the liver with age. The DNA-protein relationship increases in active chromatin mainly due to the accumulation of the histone H1. According to Khesin (1975), histones which are rich in lysine, including the histone H1, possess repressive properties. When their content increases in active chromatin, the chromatin may be repressed and the number of the RNA-polymerase connection sites may be reduced. This indicator does not change, but the RNA:DNA ratio increases in repressed chromatin. The level of incorporation of ^{14}C-orotic acid (the precursor of RNA) drops in both fractions. These data have been coroborated by Klimenko and others (1978).

Thus, the changes in the regulatory apparatus of the genome are revealed in the shifts in the relationships between protein and DNA as well as between active and repressed chromatins.

The reliability of the genetic apparatus is largely determined by the existence of the gene redundancy. For instance, the DNA of mammals has fragments which are represented by 10^5–10^6 copies. According to the "master-slave" hypothesis, there are principal genes, which participate in recombinations, and their copies, which are regulated by the principal gene. According to Vilenchik (1970), the function decreases and, what is more, the postmitotic cells die when the amount of a definite type of functionally active genes changes substantially in them. The regulatory links, which determine the synchronism in the activity of redundant genes, change with age. This sharply reduces the reliability of the genetic apparatus. The disturbance in the unique genes is believed to be the principal molecular genetic mechanism of aging.

Mechanisms which protect genetic information from damages play an important part in vitauct. One of them is the localization of the genetic apparatus in the nucleus, which is isolated from many effects of the medium that is separated from the cytoplasm of the nuclear envelope. According to Cutler (1978), it is important to protect the genetic apparatus of sex cells from damages in order to preserve hereditary information.

The regulatory part of the genome, which occupies up to 95 per cent of DNA, is very active in vital activity. It is protected from the intracellular effects least of all and is subjected to age changes most of all. This part of the genome can change and become disturbed by itself. "Errors" in protein synthesis can originate in it, causing a change in the regulation of the whole genome. Such errors can originate in two types of proteins: (a) structural proteins, which ensure metabolism, and (b) proteins which participate in the processing of genetic information and in genome regulation. Errors in the first group of proteins can disappear as a result of biological elimination, while those in the second group can disturb substantially the regulation and transfer of genetic information.

The appearance of errors in protein biosynthesis could lead to the catastrophic destruction of all the cells. However, Shelbrake (1974) believes that when division is asymmetric, one of the daughter cells could inherit the defective molecules and perish, while the other would preserve a high level of vital activity. This could be an adaptive mechanism with whose participation the organism would rid itself of the damaged structures.

In several works, we presented facts to corroborate the leading role which the age changes in genome regulation play in the shifts in protein biosynthesis (Frolkis, 1966, 1970, 1975, 1977). Some recent data should be mentioned in this respect. The correlation of the synthesis rates of various RNA classes changes with age. For instance, if the relative specific radioactivity of the preribosomal RNA (pre-rRNA) of the hepatocyte nucleus is taken as one, the ratio of the relative specific radioactivity of pre-rRNA, a mixture of pre-RNA and pre-messenger RNA (pre-mRNA), pre-mRNA and heterogeneous nuclear RNA (heterogeneous nRNA) would be $1:1:1:1$ in newborn rats, $1:2:1:1$ in rats 1 month old, $1:3:2:2$ in rats 3–4 month old, $1:3:2:3$ in rats 8–10 month old, $1:2:1:1$ in rats 24–26 month old, and $1:3:4:2$ in rats 39–40 months old. Moreover, the correlation between the specific forms of RNA in a single class, e. g. the correlation between the transfer RNA's (which transfer various amino acids), changes with age. According to Gaubatz and Cutler (1978) as well as Strehler and Chang (1979), the number of ribosomal DNA copies, which are responsible for rRNA synthesis, decreases by 40–50 per cent in the brain of old persons and animals. Cutler (1973) showed that the number of varieties of newly synthesized RNA decreases with age.

The age changes in the synthesis of various classes of RNA are also manifested clearly when the relative specific radioactivities of individual RNA fractions are compared. For instance, about three-quarters of the DNA regions being transcribed in the eukaryotic cells are known to correspond to heterogeneous nRNA, whose most probable function is participation in the synthesis of other classes of RNA. The genome gradually became more complex and the DNA regions corresponding to heterogeneous nRNA had increased with the appearance of various features of differentiation during evolution. According to Vilenchik (1970), a decrease in the rate of heterogeneous nRNA synthesis is an important link in the age changes in the genetic apparatus. An analysis of the data obtained in the researcher's laboratory shows that the synthesis of heterogeneous nRNA reaches its peak in young and mature animals, while it diminishes by old age.

The age changes in genome regulation ultimately cause irregular changes in protein biosynthesis. Opinion is still divided as to the direction of the changes which occur in protein biosynthesis with age. According to Barrows (1966), protein biosynthesis does not change at all in old age.

Our data show that protein biosynthesis changes heterochronously in various organs. This corroborates the complexity of the aging process and the origin of primary and secondary changes during its course. However, the specific changes in protein cannot be determined on the basis of a change in its overall renewal. Owing to the changes in genome regulation, various changes (which occasionally occur in different directions) in the synthesis of individual proteins are hidden behind, for instance, the invariable level of the renewal of total protein. The changes in that synthesis are an expression of the changes in genome regulation.

Much data show that the changes in the synthesis of various proteins of the blood, liver, myocardium and brain is irregular. The isoenzymic spectrum of many enzymes changes with age. The shifts which occur in genome regulation with age may be so great that they cause a change in the correlation of the polypeptide chains in the protein molecule. The shifts in the hemoglobin molecule are a case in point. The content of fetal hemoglobin, which consists of two alpha- and gamma-polypeptide chains, i. e. α^2 and γ^2, unlike that of the hemoglobin of the adult species of the type α^2 and b^2, grows with age. All this is connected with a change in the regulation of transcription from various cistrons.

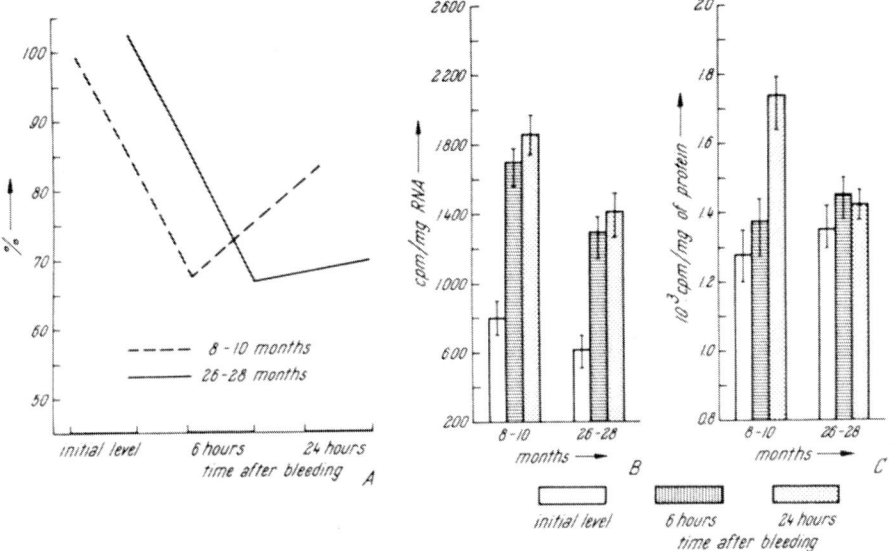

Fig. 65. Change in the content of total protein in blood serum (A), the renewability of total RNA (B) and the intensity of the incorporation of ^{14}C-hydrolyzate of the chlorella protein into the total proteins of the liver (C) 6 and 24 hours after bloodletting in rats which are 8–10 and 26–28 months old

Substantial disturbances of genome regulation during aging may probably activate genes, which have been "silent" all their life. This will cause the appearance of protein which has been synthesized earlier in the cell. Various disturbances in the activity of the cell, including its death, may originate in conformity with its type. It is believed that some new antigens may appear, subsequently changing the immune reactions. According to certain researchers, there are "suicide genes" whose activity causes the destruction of the cell and the organism at a definite stage of development. According to Denckla (1974), hormone synthesis, which suppresses tissue respiration, is activated in old age.

Thus, the age changes in genome regulation can cause many changes in protein biosynthesis in old age, ranging from initial changes, which are revealed only during intensive activity, to gross changes, which cause the death of a cell. Another important fact is that the changes in genome regulation curtail the potentialities of the protein biosynthesis systems, thus limiting the functional abilities of the cell, the tissue and the organ. We have shown that protein biosynthesis and the energy processes of cardiac hypertrophy do not intensify adequately in the case of cardiac hyperfunction in old rats (Frolkis, 1975). This is one of the causes of the more rapid and fatal development of cardiac insufficiency in old animals. The data obtained by Novikova, our fellow worker, on a change in some indices of protein metabolism in mature and old rats after the loss of blood are given in Fig. 65 A, B, C. When the plasma proteins are lost, their biosynthesis intensifies in the liver and, consequently, the protein pattern of blood is restored. This important adaptive mechanism is weakened in old animals, and the restoration processes occur less intensively in them.

Hormonal Regulation of the Genetic Induction of Enzymes

The genetic induction of enzymes is an important molecular adaptive regulatory mechanism and a significant manifestation of vitauct. Owing to enzymic synthesis, the cell adapts itself to the changed conditions of existence and the changed level of activity, thus preserving and enhancing its viability. If it were not for this, the prolonged changes in the function and metabolism would have inevitably increased the disharmony between the abilities of the cell and the requirements of the organism or the environment, thus causing the death of the cell. Enzymic induction can be of either a substrate or a hormonal nature. Both types of induction are based on the shifts in genome regulation and the activation of the transcription of definite genes. The age changes in the genetic induction of enzymes are being thoroughly studied (Frolkis, 1970; Adelman, 1975; Kanungo, 1975; Parina, Kaliman, 1979). However, it has been noted that the age dynamics of enzymic induction does not have a single pattern. Adelman (1975) singles out several types of age changes in enzymic adaptation: (1) those involving enzymes with an increased lag-period of their induction in old age but with the same growth of activity during different age periods; (2) those involving enzymes with the same duration of the lag-period of adaptation and with the least growth of activity in old age; (3) the combination of these types, and (4) the complete identity of enzymic induction during various age periods.

Obviously, any classification is arbitrary. This is also true of the above-mentioned one. Of course, there are other types of changes in the nature of enzymic adaptation in old age. The inductive synthesis of some enzymes can be more intensive in old age than during other age periods. According to Parina and Kaliman (1979), the activity of aspartate aminotransferase grows more in Wistar rats 24 months old (by 153 per cent) than in thos 1, 3 and 12 months old (by 128, 125 and 124 per cent, respectively) when the amount of casein increases in their food. Shabanova and Amiri (1975) have shown that the activity of hexokinase in the liver of old rats, which ate food with a high content of starch for 5 days, had increased by 82 per cent, while it increased by 34 and 50 per cent, respectively, in rats 1 and 3 months old. During starvation, the activity of glucose-6-phosphatase increased by 213 per cent in the liver of rats 24 months old, by 146 per cent in that of rats 12 months old, by 151 per cent in rats 3 months old, and by 202 per cent in rats 1 month old. The unchangeability and even the growth of synthesis of several enzymes are an important adaptive regulatory mechanism in old age.

The induction of microsomal oxidation is an important system of inductive enzymes. We have already seen that the existence and evolutionary development of this system, its relatively high stability and reliability throughout life, and its clearly expressed inductive ability are an extremely important manifestation of vitauct, which protects the organism from the action of endogenous and exogenous toxic substances. The powerful system of microsomal oxidation counteracts the inevitable appearance and accumulation of metabolites, which are occasionally toxic and which undoubtedly influence the course of the organism's aging. According to our data (Frolkis, Paramonova, 1980), the activity of the basic enzymes of this system does not change substantially in old age. However, the ability to induce the enzymes of the microsomal oxidation system differs in animals of different age. The inductive synthesis of microsomal oxidases is the most active in young animals (Müller, Klinger, 1978). When phenobarbital is administered, the lag-period of the action of the inducing agent is longer and the maximum inductive effect occurs later in old rats than in young ones (Adelman, 1971). The administration of phenobarbital reduces hexenal sleep in young rats, but does not change it in old ones (Rozanova *et al.*, 1978).

Experiments with the regenerating liver of young and old rats have shown that the population of the newly formed cells (after partial hepatectomy) can respond to the effect of the inducing agent to the same extent as the hepatic cells of intact animals of the same age (Baird *et al.*, 1976). In this case, the reaction and its extent in old rats which were subjected to hepatectomy are the same as in intact animals (Adelman, 1971).

According to Birnbaum and Baird (1978), hexenal sleep decreases and the activity of oxazole hydroxylase and NADPH cytochrome c reductase as well as the content of cytochrome P450 increases to the same extent in rats of different age. Moreover, the activity of the NADPH cytochrome P450 reductase increases five times in young rats and eight times in old ones, and the activity of ethylmorphine-N-demethylase increases twice and 3.5 times, respectively, when the polychlorobiphenyl Arochlore-1254 is administered (Birnbaum, Baird, 1978). The authors concluded from these data that the change in the effects of several pharmacological agents in old animals is connected not with the functional state of the system of the microsomal oxidation of the liver, but with several extrahepatic factors, such as the sensitivity of the central nervous system to the action of narcotics, etc. According to Paramonova (1981), the administration of barbiturates for 3 days to rats 1, 3, 6 and 25 months old increases the activity of aminopyrine-N-demethylase of the microsomes of the liver by 3.6, 2.2, 2.3 and 1.4 times, respectively, while the content of the cytochrome P450 is increased by 8.3, 4.4, 2.7 and 1.7 times, respectively (Fig. 66A, B, C). The content of microsomal protein is subjected to similar changes which are expressed less.

The induction of the microsomal oxidases of the liver reduces the duration of narcotic sleep. This reduction is expressed more clearly and occurs earlier in young rats than in mature and old ones. Thus, the ability to induce enzymes is reduced in old rats in spite of the fact that the age differences between mature and old animals in both the content and activity of microsomal oxidases are absent.

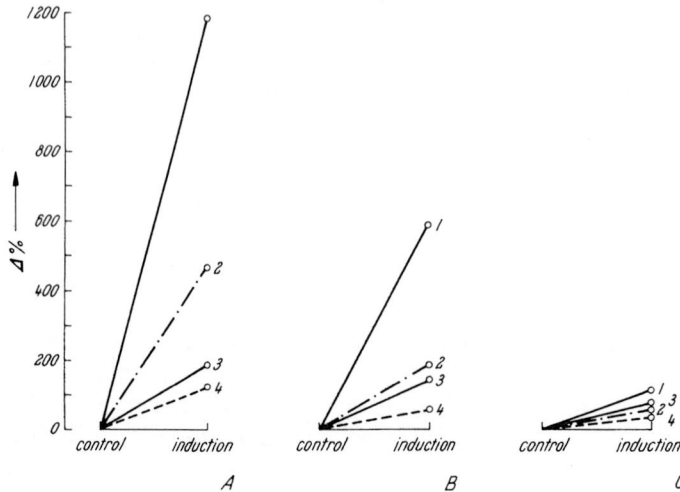

Fig. 66. Influence of the 3-day administration of barbiturates on the content of the cytochromes P-450 (A) and B$_5$ (B) and the aminopyridine demethylase activity of the hepatic microsomes (C) in rats of different age: 1 rats 1 month old; 2 rats 3 months old; 3 rats 6 months old; 4 rats 25 months old

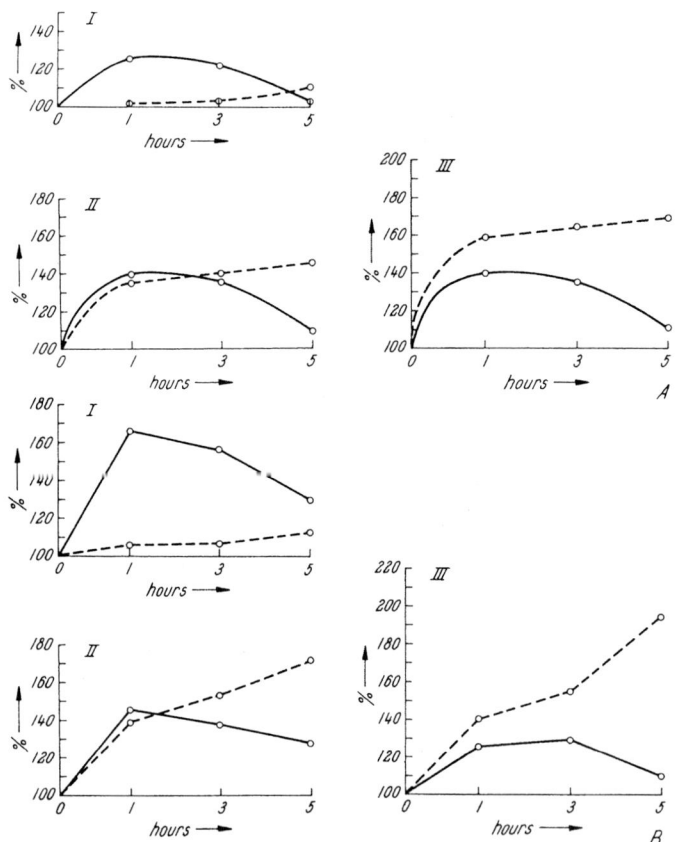

Fig. 67. Change in the activity of tyrosine aminotransferase, depending on the doses of tyrosine (A) and hydrocortisone (B) in mature rats and old rats. A I administration of 1–5 mg/kg of tyrosine; II administration of 10 mg/kg of tyrosine; III administration of 150 mg/kg of tyrosine. B I administration of 10 mg/kg of hydrocortisone; II administration of 30 mg/kg hydrocortisone; III administration of 50 mg/kg of hydrocortisone. Initial enzymic activity is taken as 100 per cent. The dashed line stands for mature rats, and the continuous line, for old rats

Many contradictions in the characterization of the genetic induction of enzymes could be eliminated if this process were studied with the aid of a wide range of loads and were described as a dose-dependent one. We have shown this by studying the induction of tyrosine aminotransferase. Fig. 67A, B shows that the increment of enzymic activity is higher in old rats when small doses of tyrosine are administered, that the age differences are levelled out when medium doses are administered, and that the growth of enzymic activity is maximal in mature animals when large doses are administered. In the last case, there is no additional growth of enzymic activity in old animals. Hence, the possible range of adaptations of the enzyme decreases and its potentialities become limited as the organism age. However, this regulatory system loses its stable state easier in old age. Such relationships have also been shown by taking the induction of tryptophan pyrrolase as an example. Of course, this regularity does not apply to the induction of all enzymes in old age. It substantiates the need to use the principle of force relations in order to characterize this system, which is being regulated.

Hormones play an extremely important role in the mechanism of the genome's supracellular regulation. Neurohormonal control of the activity of the genetic apparatus of the cells ensures the unity of the "general" and the "local" in achieving the adaptive effect of the whole organism. Hormones are cardinal in genome regulation and in the formation of the organism at the earliest stages of ontogeny. Hormones play the leading role in the structural and chemical organization of the oocyte, in the transition from one larval stage to another in insects, in the maturation of oocytes, and in other processes. The development of the fertilized oocyte is upset at the initial stages of its formation when the formation of the local hormones is disturbed and their action is blocked. The hormonal regulation of the genetic apparatus is important at the later stages of ontogeny.

The hormonal regulation of the genome is largely a preventive process, i. e. it mobilizes the mechanisms of the activation of protein biosynthesis; these mechanisms are later needed for the activity and structural restoration of the cells. This is the significance of the participation of the hormones in the most fundamental adaptive mechanisms. A change in and the disturbance of the mechanisms of hormonal regulation are among the main causes of both a change in the regulation of the genome and the aging of the cells.

The effect of the hormones on various links of protein biosynthesis is now being thoroughly studied. Apparently, there are several ways in which the hormone exerts its regulating influence on the genetic apparatus of the cells. One of them is connected with the action on the membrane hormonal receptors, the activation of the appropriate cyclases and the synthesis of cyclic nucleotides (Johnson, Hadden, 1977). It has been shown that a link can be formed between 3,5-AMP and a protein of low molecular weight. This complex interacts with the promotor part of the operon and activates the transcription of the appropriate mRNA. Another way in which cyclic nucleotides exert their influence is through the system of protein kinases, which realize the phosphate modification of proteins, including definite histone and non-histone proteins.

Consequently, the activity of both transcription and RNA synthesis changes. The phosphorylation of the non-histone proteins is believed to cause the breakdown of the complex consisting of the repressor and the genome regulator. This depresses the DNA locus and stimulates RNA synthesis.

Protein biosynthesis is stimulated by steroid hormones in a different way. The protein receptors of the steroid hormones are known to be in the cytosol of the cells. They are believed to consist of various subunits which link the hormones in different concentrations. The complex consisting of protein and steroid hormones in the nucleus of the cells becomes bound mainly with the acid proteins of chromatin. Consequently, several modifications occur in chromatin, i. e. DNA methylation is stimulated, the RNA polymerases of the nucleus become more active, the content of euchromatin increases and that of heterochromatin decreases, the RNA polymerase reaction is activated, especially at the elongation stage, polypeptide synthesis is stimulated, and so forth. Ultimately, this intensifies the synthesis of definite proteins and induces the enzymes (Sergeev et al., 1971; Protasova, 1975). Alanine, asparagine, tyrosine, histidine, phenylalanine aminotransferases, glucose-6-phosphate dehydrogenase, transketolase, malate and glycerophosphate dehydrogenases, tryptophan oxygenase, glucose-6-phosphatase, fructose-1,6-diphosphatase and other enzymes are activated already a few hours after glucocorticoids are administered.

Thus, the hormonal induction of the enzymes is an extremely important mechanism of development at the earliest stages of ontogeny. This type of regulation of protein biosynthesis is important when the organism is being formed and when it grows and ages, while its change is an important link in the mechanism of vitauct and aging. It has been shown that the substrate induction of several enzymes also has a hormonal mechanism. After adrenalectomy, for instance, tyrosine does not cause the growth of tyrosine aminotransferase activity. Hence, an important regulatory mechanism, i. e. that which links up the substrate, the hormone and genic activity, has become consolidated during evolution.

The hormonal induction of the enzymes changes with age. The nature of the change in the induction of different enzymes varies, since it is determined by the state of a genetic locus as well as by the amount of the hormone and its penetration into the cell. The available data on the hormonal induction of enzymes during aging are diverse. This is because animals of different strains were used in experiments and the hormone doses varied. According to Gregerman (1959), the activity of tyrosine aminotransferase grows approximately to the same extent in Wistar rats 1 and 2 years old when corticosterone is adminstered to them, while according to Adelman and Freeman (1972), the increment of enzymic activity is somewhat higher in old Sprague-Dowley rats when the hormone is administered. According to Finch and others (1969), this activity grows somewhat more in young animals (C57BL/6J mice). According to our data, the age differences vary, depending on the dose of the hormone (Frolkis, Mandelblat, 1970; see Fig. 42). The regulation of the biosynthesis of various enzymes changes differently with age: the genetic induction of various enzymes changes differently and occasionally in different directions in response to the administration of the same hormone.

A decrease in enzymic induction is observed not only in old age, but also at the preceding stages of ontogeny. According to Parina and Kaliman (1979), for instance, fructose-1,6-diphosphatase, phosphoenol pyruvate carboxykinase, serine hydratase, aspartate aminotransferase, alanine aminotransferase and other enzymes are activated more in rats 1 month old than in rats of other ages when hydrocortisone is administered. According to Shabanova and Amiri (1975), tyroxine induces aldolase only in immature rats. Thus, the intensity of the genetic induction of enzymes changes throughout ontogeny. Every stage of individual development has its own pattern of both the activity of the enzymes and their ability to undergo induction.

Interestingly, the substrate and hormonal inductions of the enzymes change differently as the organism ages. By old age, the hormonal induction of several enzymes changes more than the substrate one. This is connected to a certain extent with the clearly expressed shifts in the reception of the hormonal effect. The data presented by Bulankina (1973) are interesting in this respect. She studied the age changes in the genetic induction of alanine transferase in the liver after the administration of hydrocortisone and the excessive consumption of protein, which intensifies enzymic activity by itself. An analysis of the combined and separate effects of both factors on enzymic activity has shown that the effects overlap in young and mature rats. When these factors are combined in rats 24 months old, the relative increment of the activity of alanine transferase is the sum of the increments produced by the independent action of each of them. Parina and Kaliman (1979) have emphasized that these data indicate the existence of certain common links in the mechanism of enzymic induction of each factor in young and mature rats. The spheres of action of both factors are separated clearly in old rats. Therefore, the effects of the separate action of these factors are summed up when the factors are combined. This is probably connected with the age shifts in hormonal reception.

The nature of the changes in inductive synthesis is largely determined by the state of either the effector link of the genome itself or the receptors which are sensitive to the action of a hormone. This is evident from the fact that the induction of various enzymes changes differently with age when the same hormone is introduced. We compared the effects of hydrocortisone on the induction of tyrosine aminotransferase, tryptophan pyrrolase, glucose-6-phosphatase, and fructose-1,6-diphosphatase. When small doses of hydrocortisone are administered, the shift in the activity of tyrosine aminotransferase and tryptophan pyrrolase is more pronounced in the liver of old rats, while the shift in the activity of glucose-6-phosphatase and fructose-1,6-diphosphatase is more pronounced in the liver of mature rats.

An important fact is that organs have their specifics, especially with respect to the hormonal induction of enzymes. The induction of glucose-6-phosphatase and fructose-1,6-diphosphatase is different in the liver, the kidneys, the spleen and the heart with aging (Muradian, 1977a).

The inductive synthesis of enzymes changes with age under the effect of other hormones with a different site of action and with a membrane localization of the receptors. For instance, Litoshenko (1977) has shown that insulin causes less pronounced shifts in the activity of total hexokinase and in its individual isoenzymes in old animals. This mechanism can limit the insulin regulation of carbohydrate metabolism in old age.

Adelman (1975) discusses the change in hormonal induction in old age and believes that there are several mechanisms in this respect. They are (1) changes at the stage of the hormone-receptor interaction, including shifts in the affinity of the receptor for the hormone, a change in the number of available and functioning receptors (although, according to Roth [1979], and affinity of the receptors for glucocorticoids and their ability to bind them do not change in old age), and a change in the ability to activate transcription; (2) a change in the concentration of the hormone in the blood due to shifts in the secretion of the hormone and its removal from the blood, and (3) a change in the physiological effectiveness of the hormones. However, these assumptions seem to lack the most important factor, i. e. a change in genome regulation, which is the ultimate process that makes it possible to read genetic information. The changes in the genetic induction of various enzymes would be more or less of a single type if the mechanism of the age changes in induction were connected mainly with the shifts in the concentration of the hormone and with its effectiveness. However, they differ in not only the extent of the shift, but also direction. In some cases, Adelman describes the sharp decrease in enzymic induction in animals older than 1 month that cannot be explained by shifts in the concentration of the hormone or by a change in its effectiveness.

Many hormones influence the activity of not merely one gene, but a set of genetic loci, and they change the biosynthesis of many proteins. This is achieved mainly by their effect on the main structural mechanism which regulates the genetic apparatus: the chromatin complex. In their works, Khilobok and Goldstein compared the changes in the correlation between active and repressed chromatin as well as their transcribing ability under the action of hydrocortisone and insulin (Fig. 68 A, B). One of these hormones acts through the membrane receptors, while the other, through the receptors on chromatin. It has been found that great differences exist in the reaction of chromatin in old age, and that they are expressed to a different extent under the action of insulin and hydrocortisone. Under the action of hydrocortisone, the maximum incorporation of the label into active and inactive chromatin is observed earlier in old animals than in mature ones. Other relationships originate when insulin is administered: its maximum incorporation and intensity are higher in mature rats.

It follows that genome regulation changes with age. This inevitably disturbs the reaction of the genome to the action of the most important regulatory factors: hormones. The concentration of hormones and occasionally their state change under physiological conditions. When this is combined with the shifts in the regulatory system of the genome, the age changes in protein biosynthesis become very diverse. The regulation of transcription is one of the main mechanisms of hormonal induction. In our laboratory, Muradian (1977b) studied the effect of hydrocortisone on the synthesis of various classes of RNA. He showed that there were definite differences in the synthesis of pre-rRNA and pre-mRNA fractions. The stimulation of pre-mRNA synthesis was far more pronounced in the liver of adult rats, while the growth of pre-mRNA transcription did not differ substantially in animals of different ages. Hence, the differences in the reaction of the genome to the hormone are revealed in the specifics of transcription. Thus, the age specifics of protein biosynthesis in the aging organism can be determined largely by the shifts in both the concentration and activity of the hormones and by the reaction of the genome regulation system to these shifts.

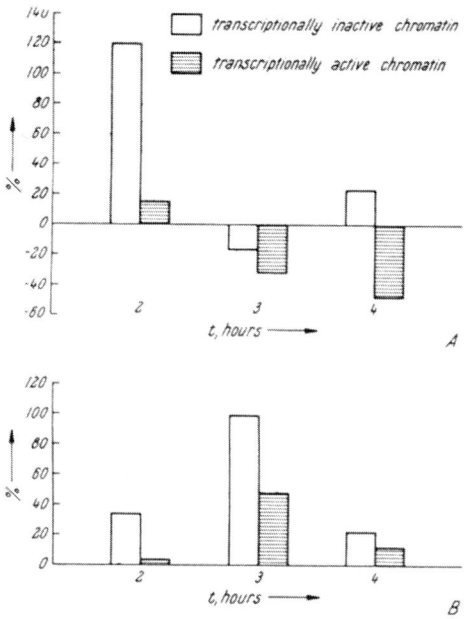

Fig. 68. Percentage of the change in the intensity of RNA synthesis in the chromatin of the liver of mature rats (A) and old rats (B) under the influence of four units of insulin

The possibilities of that system cannot be fully characterized by assessing the reaction to a single dose of a hormone. The genome is often controlled by prolonged, repeating hormonal stimuli under natural conditions of existence. Moreover, life and time inevitably create the conditions for the constantly repeating effects of the regulatory factors on the tissues and cells. Therefore, it is necessary to ascertain the potentialities of the appropriate protein-synthesizing system. According to Salganik (1972), the hepatic cells lose their ability to react to the action of an inductor by intensifying RNA synthesis and promoting enzymic activity when the inductor is administered for a long time. This "break" in the ability of the cells to undergo induction and the "exhaustion" of the genic regulatory system are prolonged.

We have shown in our works (Frolkis, Mandelblat, 1970; Frolkis, 1970, 1975; Frolkis, Muradian, 1976; Frolkis et al., 1979a) that the potentialities of the genic regulatory system decrease in old age. It can be seen in Fig. 69A, B that the long administration of hydrocortisone causes the clearly expressed growth of the activity of tyrosine aminotransferase, glucose-6-phosphatase and fructose-1,6-diphosphatase. Enzymic activity begins to decrease when the

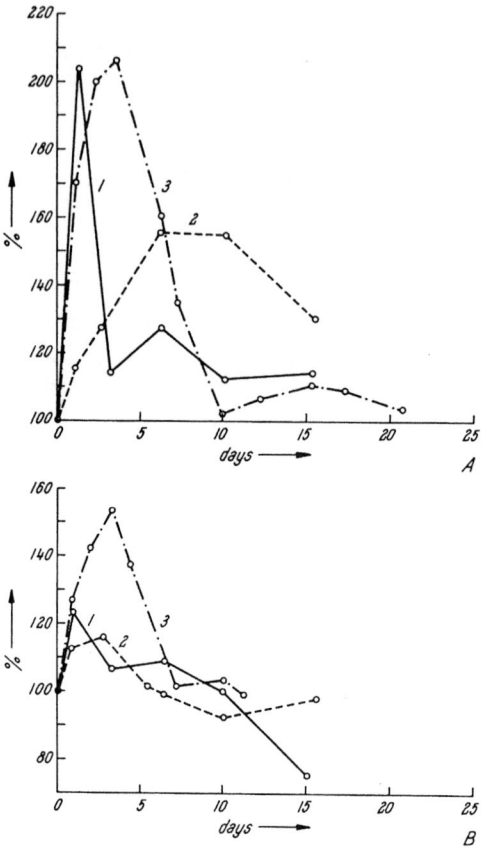

Fig. 69. Influence of the multiple administration of hydrocortisone (daily, 35 mg/kg) on the activity of fructose-1,6-diphosphatase *(1)*, glucose-6-phosphatase *(2)* and tyrosine aminotransferase *(3)* in the liver of mature rats *(A)* and old rats *(B)*

hormone is administered for a long time. This is expressed more clearly in old animals. Even when the hormone is continuously administered, the activity of tyrosine aminotransferase returns to the initial level by the 7th day in old rats. The activity of glucose-6-phosphatase and fructose-1,6-diphosphatase is also restored earlier in old rats than in mature ones. Hence, with age, the system which regulates the synthesis of definite proteins weakens and becomes "exhausted" sooner. It becomes less reliable and cannot ensure a high and stable level of protein biosynthesis when hormonal stimulation is prolonged. Such a situation may occur also under physiological conditions. Therefore, it is quite right to maintain that the limitation of the potentialities of the genic regulatory system is one of the most important mechanisms of the development of functional insufficiency and aging. The characterization of the stages of the process that precede protein synthesis indicates the decisive role which the change in protein synthesis plays in the given phenomenon of the "exhaustion" of the genetic induction of enzymes.

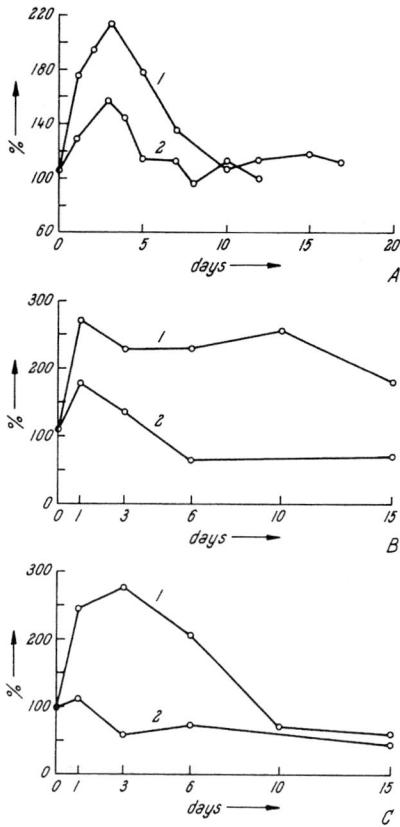

Fig. 70. Influence of the multiple administration of hydrocortisone (daily, 35 mg/kg) on the specific radioactivity of the preribosomal *(A)*, premessenger *(B)* and heterogenous nuclear *(C)* RNA in the liver of mature rats *(1)* and old rats *(2)*

Salganik (1972) has shown that the decrease in the rate of RNA synthesis is one of the main causes of the "exhaustion" of the inductive mechanisms of the cell. Our data on the change in the specific activity and the relative specific activity of the RNA fractions when hydrocortisone is administered for a long time also show that the transcription apparatus is suppressed during prolonged hormonal induction (Fig. 70A, B, C). The dynamics of this process differs in various RNA fractions. For instance, the specific radioactivity of the nuclear RNA fraction sharply increases in adult rats during the 1st day after the administration of the hormone. This increase continues with slight fluctuations until the 6th day. By the 10th day, specific radioactivity is on a high level only in the preribosomal and cytoplasmic fractions, while the radioactivity of the pre-mRNA and pre-rRNA mixture diminishes substantially. By the 15th day of the administration of the hormone, the specific radioactivity of pre-rRNA also begins to diminish, while that of pre-mRNA drops below the initial level. The inductive effect of pre-mRNA is "exhausted" more rapidly than that of pre-rRNA probably because the latter is represented in the mammalian genomes by redundant copies, while the messenger RNA is represented by several or single DNA loci and apparently carries a greater functional load.

Just as in a series of experiments involving the determination of enzymic activity, the specific radioactivity and the relative specific radioactivity of the RNA fractions in the liver of old rats grow to a much smaller extent under the effect of hydrocortisone, while the "break" in stimulation occurs earlier. In this age group, the specific radioactivity of pre-mRNA decreases earlier than that of pre-rRNA. As the organism ages, the activation of RNA fractions synthesis in liver cells following prolonged administration of hydrocortisone decreases.

The changes in genome regulation during prolonged genetic induction are so great that they can be observed when the chromatin properties are being studied (Goldstein et al., 1977).

Thus, the insufficiency of the genic regulatory system is revealed earlier under the conditions of prolonged tension in old age, and this makes the plastic insurance of the function more limited. The limitation of the potentialities of the protein-synthesizing system circumscribes the functional abilities of the cell. Hence, the attenuation of the restoration processes in the genic regulatory system is an extremely important cause of a decrease in its abilities during aging. Evidence of this was found in a special experiment. In the investigations carried out by Folbort's school (1968), restoration of the response to a load following exhaustive activity was the objective criterion of the restoration of the system. In a special series of experiments, the administration of the hormone was tested after a 3-day break in an "exhaustive" load (the daily administration of hydro-cortisone) on the tyrosine aminotransferase synthesis system. It was found that the ability to synthesize the hormone was restored very poorly in old animals: in mature rats, the increment of the activity of the hormone was 80 per cent of the initial level, while in old rats, it was 38 per cent. We have every reason to believe that such shifts originate not only during the hormonal stimulation of protein biosynthesis. A prolonged load on the function of both the cell and an organ is knwon to cause their hypertrophy, which is based on intensified protein biosynthesis (Meerson, 1978). This is an extremely important adaptive regulatory mechanism which makes it possible to maintain the function on a high level for a long time. It is expressed clearly during myocardial hyperfunction. We have shown in a series of works that protein biosynthesis is activated to a smaller extent and that hypertrophy due to a greater load on the myocardium is developed less in old age, and this is an extremely important cause of cardiac insufficiency (Frolkis et al., 1976d, 1977). In old age, the genetic induction of various enzymes changes differently: that of some enzymes either does not change or decreases, while that of others grows. Parina and Kaliman (1979), for instance, have shown that glucose-6-phosphatase is induced to the greatest extent in the liver of old rats. Parina and others (1976) have observed that the activity of hexokinase does not change in Wistar rats 1 month old, while it sharply grows in old ones under the action of insulin. It is interesting to study the hormonal induction of isoenzymes, which makes it possible to determine the state of regulation of a definite genetic locus. In studying the effect of tyroxine on the isoenzymic range of lactate dehydrogenase, Kaliman and Amiri (1977) have shown that different changes occur in various organs of rats with age. Tyroxine does not cause any substantial shifts in the correlations of the isoenzymes as well as the H and M subunits in the heart and kidneys of old animals, while these shifts are even more pronounced in the muscles of these animals.

Fig. 67 shows Mandelblat's and our data on the age specifics of the genetic induction of tyrosine aminotransferase. Interestingly, the situation caused by the administration of tyrosine is repeated when various doses of hydrocortisone are administered. When the doses of the hormone are small, the increment of enzymic activity is the greatest in old rats, and when the doses are large, it is the greatest in adult rats, while the age differences are levelled out in the case of medium doses.

Noteworthy is the fact that large doses cause a far smaller growth of enzymic activity in comparison with medium and small doses. When large doses are administered, the "disengagement phenomenon" originates. We have shown this by taking the systemic reactions as an example. The phenomenon is revealed under the action of steroid hormones, which penetrate inside the cell and which directly contact the chromatin receptors.

Hypothalamohypophysial-Adrenal System of the Regulation of the Genetic Apparatus

Any hormone is one of the links of the complex self-regulatory system. A systemic approach should be made in order to understand the mechanisms of the neurohumoral regulation of protein biosynthesis in the cell under the conditions of an intact organism. In other words, a study should be made of the shifts which occur when the activity of the whole regulatory system changes. However, the presently available factual material is based on a study of only one link of the system: the hormone-tissue-target link.

The hypothalamohypophysial-adrenal cortex-target-tissue system is especially significant in the realization of the most important adaptive reactions. The formation of the hypothalamohypophysial region of the brain during the antenatal and postnatal periods is known to determine the formation and development of the whole endocrine situation of the organism that controls the processes of protein biosynthesis and morphogenesis. The age changes in hypo-thalamohypophysial regulation are believed to be an extremely important mechanism of the intact organism's aging. It has been shown that the hypo-thalamohypophysial regulation of the activity of individual endocrine glands as well as the cardiovascular and respiratory systems and the participation of this system in stress reactions change with age. However, not enough interest is being taken in the hypothalamohypophysial regulation of protein biosynthesis.

In several researches which we carried out together with Bezrukov and Muradian (Frolkis et al., 1976a; Muradian, 1977), we studied the effect of various links of the hypothalamohypophysial-adrenal system on both the synthesis of various RNA classes and the genetic induction of the synthesis of glucose-6-phosphatase and fructose-1,6-diphosphatase. In these experiments, we tried to ascertain the link in the system of both the hypothalamohypophysial-adrenal system and the genetic apparatus of tissues that limits its potentialities during aging. The changes in the synthesis of the RNA of various classes and in enzymic induction were compared when various links of the system were successively stimulated, i. e. when hydrocortisone and corticotropin were administered and the hypothalamus was stimulated. Data have already been given on the changes which occur in the activity of the enzymes of glyconeogenesis and RNA synthesis when hydrocortisone is administered.

Hydrocortisone produces a different stimulating effect on RNA synthesis in various structures of the genetic apparatus. Consequently, not only the RNA polymerase activity of several subnuclear hepatic structures, but also the correlation between various classes of the RNA that is being newly synthesized change when hydrocortisone is administered. For instance, when the specific radioactivity of pre-rRNA is taken as one, the ratio of the specific radioactivities of pre-rRNA, a mixture of pre-rRNA and pre-mRNA, pre-mRNA and heterogeneous nRNA is 1 : 3 : 4 : 4 on the 1st day, 1 : 3 : 6 : 3 on the 3rd day, 1 : 2 : 5 : 5 on the 6th day, and 1 : 1 : 1 : 4 on the 15th day after the administration of hydrocortisone to mature rats as compared with 1 : 3 : 5 : 4 in the control animals; it is 1 : 2 : 3 : 3 on the 1st day, 1 : 2 : 2 : 6 on the 3rd day, 1 : 2 : 5 : 3 on the 6th day, and 1 : 2 : 2 : 3 on the 15th day after the administration of the hormone to old rats as compared with 1 : 4 : 4 : 3 in the control animals of the same age.

Corticotropin activates the adrenal cortex when the organism's activity is systemic. In another series of experiments, we studied the shifts in both the synthesis of various RNA classes and enzymic activity when 20 U/kg of corticotropin was administered. Using rats of the same strain and the same corticotropin preparations, Bekker and Lisitskaya have shown that the hormone doses, which cause the maximum secretion of glucocorticoids by the adrenal cortex, are about 20 U/kg. The latent period of the induction of glucose-6-phosphatase and fructose-1,6-diphosphatase in the kidneys and the liver, being engendered by the administration of corticotropin, grows with age. When the hormone is administered for a long time, the inductive effect is higher, while "exhaustion" sets in later in the liver and the kidneys of young rats. Approximately the same changes occur in both the synthesis of various RNA classes and enzymic induction when hydrocortisone and corticotropin are administered. It follows from the identical activation of the genetic apparatus that the adrenal cortex is not a link which limits the regulatory abilities of the hypothalamohypophysial-adrenal system. In other words, when corticotropin is administered, the age changes in the mechanisms of the activation of the genetic tissue-target apparatus are determined not so much by the response of the adrenal cortex as by the age changes in the tissues.

In an intact organism, the regulatory system is "triggered" by hypothalamic structures. In our experiments, we studied the effect of the single and repeated stimulation of the hypothalamus on the inductive synthesis of several enzymes (tyrosine aminotransferase, tryptophan pyrrolase, glucose-6-phosphatase and fructose-1,6-diphosphatase) as well as the synthesis of various RNA classes. According to Dunn and Critchlow (1971) as well as Konovalova (1974), the ventromedial nucleus is one of the main structural zones of the hypothalamus that can stimulate the hypophysial-adrenal system to the greatest extent. In our experiments, we implanted bipolar electrodes into the ventromedial nucleus of the hypothalamus of rats. The hypothalamus of the freely moving animals was stimulated by rectangular impulses of the current (the frequency was 100 impulses per second, an impulse lasted one millisecond, and stimulation took 10–15 minutes). The polarity of the current was changed every 30 seconds. The force of the stimulation current was selected by intensifying it until clear-cut changes in behaviour (alertness, sniffing and agitation) appeared. The current was 50–120 μA for mature animals and 80–110 μA for old ones.

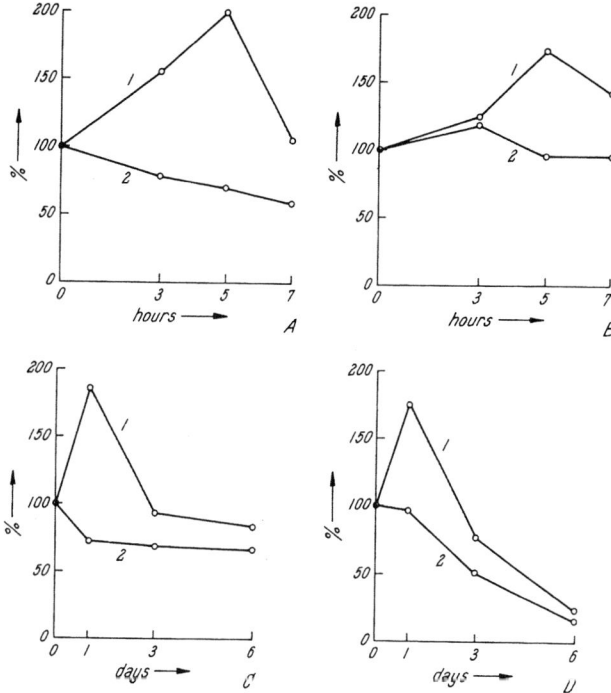

Fig. 71. Influence of the single (A, B) and multiple (C, D) stimulation of the hypothalamus on the activity of glucose-6-phosphatase (A, C) and fructose-1,6-diphosphatase (B, D) in mature rats (1) and old rats (2). The abscissa in A, B shows the time after stimulation, and the abscissa in C, D shows the number of days of hypothalamic stimulation. The ordinate stands for enzymic activity (%)

The single stimulation of the hypothalamus causes changes in the activity of glucose-6-phosphatase, fructose-1,6-diphosphatase (see Fig. 71A, B, C, D), tyrosine aminotransferase and tryptophan pyrrolase that are less pronounced in old animals than in mature ones. Hence, the effect of the hypothalamus on the mechanisms which are responsible for the genetic induction of enzymes is far weaker in old age.

Situations of the repeated and prolonged activation of the hypothalamus occasionally occur when the organism exists under natural conditions.

According to some authors, the frequently repeating stresses, which are realized through the hypothalamohypophysial pathways, are one of the main causes of the intact organism's aging. The age changes in the hypothalamic regulation of RNA biosynthesis are clearly manifested only when stimulation is performed many times. In old animals, the synthesis of both the RNA fractions and the enzyme proteins are suppressed more rapidly when stimulation is repeated (see Fig. 71). These age differences are expressed differently in various RNA classes. For instance, the specific radioactivity of pre-mRNA in the liver of adult rats greatly increases (by 163 per cent) on the 3rd day of hypothalamic stimulation, while it returns to the initial level on the 6th day of stimulation. In old rats, the specific radioactivity of pre-mRNA drops below the initial level even during the 1st day of stimulation, and it remains on a low level during the whole period of investigation. When the hypothalamus is repeatedly stimulated, substantial age distinctions are observed also in the heterogeneous nRNA fraction, whose specific radioactivity is maintained on a higher level in mature animals. However, such differences have not been observed in both the pre-rRNA fraction and cytoplasmic RNA.

The complex system of neurohumoral regulation becomes involved in the reaction when the hypothalamus is stimulated. We have every reason to believe that the given shifts which occur in RNA synthesis when the hypothalamus is stimulated are connected with the changes exactly in that link. Firstly, when hydrocortisone or corticotropin is administered for a long time, RNA synthesis becomes less intense and enzymic induction occurs much later than when the hypothalamus is stimulated. For instance, when the hypothalamus is stimulated many times, the intensity of the synthesis of various RNA classes and inducible enzymes drops below the initial level from the 3rd to the 6th day of stimulation, while functioning remains on a high level until the 10th or even the 15th day when the genetic apparatus of the hepatic cells is stimulated many times by the administration of hydrocortisone or corticotropin. Secondly, we have shown that the content of corticosterone, ascorbic acid and cholesterol decreased in the adrenal glands of adult animals when the hypothalamus was stimulated. These indices virtually did not change in old rats. Hence, the "exhaustion" effect of hypothalamic stimulation originated in them when the functional state of other links of the hypothalamohypophysial-adrenal system was on a sufficiently high level. The stimulation of the hypothalamus may also influence protein biosynthesis in the target tissues through the cholinergic and adrenergic neural mechanisms. The weakening of neural control, which has been shown by our fellow workers on the basis of various objects, probably plays a definite role in the mechanisms of the given changes in hypothalamic regulation.

These data show that the hypothalamus participates in the regulation of the synthesis of various RNA classes in the target tissues. The hypothalamic regulation of this synthesis changes with age. This can largely be due to the changes in the biosynthesis of RNA and protein in the hypothalamus itself and in tissues which participate in the transfer of hypothalamic effects. A comparison of the dynamics of the specific radioactivity of the RNA classes and the intensity of enzymic induction when individual links of the hypothalamo-hypophysial-adrenal system are stimulated suggests that the potentialities of the mechanisms of the prolonged hypothalamic stimulation of the synthesis of RNA and protein are less than the ability of the target tissues to maintain the stimulation of the genetic apparatus for a long time. Since the repeated activation of the hypothalamus is always found under natural conditions of existence, it can be concluded that the given age decreases in hypothalamic control over the genetic apparatus plays an important role in the change of the adaptive reactions in old age and is an important mechanism of the intact organism's aging. The changes which occur with age in hypothalamic regulation can be a cause of the changes in protein biosynthesis in several target tissues.

We believe that the data on the specifics of the hypothalamohypophysial-adrenal regulation of protein biosynthesis are of fundamental significance in understanding the mechanisms of the intact organism's aging. They show that when the organism is intact, the limitation of both the plastic ensurance of the functions and the possible activation of the genetic apparatus of the tissues may be connected with shifts in other links of the self-regulatory system as well as shifts in the links which are far away from the target tissues, particularly the shifts in the central and hypothalamic mechanisms. In other words, as the organism ages, situations often occur when the genetic apparatus of the tissues "still can" react to the regulatory stimuli, while the centres do not realize this possibility. The rapid "break" in regulation and the "exhaustion" of the activity of the regulatory system during prolonged stimulation not only reveal important changes in the system during aging, but also can cause the disturbance of the regulatory mechanisms. Hence, it may be possible to influence the genetic apparatus by constant stimulation throughout life. We are now working on the establishment of a link between the species life span and the rate of development of the given changes when the genetic apparatus is stimulated by hormones for a long time. The species specificity of the genic regulatory system is believed to determine the possibilities of its prolonged functioning.

The control mechanisms greatly change with age, and this is one of the most important factors in the genesis of aging. Many changes in genome regulation are secondary with respect to the shifts in neurohumoral regulation.

11. Neurohumoral Regulation of the Energy Processes

Life is the unity of three flows: the flow of matter, the flow of energy and the flow of information.

Any manifestation of the organism's vitality requires a definite amount of energy. Energy expenditures and the work done in maintaining and developing biological orderliness are the essence of anti-entropy and vitauct that occur throughout ontogeny.

The hypotheses according to which aging was regarded as a unidirectional entropic process had been advanced at various stages of development of the biology of aging. Rubner (1908) was among the first to try to link the species life span with the expenditures of the energy potentials. Zotin (1974) regards development and aging as the gradual approach of the organism to the final stationary state, i. e. to death owing to constant thermal production and the diminution of the organism's energy potential. Fixed correlations between the species life span and energy expenditures are absent because of the role which the non-entropic processes and the vitauct mechanisms play in this respect.

At present, there is much factual material on definite mechanisms which reduce the reliability of the systems that provide the cells with energy in old age and on the adaptive mechanisms which are simultaneously switched on due to the self-regulation mechanisms.

Oxidative and Glycolytic Phosphorylation During Aging

The oxidative processes determine the energy potential of the cell and ensure the gradual, stepwise liberation of energy. Thus, energy is prevented from being greatly scattered and the cell is protected from the destructive action of thermal energy. In spite of these adaptive mechanisms, thermal disturbances, though limited by the perfect mechanisms of energy supply, inevitably occur throughout life and influence all the aspects of the vital activity of the cells, becoming one of the causes of cellular aging.

The mechanism which supplies various aspects of life with energy is more or less universal in spite of the diverse manifestations of the organism's activity and the diverse forms of adaptation to the environment. Most of the energy, being stored up by the cell in an easily usable form, i. e. in the form of ATP, is produced during oxidative and glycolytic phosphorylation. Some energy is stored up in the form of creatine phosphate, which is now believed to play an important role in the transport of energy.

According to most authors, tissue respiration, being expressed by the value of the oxygen consumption of the tissues (Qo_2), becomes less intense with age.

Table 9. *Intensity of tissue respiration (Qo_2) in the heart and the liver of rats of different ages*

| | Heart | | | | | Liver | | | | |
| | 8–12 months | | 28–32 months | | | 8–12 months | | 28–32 months | | |
	Qo_2 (M±m)	"extra" Qo_2	Qc_2 (M±m)	"extra" Qo_2	Age difference (p)	Qo_2 (M±m)	"extra" Qo_2	Qo_2 (M±m)	"extra" Qo_2	Age difference (p)
Absent	4.0 ±0.27	–	1.81±0.36	–	<0.001	2.80±0.17	–	1.86±0.10	–	<0.001
Lactate	7.14±1.63	3.14	4.59±0.70	2.78	>0.05	5.06±0.17	2.26	4.61±0.59	2.75	>0.05
Glucose	4.24±0.47	0.24	1.83±0.52	0.02	<0.001	–	–	–	–	–
Succinate	8.13±0.73	4.13	7.41±0.81	5.60	>0.05	8.76±0.50	5.96	6.36±0.6	4.50	<0.01
α-Ketoglutarate	9.04±1.04	5.04	6.21±0.75	4.40	<0.05	4.75±0.67	1.95	3.05±0.51	1.19	<0.05

It has been shown that this value diminishes in the homogenates and sections of the cardiac muscle, the spleen, the intestine, testicles, the liver, the blood vessels, and the cerebral cortex.

The intensity of respiration diminishes most of all in the cardiac muscle with age. This diminution is observed when both endogenous respiration and respiration in the presence of oxidative substrates are being determined (Table 9). An exception is the oxidation of succinate. When it is used, oxygen consumption in the heart of old rats does not differ from that in the heart of adult rats.

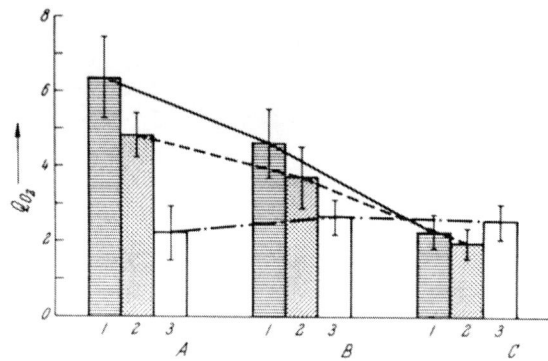

Fig. 72. Age specifics of a change in the intensity of the respiration of the myocardium of white rats when the oxygen content in the gas mixture differs. *A* rats 1 month old; *B* rats 8–12 months old; *C* rats 26–30 months old. *1* 93–95 per cent of oxygen; *2* 21 per cent of oxygen (air); *3* 2–3 per cent of oxygen in the gas mixture

According to our data, the diminution of Qo_2 in the liver is less pronounced in old age, while some researchers did not detect it at all (Rafsky *et al.*, 1952; Barrows *et al.*, 1958).

The potentialities of the activation of the intracellular systems of oxygen supply diminish with age. In a special series of experiments, we compared the oxygen consumption of the myocardial tissue of rats of different ages when the oxygen content varied in the medium (2–3, 21 and 93 95 per cent). Fig. 72A, B, C shows that the highest ratio between the intensity of tissue respiration and the partial pressure of oxygen is observed in rats 1 month old, while the lowest ratio, in old rats.

Nikitin (1963) divides all the tissues into three groups according to the intensity of oxygen consumption and the extent of its diminution. The first group comprises organs with a high level of respiration intensity (the kidneys, the heart, the spleen, the liver and the brain) and is characterized by the great diminution of oxygen consumption with age. The second group (the muscles, the intestine and the salivary glands) is characterized by the rapid diminution of tissue respiration at the initial stage and the slow rate of its diminution at the subsequent stages of ontogeny. The third group comprises the organs with low oxygen consumption (the skin and the cartilage) and an inconsiderable diminution of tissue respiration when old age is reached.

Heat "strokes," the appearance of metabolites, and the accumulation of free radicals during energy processes can damage the cell and promote its aging. A decrease in the intensity of oxidative processes during aging may be of adaptive significance.

The processes of respiration and oxidation are known to occur in mitochondria. Therefore, the age specifics of the oxidative processes are now being studied directly in the mitochondrial preparations from the organs and tissues. These studies have confirmed the concept that the oxidative processes decrease with age. However, the results turned out to be contradictory in some cases. For instance, Gold and others (1968) did not discover any age-dependent changes in the oxidation of beta oxybutyrate by the myocardial mitochondria, while Chen and others (1972) observed a sharp decrease in the intensity of oxidation of this as well as other substrates (glutamate + malate, glutamate + pyruvate, pyruvate + malate). However, these authors did not detect any decrease in the oxidation of succinate and alpha ketoglutarate, although Frolkis and Bogatskaya (1974) have shown that it decreases. A decrease in the respiration of cardiac mitochondria by 20–50 per cent in old rats as compared with adult ones was discovered also when the derivatives of fatty acids, e. g. palmitoyl carnitine, octanoate and the palmitoyl coenzyme A, were used as the oxidative substrates (Hansford, 1978). Thus, most of the data show that the oxidative activity of mitochondria diminishes with age.

However, an interesting fact is that the age differences in the intensity of tissue respiration are less pronounced when the oxidative substrates are added. A decrease in the content of the coenzyme A may be of the possible causes of the lack of oxidative substrates in old age (Nikitin, Martynenko, 1963). The incorporation of acetyl coenzyme A into the tricarboxylic acid cycle is reduced when there is a shortage of the coenzyme A. Consequently, the oxidative processes in the cycle may become less intense.

The substrates used by cells for energy purposes are redistributed in old age. According to Pashkova (1965), the ability of the myocardial tissue to oxidize fatty acids greatly decreases in old age. For instance, if the oxidation of caprylic acid by the myocardium is taken as 100 per cent in rats 1 month old, it is 70.9 per cent in rats 1 year old and 35.4 per cent in rats 2 years old. In the first group of rats, the cardiac muscle is capable of oxidizing 3.2 μmoles of caprylate and 2 μmoles of glucose in 1 hour, while in the last group of animals, it is capable of oxidizing 1.1 μmole of caprylate and 2 μmoles of glucose during the same length of time. If it is assumed that these substances are completely oxidized and produce the maximum ATP output, 256 μmoles of ATP are formed in rats 1 month old (196 μmoles due to fatty acids and 60 μmoles due to carbohydrates) and only 158 μmoles are formed in old rats (68 μmoles due to fatty acids and 90 μmoles due to carbohydrates).

A change in the structure and properties of mitochondria may be one of the reasons why their oxidative activity decreases with age. Mitochondria which have been isolated from the tissues of old animals are more sensitive to damaging influences and are less stable than those of young animals (Dietrich, Yero, 1965). Changes occur in the dimensions of these organelles and in the ratio of the volume of their matrix to the area of the membranes (Travis, Travis, 1972;

Tribe, Ashhurst, 1972; Herbener, 1976). It has been observed that the average volume of mitochondria and the amount of large mitochondria with a "foamy" vacuolated matrix increase in the liver and the heart of old mice (Wilson, Franks, 1975). The swelling of mitochondria, which occasionally even became hollow formations, was observed in the neurons of the cerebral cortex of old cats (Aksenova, 1971). Besides a decrease in the ratio of the area of cristae to the volume of mitochondria, the relationship of the lipid fractions in mitochondria changes mainly because the content of cholesterol increases in them (Grinna, 1977). Naturally, this can affect the permeability of the membranes of these organelles with respect to the oxidative substrates and oxygen, thus strongly influencing the oxidative activity of mitochondria.

The amount of mitochondria per unit mass of tissue decreases with age in the liver of rats, mice and man as well as in the heart of rats and mice (Herbener, 1976; Grinna, 1977; Abu-Erreish, Sanadi, 1978). This reduces tissue respiration, since its extent correlates with the concentration of mitochondria in the tissue. The shifts in the biosynthesis of mitochondrial proteins can be of great importance in the age changes which occur in energy metabolism. The investigations carried out by Litoshenko (1977, 1979, 1981) have shown that the replication of mitochondrial DNA in the liver and the synthesis of proteins which are coded by the mitochondrial genome slow down with age. These proteins play an important role in energy generation, since they are all in the composition of the inner mitochondrial membranes, including the respiratory chain and proton ATPase. However, the synthesis of total mitochondrial proteins virtually does not change with age. This phenomenon is due to the preservation of the synthesis of mitochondrial proteins which are coded by the nuclear genome and are synthesized on the cytoribosomes. Those proteins constitute about 90 per cent of the total proteins of mitochondria. These data correlate well with the results of cytological investigations in which it has been shown that the dimensions of mitochondria and the ratio between matrices and inner membranes grow with age (Wilson, Franks, 1975).

Thus, the shifts which occur in mitochondrial protein biosynthesis with age should, in spite of their adaptive nature (which is manifested in the maintenance of the mitochondrial mass at least in the liver), cause the "energy insufficiency" of cells in old age as a result of a decrease in the synthesis of proteins which directly perform the function of energy generation.

A change in the activity of the enzymes of the Krebs cycle and the respiratory chain may also be one of the reasons why the oxidative ability of mitochondria decreases in old age. The activity of these enzymes changes to a different extent and occasionally in different directions in various tissues with age. For instance, some authors maintain that the activity of malate dehydrogenase increases in the mitochondria of the heart of old rats (Limas, 1975), while others hold that it either decreases (Singh, 1973) or remains unchanged (Schmukler, Barrows, 1966; Razumovich, 1972). However, the activity of isocitrate dehydrogenase does not change in the mitochondria of the heart of old rats, but it increases in the mitochondria of the liver, while the activity of alpha-ketoglutarate dehydrogenase grows in the mitochondria of both tissues (Razumovich, 1972).

At the same time, the activity of the succinoxidase system, including succinate dehydrogenase and the whole respiratory chain, beginning with ubiquinone, grows in the liver, the skeletal muscles and other organs with age (Lowrie, 1953; Sazonova, 1959; Barrows, 1960; Uzbekov, 1967). The activity of succinoxidase is especially high in the mitochondria of an old heart (Frolkis, Bogatskaya, 1974). This activity grows from $135.9 \pm 4.5 \mu g$ of oxygen per milligram of mitochondrial protein per hour in rats 6–12 months old to $212.2 \pm 8.3 \mu g$ in old rats. Hence, the respiratory chain of the mitochondria of an old heart does not limit the respiration rate when succinate is the oxidative substrate.

The amount of pyridine coenzymes grows in old age. Their content is 10–30 per cent higher in the liver and the skeletal muscles of old rats (Voitenko, Bogush, 1969; Frolkis, 1970) and 12 per cent higher in the heart of old rats (Bogatskaya, 1968) than in those of adult rats. Along with this, the concentration of pyridine coenzymes grows in old age mainly due to their reduced forms (NADH and NADPH). Consequently, the NAD/NADH ratio decreases, indicating that NADH oxidation is disturbed, namely, that changes occurred at the very beginning of the respiratory chain. At the same time, the topography of the distribution of the pyridine coenzymes inside the cell changes with age, i. e. their content grows mainly in the cytoplasm and diminishes in the mitochondria. The correlations which are formed indirectly show that the pool of the NAD-dependent dehydrogenases is reduced in old age and that glycolysis intensifies with age.

In old age, substantial shifts occur also in the cytochrome system, which is the last link that makes it possible to use oxygen at the last stages of biological oxidation. According to Frolkis and Bogatskaya (1965), the activity of the cytochrome system and particularly cytochrome oxidase increases per milligram of the mitochondrial protein of the heart of old rats in comparison with that of adult rats. However, when the activity of cytochrome oxidase is calculated per gram of the myocardium, it is 32.8 per cent lower in old rats than in adult rats. The fact that the activity of the cytochrome system decreases with age has been shown in the cardiac muscle of the horse (Lowrie, 1953) and in the liver of rats (Tsipriyan, 1969). Abu-Erreish and associates (1974) have discovered that the cytochrome oxidase activity of the homogenates of the myocardium and the brain of rats diminishes parallel to the activity of the homogenates of their liver and kidneys. It has also been shown (Abu-Erreish, Sanadi, 1978) that the activity of cytochrome oxidase in the myocardium of old rats decreases just as the concentration of the cytochromes $a + a_3$ and $c + c_1$. These facts indicate that the changes in the cytochrome link of the respiratory chain may play a certain role in the disturbance of energy generation in old age. However, changes in the content of the cytochrome c and the cytochrome $a + a_3$ were not discovered in the mitochondria of the human liver (Kazue et al., 1972). The myoglobin content diminishes in the myocardium of old rats. According to our data, this content comes to 1.26 ± 0.027 g per 100 g of dry tissue in rats 8–12 months old, while it is 0.95 ± 0.061 g per 100 g of dry tissue in rats 24–26 months old. Thus, various links of the respiratory chain change irregularly with age.

Definite shifts in oxidative phosphorylation occur with age. Parina and Solodinskaya (1965) have concluded that oxidation and phosphorylation are slightly separated from one another in the brain and the liver of old rats. Weinbach and Garbus (1956) did not observe such a shift. According to our data, oxidation-phosphorylation coupling in the myocardium grows in old age (Fig. 73). This increase in coupling, which we have observed in the

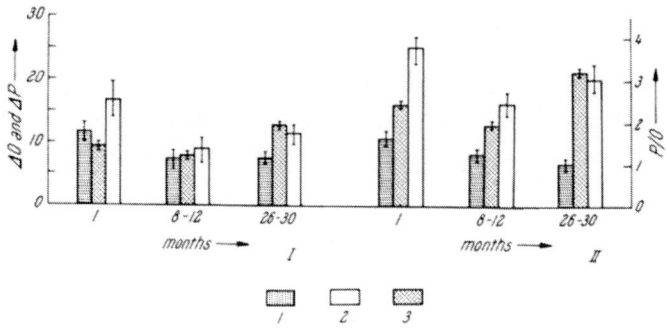

Fig. 73. Age specifics of respiration and oxidative phosphorylation in the mitochondria of the cardiac muscle of rats. *I* when succinic acid is added; *II* when ketoglutaric acid is added. *1* oxygen consumption (microatoms); *2* decrement of phosphorus (microatoms); *3* P/O ratio

mitochondria of the cardiac muscle, can be regarded as an adaptive mechanism which is intended to maintain a sufficiently high level of ATP resynthesis when oxygen consumption becomes less intense. This coupling naturally increases because of the more economical utilization of oxygen. An increase in respiration-phosphorylation coupling in old age should reduce the intensity of the free oxidation processes, as a result of which the free energy of the oxidative substrates is converted not into the energy of the ATP chemical bonds, but into heat. The mechanisms underlying the diminution of the ability of the old organism to generate a large amount of heat (in the case of muscular work, infectious diseases, the cooling of the body, etc.) probably include an increase in respiration-phosphorylation coupling. ATP is formed in the reactions of glycolytic phosphorylation in the cytosol during the breakdown of glucose (glycolysis) or glycogen (glycogenolysis) down to pyruvate or lactate. Participation of oxygen in this process is not obligatory. Although the energy effectiveness of this stage of carbohydrate conversion is rather low, it is exceptionally important as the main source of energy when there is a lack of oxygen. Age changes have not been observed in the rate of glycolytic phosphorylation in the skeletal muscle and the brain.

However, the activity of the limiting enzyme of glycolysis, i. e. hexokinase, increases almost two-fold in the liver in old age (Litoshenko, 1977). This indicates that a greater amount of carbohydrates (glucose) participate in the metabolism of the hepatic tissue and that glycolytic phosphorylation plays a greater role in supplying the hepatic function with energy as the organism ages.

Kirk (1959) has shown that glycolysis plays a greater role in supplying the muscle wall of the vessels with energy when the activity of the oxidative processes is low.

The most pronounced changes occur in the cardiac muscle with age. The intensity of glycolysis, being expressed in the value of the increment of lactate, becomes much higher in the myocardium with age (it grows from 77.2 ±1.5 mg

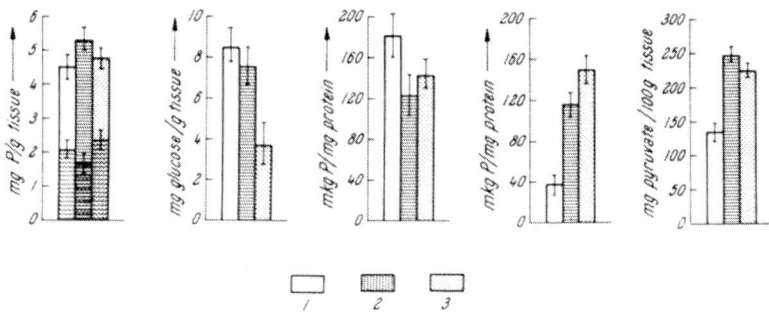

Fig. 74. Age changes in the activity of some glycolytic enzymes (from left to right). Phosphorylase – dark shading represents phosphorylase "a" activity; hexokinase, aldolase, phosphofruktokinase, lactatdehydrogenase in the cardiac muscle of white rats. *1* rat 1 month old; *2* rats 8–12 months old; *3* rats 26–30 months old. First group of columns stands for phosphorylase (dark shading represents phosphorylase "a" activity); second group, hexokinase; third, aldolase; fourth, phosphofruktokinase; fifth, lactic dehydrogenase

per cent in rats 8–12 months old to 103.7 ±1.7 mg per cent in rats 28–32 months old). Glycogenolysis grows even more rapidly (from 82.8 ±1.9 mg per cent to 149.9 ± 2.4 mg per cent, respectively). At the same time, the activity of glycolytic enzymes changes (Fig. 74). When glycolytic phosphorylation is activated in the tissues, the content of the carbohydrate reserve (glycogen) decreases and the peroxidized products of the glycolytic stage of their conversions, i. e. pyruvate and lactate, accumulate. The age-related suppression of the oxidative conversions of pyruvate and lactate results in their further accumulation. Consequently, pH and the redox potential of the tissues may shift and, consequently, metabolism and the functions may be greatly disturbed.

The share of glycolytic phosphorylation increases in the energy supply of tissues so as to maintain energy homeostasis. This increase is one of the links in the chain of the adaptive reactions which develop with age. At the same time, the mobilization of this adaptive mechanism (which usually participates in ensuring greater energy consumption) under the conditions of rest in old age indicates that the range of the adaptive abilities of the aging organism diminishes.

The pentose phosphate cycle, which participates in the organism's energy balance, is one of the ways of oxidizing glucose. This process ensures carbohydrate oxidation, bypassing glycolysis and the Krebs cycle. More than two-thirds of the NADPH molecules are formed during the enzymic reactions of the pentose phosphate cycle. These molecules are indispensable in the

Table 10. *Content of adenosine phosphate and the renewal of ATP in the tissues of rats of different ages*

Tissue	Age (months)	ATP	ADP	AMP	Relative activity of ATP	Reference
		μmole/g of wet tissue			impulses per minute per gram of wet tissue	
Heart	8–12	1.34 ± 0.04	1.73 ± 0.08	–	0.42 ± 0.02	Bogatskaya, 1963
	28–32	1.03 ± 0.04	1.98 ± 0.05	–	0.24 ± 0.01	
Heart	6– 8	1.41 ± 0.13	0.89 ± 0.02	0.71 ± 0.02	0.32 ± 0.02	Kulchitsky,
	24–26	1.10 ± 0.05	0.65 ± 0.04	0.92 ± 0.05	0.15 ± 0.02	1971, 1977
Heart	6– 8	1.36 ± 0.05	0.74 ± 0.03	0.57 ± 0.05	–	Golovchenko,
	24–26	1.12 ± 0.04	0.76 ± 0.04	0.48 ± 0.05	–	Potapenko, 1978
Brain	6– 8	1.60 ± 0.18	0.38 ± 0.04	0.34 ± 0.05	–	*Ibid.*
	24–26	1.09 ± 0.02	0.27 ± 0.01	0.30 ± 0.01	–	
Liver	8–10	1.38 ± 0.03	0.64 ± 0.02	0.75 ± 0.02	–	Novikova, 1964
	26–28	1.10 ± 0.02	0.48 ± 0.01	0.92 ± 0.03	–	
Skeletal muscles	8–10	0.73 ± 0.02	–	–	0.46 ± 0.02	Epstein, 1963
	30–32	0.56 ± 0.03	–	–	0.36 ± 0.02	

synthesis of fatty acids, cholesterol, the steroid hormones, etc. Moreover, ribose-5-phosphate, being the component of nucleotides and nucleic acids, is formed during the reactions of the pentose phosphate cycle. The activity of individual enzymes of the cycle changes with age. The activity of transketolase and glucose-6-phosphate dehydrogenase decreases in both the brain and the kidneys. The activity of these enzymes grows somewhat in the liver, but virtually does not change in the cardiac tissue.

The effectiveness of the entire system of providing the cell with energy is determined by the course of ATP synthesis. Table 10 shows our fellow workers' data on the changes in ATP and the products of its dephosphorylation, i. e. ADP, AMP and creatine phosphate (CP) in various organs. As the amount of ATP decreases, it is renewed more slowly in the heart and the skeletal muscle. A decrease in both the content and renewal of ATP shows that the rate of energy generation diminishes with age. This decrement is bound with changes in oxidative phosphorylation. At the same time, the processes of ATP hydrolysis are activated in several organs. According to Khilko and Grabina, for instance, the ATPase activity of myosin increases in old rats (from 23.0 ± 2.8 μgP/mg of protein in rats 8–10 months old to 35.7 ± 3.9 μgP/mg of protein in rats 26–30 months old).

The sulfhydryl groups of the active centre of myosin are very important in the mechanism which realizes the ATPase activity of myosin. According to Khilko (1965), the content of these groups in native myosin is the highest in old animals. Our coworker Bogatskaya showed that in the myocardium the ATPase activity of individual cellular fractions changes differently with age. For instance, this activity of mitochondria is 33.2 ± 1.12 μg P/mg of protein in rats 8–10 months old and 42.2 ± 4.1 μg P/mg of protein in rats 26–30 months old.

This activity of the myofibrillar nuclear fraction is $6.1 \pm 0.68\,\mu g$ P/mg of protein in mature rats and $14.6 \pm 1.4\,\mu g$ P/mg of protein in old rats. The ATPase activity of the homogenate of the heart noticeably decreases. Bulos and others (1975) discovered that the ATPase activity of mitochondria increases in the flight muscles of old flies. In the previous chapters, we have already seen that the activity of K^+, Na^+ and ATPase of the membrane of the neurons and hepatic cells decreases in old age.

ATP dephosphorylation occurs with the participation of adenosine triphosphatase and makes it possible to use the energy of the macroergic bonds. The different changes in the activity of ATPase of various localizations show that the energy is utilized non-uniformly for different necessities of the cell in old age. The growth of the ATPase activity of both mitochondria and the myofibrillar nuclear fraction is probably of adaptive significance. It makes it possible to utilize energy more fully for maintaining the contractility of the muscle tissue.

The content of CP as well as its renewal rate decreases to a greater extent than the content of ATP in the heart and the skeletal muscle with age (Frolkis *et al.*, 1966; Razumovich, 1972). In the cardiac muscle of old rats (Frolkis, Bogatskaya, 1965), for instance, the amount of CP is almost halved (it decreases from 7.54 ± 0.13 mg per cent in rats 8–10 months old to 3.9 ± 0.27 mg per cent in rats 28–32 months old). This is in accord with the data on the retardation of the processes of CP resynthesis in the skeletal muscles of old rats (Ermini, Verzar, 1968). A change in CP metabolism is probably one of the factors which limit energy supply in old age. Great importance is now being attached to CP in the intracellular transport of energy. In this respect, reference should be made to the data on a decrease in the activity of creatine phosphokinase in the myocardium of old rats.

In old age, the specific creatine kinase activity of the myocardium decreases by 35.4 per cent in comparison with mature rats. Four isoenzymic forms of creatine kinase have been discovered in the heart of adult and old rats. They are: MC (mitochondrial type), MM (muscular type), MB (mixed type), and BB (brain type). An analysis of electrophoretic data has shown that the content of isoenzymes is 27.3 ± 1.09 per cent, 36.1 ± 0.53 per cent, 28.3 ± 0.77 per cent, and 8.3 ± 1.32 per cent, respectively, in the heart of mature rats, and 26.0 ± 1.15 per cent, 34.5 ± 0.53 per cent, 28.5 ± 0.38 per cent, and $11.0 \pm \pm 0.73$ per cent, respectively, in the heart of old rats. Thus, the relationship of the isoforms of creatine phosphokinase does not change substantially with age. Less pronounced shifts which occur in the level of ATP with age can be associated with its exceptional role as a universal source of energy and as the regulator of cellular metabolism. Therefore, all the adaptive mechanisms which are in the cell, especially those which draw on CP reserves, are utilized in order to maintain ATP on a constant level. However, this reduces the extent of adaptation of energy metabolism to the changing conditions under which the cells and tissues function. The energy requirements of these cells and tissues are the basis on which energy metabolism is regulated. Therefore, even slight changes in the amount and correlation of adenosine phosphates can upset the course of various metabolic reactions, especially energy metabolism, thus influencing the aging rate. The disturbances in the mechanisms of the intracellular transport of energy apparently plays an important role in limiting the energy potential of the cells.

The relative concentrations of ATP, ADP and AMP control not only the rates of glycolysis and respiration, but also virtually all the processes in which the energy of the macroergic phosphate bonds is either generated or consumed.

The ATP : ADP ratio changes with age (Table 10). The age shifts are inconsiderable in the liver and the brain. That ratio, however, is greatly reduced in the cardiac muscle. The originating relationships explain why glycolysis is activated in the heart of old rats and why such changes are absent in the brain tissue.

The energy state of the cell as a whole and the direction of its energy exchange can be seen from the value of the energy charge (Atkinson, 1968), which is calculated by the formula:

$$\frac{1}{2} \cdot \frac{ADP + 2ATP}{AMP + ADP + ATP}$$

When the rates of the synthesis and hydrolysis of ATP are equal, the charge of the adenosine phosphate system is approximately 0.85. The smaller is this value, the more strongly are the ATP formation processes activated and the ATP utilization processes inhibited, and vice versa. The data in Table 10 show that the value of the energy charge diminishes somewhat in the heart and the liver of adult animals, indicating preexisting tension in the process of ATP generation. Such a situation probably occurs most frequently under physiological conditions, since energy must be consumed constantly so that the cells can function. Therefore, ATP utilization is the most important regulator of energy metabolism. The value of the energy charge diminishes with age. This is expressed especially clearly in the heart and the liver, while the value is quite high in the brain of old animals. These differences are connected with the functional specifics of the tissues.

Thus, energy metabolism becomes more intense in old age because of an increase in the disproportion between the energy consuming processes and the ATP generating processes. This tension, whose integral indicator is a decrease in the value of the energy charge, determines the adaptive mechanisms, which are exhibited at various levels of the regulation of energy metabolism. Several vitauct phenomena occur with age, including the activation of glycolytic phosphorylation, the intensification of respiration-phosphorylation coupling, and the activation of several enzymes of glycolysis and the Krebs cycle, i. e. adaptive shifts which are aimed at increasing the energy charge of the old organism's cells.

Thus, the adaptive opportunities of the energy processes are already mobilized under ordinary conditions in old age. That is why the inadequacy, in old age, of the energy supply of the organs is revealed more quickly when greater functional demands are made and loads are applied. This is especially evident when studying cardiac activity.

Cardiac insufficiency develops more frequently in old age. In our experiments, which were carried out together with Bogatskaya, Kozinets and

Table 11. *Change in energy metabolism during stable hyperfunction and hypertrophy in adult and old rats*
(on the 14th day after aortic coarctation)

Age (months)	Control							14 days after aortic coarctation						
	ATP	ADP	AMP	CP	Inorganic phosphate	Glycogen mg/g	Lactate μM/g	ATP	ADP	AMP	CP	Inorganic phosphate	Glycogen mg/g	Lactate μmole/g
	μmole/g							μmole/g						
	M±m							M±m						
6—8	1.50	0.84	0.70	3.60	7.40	5.19	1.62	1.67	0.80	0.57*	3.88	8.06	6.30*	1.85
	0.05	0.03	0.04	0.02	0.23	0.10	0.09	0.06	0.04	0.03	0.19	0.30	0.12	0.16
24—26	1.31	0.75	0.84	2.60	10.25	3.21	3.63	1.21*	0.88	0.61	2.13*	12.86*	2.21*	5.86*
	0.02	0.04	0.05	0.26	0.60	0.16	0.26	0.01	0.03	0.05	0.08	0.36	0.06	0.30

* statistically reliable difference ($p < 0.05$)

Shevchuk, were studied the changes in the energy processes in the myocardium when aortic coarctation was simulated. During the first 5 or 6 days, the number of old animals which died of cardiac insufficiency as a result of such coarctations was 4.5 times higher than that of the mature ones. Table 11 shows that the disturbances of several indices of the energy metabolism in the heart are more pronounced in old rats than in mature ones. In spite of the vitauct processes, the potentialities of the systems which provide the functions with energy are limited in old age.

The insufficiency of the energy processes that grows with age may be one of the reasons why metabolism and the functions diminish as the organism ages. The molecular changes which are the cause of the aging and death of cells of various types occur in various sequences. Moreover, the disturbances of the energy processes, which are expressed diversely in the brain, the myocardium, the skeletal muscle, the liver, and so forth, differ in their significance.

Hormonal Mediatory Influences on the Energy Processes

One of the molecular mechanisms of the neurohumoral regulation of the activity of the cells and organs acts through the energy processes. Catecholamines strongly influence various links of the energy processes. They reduce the content of glycogen, activate phosphorylase, increase the content of lactic acid, change the intensity of tissue respiration, glycolysis, oxidation-phosphorylation coupling, etc.

In our work, which carried out together with Bogatskaya, Postrelko, Polyanskaya and Bezhanyan, we tried to compare various changes in different links of the energy processes, changes which were caused by greatly varying doses of catecholamines.

When small doses of adrenaline $(10 \mu g/100 \text{ g})$ are administered intraperitoneally, the intensity of the tissue respiration of the skeletal muscle, the heart, the liver and the thyroid gland does not change in adult animals, while oxygen consumption sharply increases in old animals.

However, when the dose of the hormone is increased, oxygen consumption may decrease instead of endogenous respiration increasing. For instance, when $50 \mu g/100 \text{ g}$ of adrenaline are administered intravenously, the value of oxygen consumption (Q_{O_2}) by the myocardium of rats 8–12 months old is halved $(4.00 \pm 0.27$ units before its administration and 2.03 ± 0.23 units after its administration). When such a dose of adrenaline is administered to old animals, the intensity of respiration virtually does not change in the heart.

The potentialities of the biological oxidation systems diminish with age. It has been discovered that the stimulating effect of adrenaline is more pronounced in adult animals when oxidative substrates are added to the homogenates and the mitochondrial mixture. Under the action of adrenaline $(50 \mu g/100 \text{ g})$, for instance, with addition of glucose the increase of oxygen consumption is doubled in the myocardium of rats 8–12 months old as compared with old rats. Succinate increases the endogenous respiration of the myocardium by 1.5 time in old rats and by 4 times in adult rats, while lactic acid increases endogenous

espiration by 1.5 time in rats 8–12 months old and halves the intensity of
espiration in old rats.

Many researchers associate the influence of adrenaline on the function of the
)rgans with the so-called calorie effect. The respiratory chain has free oxidation
)athways which can shunt the transfer of electrons, bypassing the stages of the
accumulation of energy that is formed during oxidative phosphorylation. It is
)elieved that adrenaline and the product of its oxidation, i. e. adrenochrome, are
he activators of free oxidation and thus change the correlation between free
)xidation and phosphorylation.

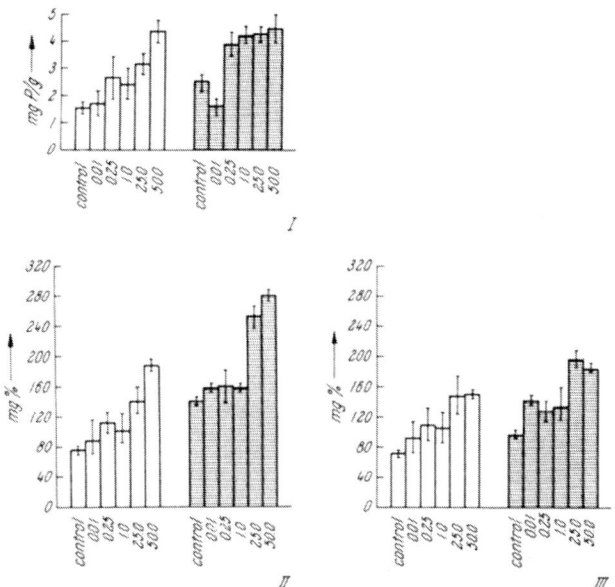

Fig. 75. Influence of various doses of adrenaline on the change in the activity of phosphorylase a
I), the intensity of glycogenolysis (II), and the intensity of glycolysis (III) in the myocardium of
animals of different ages. Light columns stand for mature rats, and shaded columns, for old rats

The administration of 50 μg/100 g of adrenaline dissociates oxidation and
)hosphorylation in animals of different age. When adrenaline is administered,
·espiration and phosphorylation changes to the greatest extent in the
mitochondria of old animals. When succinate is used as a substrate, the P/O
·atio decreases from 1.87 ± 0.15 to 1.32 ± 0.11 unit (p < 0.001) in the heart of
)ld rats, while it virtually does not change in mature animals (it decreases from
1.16 ± 0.14 to 1.10 ± 0.3 unit; p > 0.5).

All these changes in oxidative phosphorylation in the myocardium can
·educe the synthesis of macroergic compounds and increase the liberation of
:nergy in the form of heat.

In old animals, smaller doses of adrenaline intensify glycolysis as well as
glycogenolysis and activate phosphorylase (Fig. 75). For instance, glycolysis and
glycogenolysis intensify and shifts occur in the activity of phosphorylase in the

myocardium of old rats when adrenaline is administered in a dose of 0.01 $\mu g/100$ g, while such changes occur in adult rats when adrenaline is administered in a dose of 0.25 $\mu g/100$ g. The content of glycogen decreases in old animals when adrenaline is administered in a dose of 0.25 $\mu g/100$ g, while it decreases in mature animals when the hormone is administered in a dose of 1.0 $\mu g/100$ g. The age differences in the shifts are levelled out when "average" amounts of adrenaline are administered, but they are more pronounced in the myocardium of adult rats when large amounts are administered. Such relationships are revealed also when noradrenaline is administered. When this mediator of the sympathetic system is administered in a dose of 5 $\mu g/100$ g, it virtually does not change the intensity of glycolysis in rats 8–12 months old; however, it intensifies this glycolysis in old rats (from 103.7 ± 1.72 to 149.0 ± 3.9 mg per cent of lactic acid). When noradrenaline is administered in the same dose as adrenaline, it causes less pronounced changes in the intensity of tissue respiration and in oxydation-phosphorylation coupling in the myocardium and the liver.

Phosphorylase "b" (inactive form) is transformed into phosphorylase "a" (active form) under the influence of adrenaline with the participation of 3,5-AMP, whose formation is stimulated by catecholamines.

In the previous chapters, we have seen that 3,5-AMP is formed in the heart of old rats under the action of smaller doses of catecholamines. According to Kulchitsky (1977), the content of ATP, creatine phosphate and inorganic phosphorus decreases, while the content of ADP increases in the heart of adult and old rats when adrenaline is administered in a dose of 1.0 $\mu g/100$ g.

An increase in sensitivity to catecholamines in old animals can be attributed to the activation of phosphorylase and a change in the intensity of glycolysis and glycogenolysis under the action of smaller doses of adrenaline. In old persons and animals, many functional effects originate under the action of catecholamines whose doses are smaller in comparison with those administered to mature persons and animals. Interestingly, the potentialities of an increase in the activity of phosphorylase are almost exhausted when adrenaline is administered in a dose of 50 $\mu g/100$ g. Under these conditions, the activity of phosphorylase "a" may still greatly increase in adult rats. Even when adrenaline is administered together with the oxidative substrates, the possible increment of oxygen consumption by the tissue is higher in adult animals than in old ones, while in the latter, oxidation and phosphorylation are dissociated more sharply. Thus, the possible range of the changes in the energy processes is reduced under the influence of catecholamines, and the possible energy supply of the adaptive reactions of the tissue decreases. All this can be one of the molecular mechanisms of the above-mentioned decrease in both the reactivity of the tissues in old age and in the possible intensification of their activity under the influence of catecholamines. The shifts in the energy processes under the influence of catecholamines are a phasic process. In most cases, we determined great changes 3 minutes after the intravenous administration of catecholamines. At the same time, the subsequent changes are known to differ not only by the extent, but also by the direction of the shifts.

The mechanism of the effect of catecholamines on the organs, particularly the myocardium, is a complicated one. Adrenaline and noradrenaline can act directly and indirectly (i. e. in a reflex way) on the cardiac muscle. This reflex influence is largely cholinergic. Hence, the shifts in the energy processes of the myocardium, being caused by catecholamines, are a combination of direct and reflex actions. In the experiments with rats of different ages, a comparison was made of the shifts in the myocardium when adrenaline was administered both before and after the vagus nerves were cut.

In 10 minutes, the section of the vagus nerves itself reduced the anaerobic consumption of carbohydrates (by 17–20.54 per cent). After vagotomy, the administration of noradrenaline intensifies glycolysis and glycogenolysis to a smaller extent than in the control experiments. An important fact is that the smaller intensification of glycolysis and glycogenolysis after vagotomy is expressed less in old rats than in adult ones. For instance, before the vagus nerves are cut in old rats, adrenaline intensifies glycolysis by 80.9 per cent and glycogenolysis by 49.3 per cent, and after they are cut, it intensifies glycolysis by 26.57 per cent and glycogenolysis by 45.5 per cent. In adult rats, the intensity of glycolysis and glycogenolysis decreases from 52.58 and 42.39 per cent to 16.98 and 13.21 per cent, respectively. According to our data, the activity of glucose-6-phosphate dehydrogenase and succinate dehydrogenase decreases to a smaller extent in old animals than in mature ones when the vagus nerves are cut.

In assessing the results of these experiments, account should be taken of two possible mechanisms: (a) the section of the vagus nerves switches off the reflex component of the effect of catecholamines, and (b) the section of the vagus nerves changes the reactions of the myocardium itself to the action of these substances. Moreover, it should be borne in mind that the experiments were carried out with rats which had very low tonicity of the centre of the vagus nerve and, consequently, the centre acted strongly on the heart when various reflex influences were exerted.

Nevertheless, the experiments show that catecholamines have a stronger direct and a weaker indirect (reflex) influence on the heart of old animals.

Great metabolic and functional shifts occur in the tissues under the action of the thyroid hormone, which exerts wide-ranging influence on the energy processes in the cells. For a long time, many researchers supported the hypothesis that the hormone of the thyroid gland was a factor which dissociated oxidation and phosphorylation in mitochondria. In physiological situations, the mechanism of the action of the thyroid hormones on the energy processes in the cells is believed to serve the purpose of increasing the permeability of the mitochondria for the substrates and regulating mitochondrial, phosphorylative and extramitochondrial oxidation. When mitochondria swell and the permeability of their membranes changes, the formation of macroergs in the cell is upset and energy consumption is redistributed.

In our researches, which were carried out together with Bogatskaya and Verzhikovskaya, we studied the age distinctions in the energy metabolism of the heart and the liver when hyperthyroidism and hypothyroidism were reproduced in experiments with rats. The former was reproduced by administering thyroxine (10 μg/100 g) daily, while the latter was reproduced by thyroidectomy.

It was discovered that the shifts in many links of energy metabolism are expressed to a greater extent in the liver and the heart of old rats during the early stages of the development of hyperthyroidism, while at the late stages, they are more pronounced in adult rats.

We have already seen that tissue respiration increases in the heart (by 101.1 per cent) and the liver of old animals on the 4th day of the administration of thyroxine. In mature rats, oxygen consumption does not change substantially during this period of hyperthyroidism. At the same time, the possible range of changes in the intensity of the oxidative processes, being caused by the thyroid hormone, is reduced in old age. In experimental hyperthyroidism, which greatly stimulates the endogenous respiration of the myocardium of old rats, the addition of oxidative substrates increases oxygen consumption in the heart and the liver of old rats far less than in those of rats 8–12 months old. This was revealed especially clearly when succinate was added.

The earlier dissociation of oxidation and phosphorylation in the mitochondria and the intensification of glycolysis in old animals show that the animals are very sensitive to the action of thyroxine. For instance, the intensification of glycolysis was not reliable on the 4th day of the administration of thyroxine in the liver of rats 8–10 months old, but it greatly intensified on the 10–14th day of hyperthyroidism (it increased by 95.5 per cent in comparison with the initial level and by 84.2 per cent in comparison with the level which existed on the 4th day of the experiment). Different relationships are formed in old animals. In them, anaerobic glycolysis increases noticeably (by 29.8 per cent) on the 4th day of hyperthyroidism. But as hyperthyroidism develops, it increases to a smaller extent than in mature animals (it increases by 44.3 per cent in comparison with the initial level and by 11.2 per cent in comparison with the level which existed on the 4th day of hyperthyroidism).

The content of glycogen in the liver of rats 8–10 months old virtually does not change after a single administration of thyroxine. However, it greatly decreases when thyroxine is administered for 2 days (it decreases by 31.2 per cent in comparison with the level in the control group). In old animals, even a single administration of the hormone greatly reduces the content of glycogen in the liver (by 43.7 per cent).

The extent of the changes in separate links of the energy transformations during hyperthyroidism differs in the heart and the liver of animals of different ages. For instance, the glycogen content decreases more sharply in the heart of mature rats and in the liver of old rats.

During hyperthyroidism, great shifts occur in both the activity of individual enzymes and the coenzymic content in animals of different ages. Experiments have shown that the overall amount of NAD and its oxidized forms decreases more in the heart of rats 28–32 months old than in that of rats 8–12 months old on the 10–14th day of hyperthyroidism.

The age distinctions in the effect of the thyroid hormones on the glycolytic processes are due to several causes. Firstly, the thyroid hormones can directly activate some glycolytic enzymes which contain the –SH groups. Secondly, the thyroid hormones can influence indirectly the glycolytic processes through the mechanisms of intracellular regulation. The dissociation of oxidation and phosphorylation under the influence of the thyroid hormones reduces eventually the ATP level and increases the amount of ADP and inorganic phosphorus. The accumulation of these products on the basis of positive feed-back activates glycolysis.

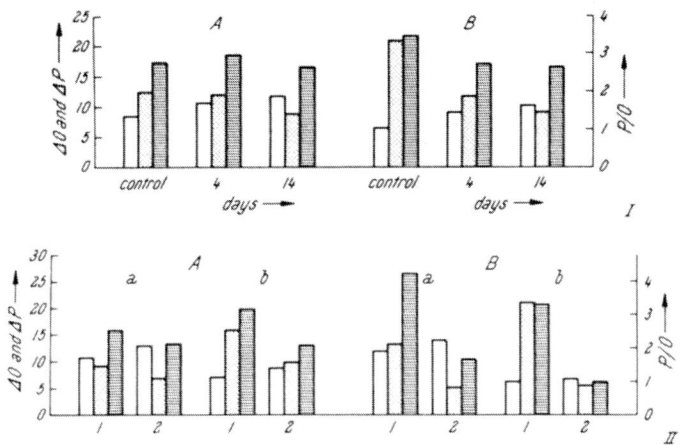

Fig. 76. Influence of thyroidin on respiration and oxidative phosphorilation in the mitochondria of the cardiac muscle *(I)* and the liver *(II)* of rats of different ages. *A* rats 8–10 months old; *B* rats 28–32 months old. Light columns stand for consumed oxygen (microatoms), cross-hatched colums, for loss of phosphorus (microatoms), and dotted columns, for the P/O ratio. *1* control; *2* 14th day of thyroidin administration. Cardiac muscle – ketoglutarate; liver: *a* succinate; *b* ketoglutarate

Using various oxidative substrates, Rachev (1979) concluded that the thyroid hormones influence various aspects of oxidative phosphorylation. As thyrotoxicosis develops, dissociation occurs first of all in the initial phosphorylative link, which is between NAD and flavoprotein. As thyrotoxicosis intensifies, the second link, i. e. the one between the cytochromes b and c, becomes dissociated, while the third phosphorylative link in the respiratory chain is not dissociated even when thyrotoxicosis is very severe.

In our experiments, we used two substrates during the oxidation of which the electrons entered various parts of the respiratory chain. When alpha ketoglutarate is oxidized, the electrons enter the respiratory chain at the level of the NAD link, and when succinate is oxidizing, they enter it at the flavoprotein level.

When alpha ketoglutarate was oxidized, oxidation and phosphorylation was not dissociated in the mitochondria of the myocardium of mature rats, while the P/O ratio sharply diminishes in old rats (Fig. 76A, B). These data show that oxidation and phosphorylation is dissociated in the region between NAD and flavoprotein in old animals. When succinate is oxidized, the P/O ratio does not change in mature rats, while it sharply diminishes in old ones. Hence, not only the first, but also the second phosphorylative site in the respiratory chain between the cytochromes b and c_1 is affected in old rats on the 4th day of the administration of thyroxine. These data confirm that the heart of old animals is very sensitive to the action of the thyroid hormones. This is in accord also with the data on the greater diminution of the activity of adenosine triphosphatase of the cellular fractions of the cardiac muscle. In rats 8–12 months old and those 28–32 months old, the activity of the homogenate adenosine triphosphatase grows by 178.3 and 356.9 per cent, that of the supernatant fluid, by 729.7 and 824.3 per cent, and that of the mitochondria, by 150.6 and 176.2 per cent, respectively.

The age differences in the change of the intensity of tissue respiration, in the dissociation of oxidation and phosphorylation, in the growth of glycolysis and in the activation of adenosine triphosphatase of various cellular fractions determine the specifics of the main ways of the formation and accumulation of energy in the cells of animals of different ages when hyperthyroidism is simulated experimentally. All these changes result in shifts in the content and renewal of the macroergic phosphorus compounds.

Hyperthyroidism (10 days of hormone administration) reduces the content of ATP in the myocardium of old animals (by 16.6 per cent) and virtually does not change that in the myocardium of mature ones (it changes the content only by 3.3 per cent). When the hormone is administered for a long time (50–60 days), the content of ATP in the myocardium diminishes much more, but then the shifts are greater in old animals than in mature ones.

However, the change in the amount of ATP cannot fully describe the direction of the shifts of the energy processes in the cell in qualitative terms. The shifts in the content of ATP in the tissues depend on both the intensity of synthesis and breakdown.

In the previous chapters, our data were given on a change in the hemodynamics and contractility of the myocardium during different periods of hyperthyroidism. In old animals, myocardial contractility and cardiac output diminish as hyperthyroidism develops. The data given in this chapter show that these functional shifts are based on the more clearly expressed disturbances of the energy processes in the heart.

Great changes occur in the energy processes in the tissues after thyroidectomy. It has long been shown that oxygen consumption of several tissues decreases a week after thyroidectomy.

According to our data, thyroidectomy reduces the intensity of oxygen consumption of the cardiac and hepatic tissues of mature and old animals. The tissue respiration of the myocardium of mature rats diminished by 47.4 per cent 2 weeks after thyroidectomy. In old rats, however, the intensity of oxygen consumption decreased by only 6.5 per cent after thyroidectomy during the same length of time. Such a nature of the changes in the extent of oxygen consumption has been observed also in the hepatic tissue after thyroidectomy. 2 weeks after the operation, the intensity of the tissue respiration of the liver decreased by 29.8 per cent in mature rats and by 14.9 per cent in old rats.

These data show that, under ordinary conditions, the hormones of the thyroid gland are somewhat more important in regulating the energy processes in the mature age range than in elderly range.

Table 12. Change in the content of ATP, ADP, AMP, CP, inorganic phosphate and lactate in the brain of rats of different ages under the influence of vasopressin (M ± m)

Age group	Experimental conditions	ATP	ADP	AMP	Inorganic phosphate	Lactate	CP
		μmole/g					μmole P/g
Adult rats	Control	1.60 ± 0.18	0.38 ± 0.04	0.34 ± 0.05	5.63 ± 0.13	3.48 ± 0.85	1.92 ± 0.18
	Administration of vasopressin	1.64 ± 0.15	0.38 ± 0.03	0.33 ± 0.02	8.30 ± 0.73	7.50 ± 0.53	1.39 ± 0.05
	p	> 0.05	> 0.05	> 0.05	< 0.01	< 0.01	< 0.05
Old rats	Control	1.09 ± 0.02	0.27 ± 0.01	0.30 ± 0.01	9.08 ± 0.47	4.50 ± 9.43	1.81 ± 0.03
	Administration of vasopressin	0.74 ± 0.04	0.36 ± 0.01	0.42 ± 0.04	14.25 ± 0.85	12.80 ± 1.58	1.12 ± 0.08
	p	< 0.001	< 0.001	< 0.01	< 0.001	< 0.01	< 0.001

Vasopressin causes great changes in the cardiac function. As we have already seen, symptoms of hypoxia and coronary insufficiency are registered on the electrocardiogram after vasopressin is administered. Moreover, myocardial contractility diminishes. Vasopressin also causes shifts in the blood supply of the brain. All this prompted us, together with Golovchenko and Potapenko, to study the age specifics of the change in the energy processes in the heart and the brain under the influence of vasopressin. The hormone was administered intravenously to rats in a dose of 0.2 unit per 100 g of weight.

Table 12 shows that the content of ATP, ADP and AMP does not change, while only the level of creatine phosphate drops as that of inorganic phosphorus grows in the brain of mature rats when vasopressin is administered. Unlike in mature rats, the content of ATP decreases and the amount of the products of its dephosphorylation, i. e. ADP and AMP as well as inorganic phosphorus, increases in the brain tissue of old rats. The content of creatine phosphate decreases more sharply in the brain of old rats under the influence of vasopressin.

The shifts are somewhat different in the myocardium when vasopressin is administered. The content of ATP increases by 15 per cent and the amount of its precursor (ADP) decreases by 13 per cent in the myocardium of mature animals. In these animals, the amount of creatine phosphate decreases by 27 per cent and that of inorganic phosphorus increases by 33 per cent.

Unlike in mature rats, the ATP level decreases by 17 per cent, the content of ADP, AMP and inorganic phosphorus increases by 10, 28 and 35 per cent, respectively, while the content of creatine phosphate decreases by 15 per cent in the heart of old rats. The content of lactate grows in the heart and the brain of rats of both groups.

According to our data, vasopressin causes dissimilar shifts in the activity of individual enzymes, which ensure the normal course of energy metabolism. For instance, vasopressin increases the activity of creatine phosphatase by almost 200 per cent in the heart of mature rats and only by 50 per cent in that of old ones.

The shifts caused in the energy metabolism of the heart and the brain when vasopressin is administered are due mainly to the disturbance of oxygen transfer as a result of the vascular spasm and the disturbance of general hemodynamics. This reduces the level of adenosine triphosphoric acid and creatine phosphate in the heart and the brain of old rats. Glycolysis is activated when the resynthesis of the energy-rich phosphorus compounds diminishes during oxidative phosphorylation. This is evident from the growth of the content of lactate in the heart and the brain of mature and old rats. The Klinkenberg ratio grows more in the heart of old rats than in that of mature ones (47.3 and 24.3 units, respectively), indicating that the activity of the factors which stimulate glycolysis grows more in old animals.

A sharp decrease in the level of creatine phosphate can be of adaptive significance, since it is connected with the activation of transphosphorylation between creatine phosphate and ADP with the formation of the ATP molecules. This is confirmed by the almost three-fold increase in the activity of creatine phosphokinase, which is an enzyme that allows transphosphorylation to occur.

This adaptive reaction is activated not so strongly in old animals. Indeed, creatine phosphokinase is activated less and the content of creatine phosphate decreases less in the heart of old animals.

Thus, there is a definite relationship between the age specifics of a change in the functions and the shifts in the energy processes which originate in the organs under the influence of hormones.

12. Neurohumoral Mechanisms of Cellular Aging

Sequence of Cellular Aging

Galilei once wrote that one of the main tasks of science is to measure the measurable and to make what cannot be measured measurable. An old and at the same time always new question is whether the rate of aging of individual groups of cells can be determined and whether, consequently, the principal mechanisms of the whole organism's aging can be assessed exactly.

In this respect, it should be taken into account that the intact organism's aging is not the sum of its individual cells' aging. From the standpoint of the adaptive regulatory theory, the organism ages as a complex biological system in which the shifts in one cellular population influence the processes of aging and vitauct in other cells. It is especially important to emphasize this, because the concept of life's limit, of biological clocks in every individual cell, is popular now.

Today, just as 50 and even 100 years ago, three questions of aging are debated: 1. How does the environment of the cell in the organism influence the course of its aging? 2. The aging of what cells is primary in the organism's aging: the dividing or the non-dividing ones? 3. What cells age earlier and influence the organism's aging to the greater extent: plasmic or metaplasmic (connective-tissue) ones?

The experiments carried out by Metalnikov (1917) and Woodruff (1929), who obtained thousands of generations of unicellular organisms, are widely known. Woodruff concluded from these experiments that old age was not an indispensable property of living matter. In this conclusion, he mixes aging, an individual's death and the possibility of infinite natural development. When unicellular organisms divide, it does not mean that their individuality is potentially immortal, but that it is possible for evolutionarily changed species to develop continuously. The research which has been carried out in the last few decades suggests that unicellular organisms pass through a cycle of individual development from one division to another. The aging processes hold an important place in this development. At a definite stage of the unicellular organisms' development, changes take place in the structure of individual organoids, a decrease is observed in the intensity of tissue respiration, sorption, the activity of the respiratory enzymes, locomotion and in sensitivity to several chemical agents, and other phenomena also occur. All can be regarded as symptoms of aging (Tokin, 1979; Smith-Sonneborn, 1979). Cellular division is activated by these age changes. It is an extremely important manifestation of vitauct, which is aimed at renewing the structures and metabolic cycles of the cell, restoring the high level of its viability and eliminating the previous age changes. As Mezin (1977) figuratively put it, life manages to fool time owing to cellular division and wins double stakes: two cells are obtained instead of one.

In a series of works by Carell (1912), Maximov (1916) and others (being regarded as classical for many years), it has been shown that the cells of multi-cellular organisms can also divide for an infinitely long time under the conditions of tissue culture. These experiments seem to show that the life span of the cells is limited due to the conditions of their existence in the organism, and when the cell tears away from these conditions, it acquires the ability to divide for a long time and sometimes even infinitely.

In the last few decades, events have obliged us to return to this problem. They involve a series of works by Hayflick (1972, 1979), which have attracted a great deal of attention. According to Hayflick, Curell made errors in this method of investigation, as a result of which inaccurate results were obtained. It was discovered that the fibroblasts of the human embryos produce a limited number of divisions (56) in culture and are then gradually degraded. This phenomenon is defined as clonal aging, or "Hayflick's limit." In Hayflick's opinion, such a limited mitotic potential is characteristic of the cells in the organism. It has been proved that this phenomenon of clonal aging exists and that there are links between the donor's age and the ability of the cells to divide *in vitro*. Moreover, it has been shown that there is a relationship between the donor species life span and the mitotic activity of the donor cells in culture. The fibroblasts taken from patients suffering from progeria produced a small number of divisions. Finally, it has been established that the serial transplantation of fibroblasts leads to their limited clonal survival in the experiments carried out *in vivo*.

Hayflick's estimates have shown that the limited mitotic potential of the cells cannot be connected with the exhaustion of the metabolite reserves. In all, 10^{15} cells are formed from one cell as a result of 50 divisions. Hence, if the metabolite is simply exhausted, it should have at least 10^{15} molecules in the ancestral cell. However, such an amount of molecules can be kept only in a volume which is much larger than that of the biggest cell in the organism.

There is now a great deal of data which make it possible to critically assess some general biological conclusions which were drawn on the basis of the above-mentioned works. These data are given in the review by Evans (1979), in a series of articles by Franks (1970) and Rowlatt (1972), and in other works. However, even if the data on clonal aging are accepted, it should be taken into account that they relate to a definite type of cells and cannot be applied to all the dividing cells of the complex organism. Moreover, the whole organism dies much earlier than "Hayflick's limit" of cell division is attained.

The relationship between the species life span and the ability to divide was established when the fibroblasts of man, the mouse, the hen and the turtle were studied. However, such relationships have not been established for many other species. In Rowlatt's opinion, the tissue culture method does not make it possible to study the differentiation of cells or whole organs for a long time.

Differences have not been observed in the life span of the culture of cells taken from mice 3 days old and old mice (Rowlatt, 1972). Many rotifers, nematodes and fruit flies are composed of postmitotic cells (except the sex cells) and their aging cannot be regarded as clonal (Franks, 1970). Planarians can multiply sexually or asexually; this includes active regeneration and division. Sexually, the organism's life span is limited (50–60 days). However, planarians can multiply infinitely asexually. Hence, the dividing planarian cells have an unlimited mitotic potential. Some sea anemones and worms can divide infinitely when their body is divided. Two or three (or even one) segments of the marine annelides can multiply infinitely until they reach the size of the whole organism. In hydras and actiniae, the cells of the body are constantly replenished from the pool of the continuously dividing non-differentiated interstitial cells. It is interesting how the glia cells age in mammals. According to Brunk and others (1973), the glia cells *in vitro* have a limited mitotic potential the alterations in them however being negligible. Krohn (1966) transplanted the skin of mice and showed that the possible transplantation periods are longer than the individual's life span.

There are non-dividing cells which can start dividing under definite conditions. They include hepatic cells, whose mitotic activity originates during tissue regeneration after partial hepatectomy. It was found that the mitotic activity which originates under these conditions does not have the above-mentioned limit. For instance, the mitotic activity of the hepatocytes does not diminish even when there are 12 hepatectomies in a year (Comfort, 1964).

All these data show that the complex organism's aging cannot be regarded as simply the limitation of the mitotic potential of its cells and as a biological clock which exists in every cell. These data indicate that the general regulatory effects inside the organism play the leading role in a given cellular population's aging. The neurohumoral and hypothalamohypophysial shifts are apparently very important in this respect. For instance, Price and Makinodan (1972) believe that the immune response decreases by only 10 per cent due to the cellular environment and by 90 per cent due to the age changes in the cells. However, the relationships are different when cells are transferred for a long time to the recipient's organism which was exposed to radiation. The cells of an old donor's spleen that have been transferred to a young recipient become capable of responding like those in young animals (Butenko, Andrianova, 1979). At the same time, the cells of a young donor lose their ability to respond fully in an old recipient. Daniel (1972) showed that when serial transplantations were made to new recipients, the skin of mice kept its viability for 7 years, while the prostate cells, for 6 years. In other words, a change in the host makes it possible to maintain tissue life for a much longer period than the life spans of the tissue donor. Harrison (1975) had been transplanting cells of the hemopoietic tissue of mice for 7 years. Interestingly, the life spans of the transplants of young and old animals were approximately the same in a young host's organism (Daniel, 1972).

The data obtained from the experiments with parabiosis, in which old and young animals were mates, show the role which the factors of humoral regulation play in cellular aging. For instance, after observing the structural changes in the liver, the kidneys and the spleen, Tauchi and Hasegawa (1977) concluded that old animals age more slowly, while young ones, more quickly under parabiotic conditions. Ludwig and Flashoff (1972) reported that the young mates increase the life span of old ones in parabiosis.

The role which the regulatory factors play in cellular aging is evident from the data on the effect which the changes in the central nervous and hormonal regulation have on the rate of cellular aging. The data presented by Cristofalo (1975) are interesting in this respect. In studying the clonal aging of fibroblasts on tissue culture, he showed that hormones (hydrocortisone) increase the number of duplications. The primary shifts in neural and hormonal control as well as general metabolic disturbances can cause secondary changes in the dividing cells. At the Ninth International Congress of Gerontology held in Kiev in 1972, Hayflick, the father of the concept of clonal aging, stated: "The likelihood that animals age because one or more important cell populations lose their proliferative capacity is very unlikely. It is more likely that those changes heralding the approach of loss of division capacity play a greater role in the expression of age changes and result in death of the individual animal well before his cells fail to divide." These shifts should be sought for in the age changes of the regulation of both metabolism and the functions and in the state of the non-dividing cells. Hayflick (1979) believes that the classes of cells which are incapable of undergoing division in the mature organism (e. g. neurons and muscle cells) play a greater role in the manifestation of age shifts than the classes of cells which are capable of undergoing division.

Cowdry (1939) proposed a classification which, in his opinion, reflects the link between the ability of the cells to undergo division and aging. The first group consists of cells whose existence begins and ends with mitosis (the basal cells of the epidermis, the spermatosome, etc.). These cells have a short life, and attempts to observe the aging processes in them have so far failed. The second group consists of cells which are more specialized and which possess the properties of differentiated mitosis. Several age changes can be observed in them, including the accumulation of hemoglobin, the transition of the hemocytoblast to the normoblast and the erythrocyte, and the appearance of carotene in the skin. The third consists of specialized cells with clearly expressed signs of aging. They exhibit the ability to undergo mitosis only under definite conditions, such as in the case of damage, and include the cells of the liver, the kidneys, and the thyroid gland. The fourth group consists of highly specialized cells which are incapable of undergoing mitosis under any conditions (the somatic muscle fibres, neurons etc.). Clear-cut features of aging develop in such cells. The main disadvantage of this classification is that the aging of individual cells is dissociated from the numerous regulatory and trophic influences in the organism and from all the intercellular relationships.

The aging of the cells in an intact organism is an intricate combination of their own age changes and regulatory and trophic influences. From this standpoint, there are three types of cellular aging, which involves (a) cells which undergo primary aging, (b) cells whose aging is the result of their own age changes and the regulatory, trophic and environmental influences which are connected with the primary aging of other cells, and (c) cells whose aging is mainly secondary under the natural conditions of existence and which is connected with a change in the set of regulatory effects, including shifts in the mechanisms of trophism, i. e. blood supply, the permeability of barriers, and so forth (Frolkis, 1971). The first group comprises nerve cells and some connective-tissue cells, the second group comprises the muscle fibres, the cells of endocrine glands, the liver and the kidneys, while the third group comprises the cells of the epidermis, the epithelia of many organs, and so forth.

The aging rate of the cells is determined not only by its above-mentioned properties, but also by its relation to one functional system or another. This is how Anokhin (1968) defined the concept of the functional system: "As a rule, the functional system is a central-peripheral formation, thus becoming a specific apparatus of self-regulation. It maintains its unity on the basis of circulation from the periphery to the centres and vice versa, although it is not a 'ring' in the strict sense of the word. The existence of any functional system is surely connected with the production of a clear-cut adaptive effect. It is this ultimate effect which determines a certain distribution of excitations and activities throughout the functional system."

Various cells eventually unite to produce a definite manifestation of vitauct, and extremely important links are established between them. The disturbance of these links affects their structure and function. Unfortunately, the systemic approach was not widely taken in the analysis of the mechanisms of aging. When it is taken, however, the sequence of aging, which covers the heterogeneous structures of one functional system, becomes clear in many respects. For instance, the functional system, which determines the reproductive function of the organism, is one of the first to be affected when the organism ages.

The data obtained by Kopieva, our fellow worker, are given in Fig. 77A, B, C. They show that, with age, changes occur in the most diverse structures belonging to one functional system, i. e. in the arcuate nucleus of the hypothalamus, adenohypophysis, the muscle cells of the uterus, and especially the ovary. The cells age within a single system. The number of polyribosomes decreases, shifts occur in the nuclear cytoplasmic relationships, and the active zones of the axodendritic and axosomatic synapses diminish in the neurocyte of an old animal's hypothalamus (Fig. 77A). Clearly expressed fenestration occurs in the capillaries, while various signs of the distrophy of the secretory cells and the vacuolization of the cytoplasm (especially the FSH cells) are observed in the hypophysis. The number of pycnotic osmiophilic cells grows sharply. The hyperplasia of the granular endoplasmic reticulum is expressed clearly in the ACTH cells (see Fig. 77B). Ultrastructural disorganization and vast zones of loosely arranged osmophilic cells, being separated from one another by broad layers of collagenous fibre bundles, are observed in the ovary. Loose, formless connective tissue grows widely in the uterus, the number of collagenic fibres increases and that of the smooth muscle cells decreases, lipids are deposited, and the amount of capillaries diminishes (see Fig. 77C).

According to our data, functional and metabolic age-related shifts are similar in various parts of the intestine, i. e. in the muscle layer, the neural apparatus and the intestine vessels, and in the acetylcholine turnover, while reactions to both sympathetic stimulation and the administration of acetylcholine and

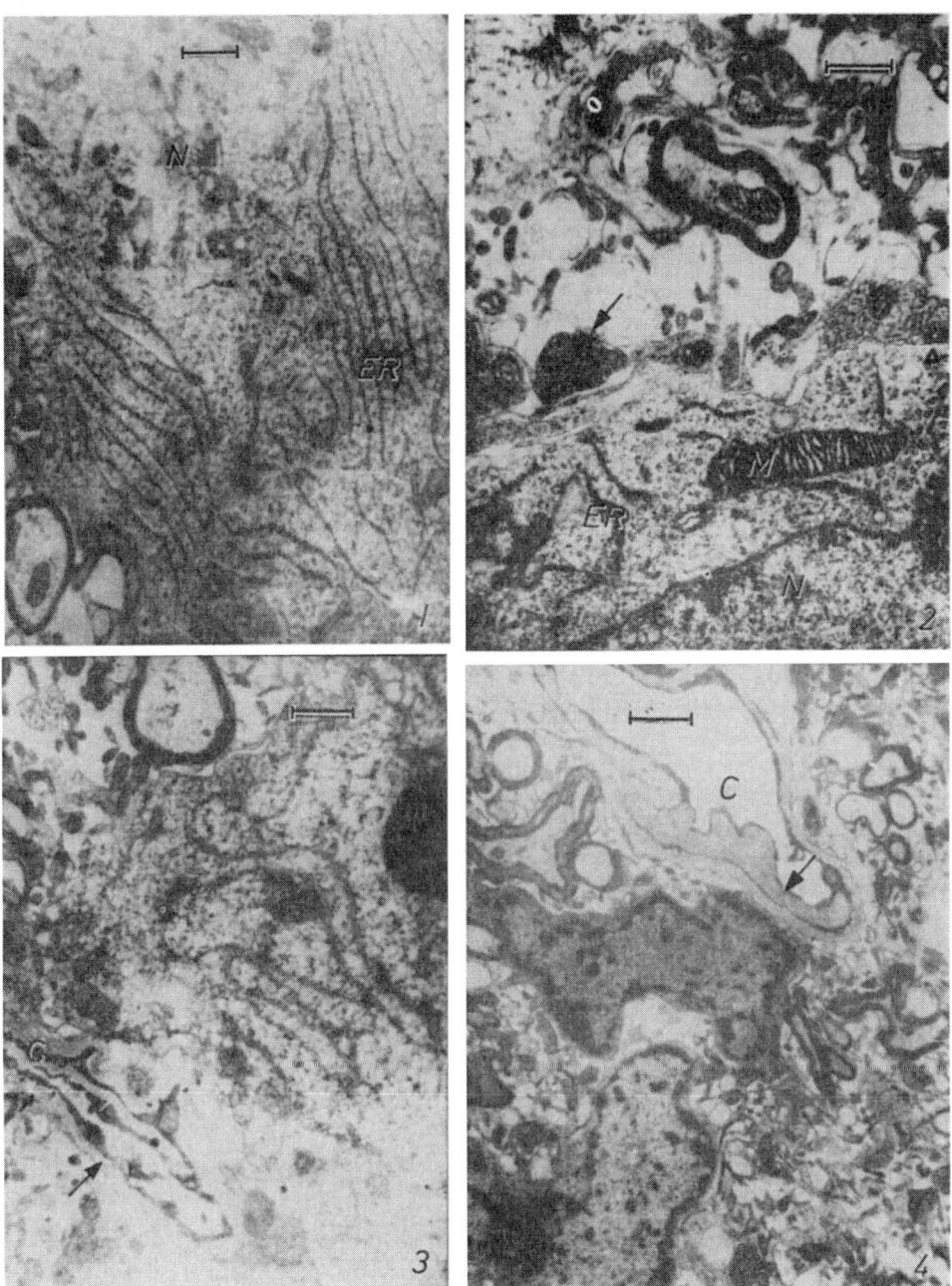

Fig. 77 A. Age changes in the hypothalamic ultrastructure. Scale: 1 μ. *1* neurocyte *(N)* of the anterior part of the hypothalamus of a young rat. The network of the slit-like cisternae of the granular endoplasmic reticulum *(ER)* is developed. *2* neurocyte of the anterior part of the hypothalamus of an old rat and a neurophile region. Mitochondrium *(M)* and the endoplasmic reticulum in the neurocyte. Axodendritic synapse (arrow) and axosomatic synapse (triangle). *3* fragment of the capillary *(C)* of the posterior part of the hypothalamus of a young rat. Basal membrane (arrows) of the capillary. *4* fragment of the capillary of the posterior part of the hypothalamus of an old rat. Thickened basal membrane (arrow)

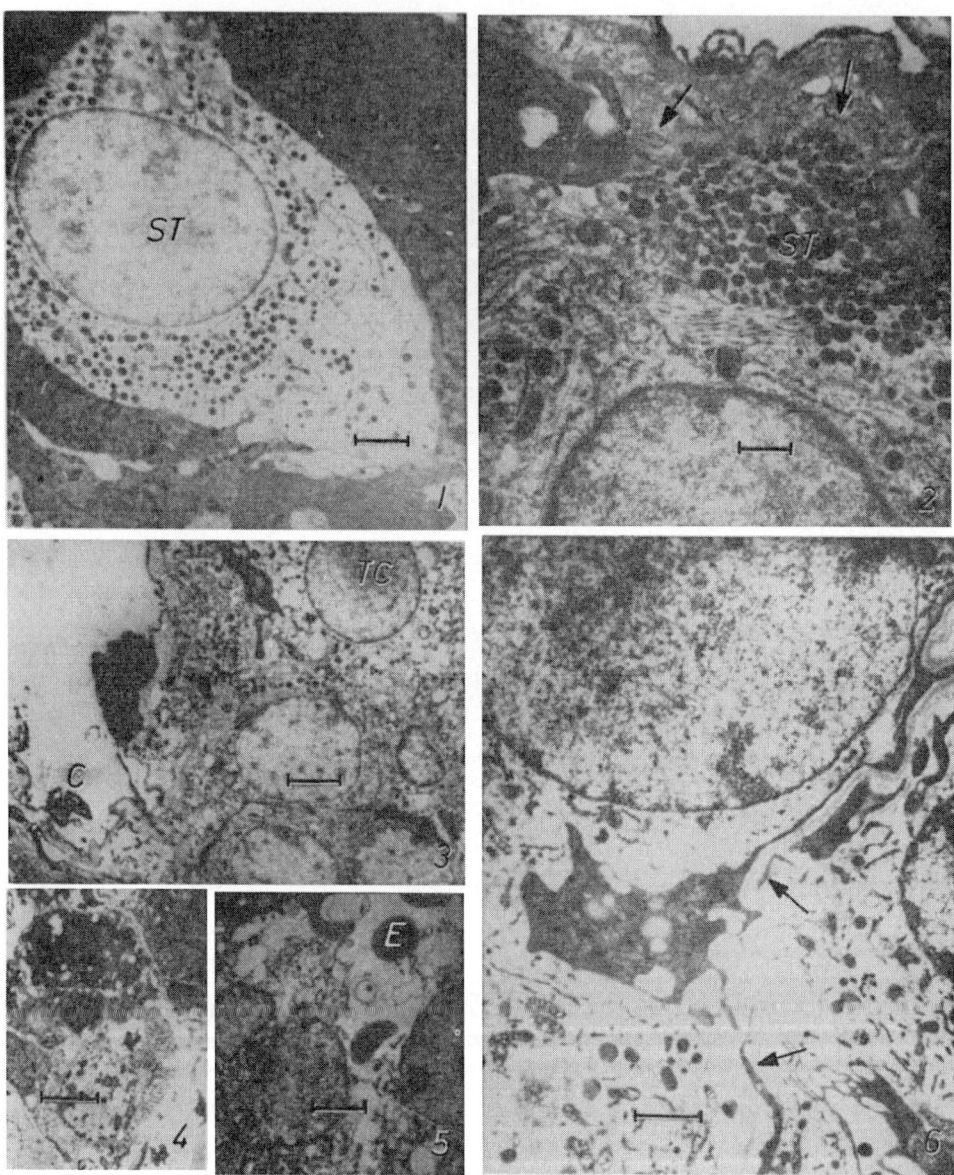

Fig. 77B. Age changes in the hypophysial ultrastructure. *1* somatotropocyte *(ST)* with a large amount of secretory granules in the cytoplasm. Adenohypophysis of a young rat. Scale: 2 μ. *2* fragment of a somatotropocyte of the adenohypophysis of a young rat; it is adjacent to periendothelial space (arrows). Scale 1 μ. *3* adenohypophysis of an old rat. A cell which resembles a thyroidectomy cell *(TC)*. Capillary *(C)*. Scale: 3 μ. *4* adenohypophysis of an old rat. Destruction of light and dark cells. Scale: 3 μ. *5* adenohypophysis of an old rat. Erythrocytes *(E)* in intercellular space. Scale: 3 μ. *6* adenohypophysis of an old rat. Periendothelial space in the parenchyma (arrows). Scale: 1 μ

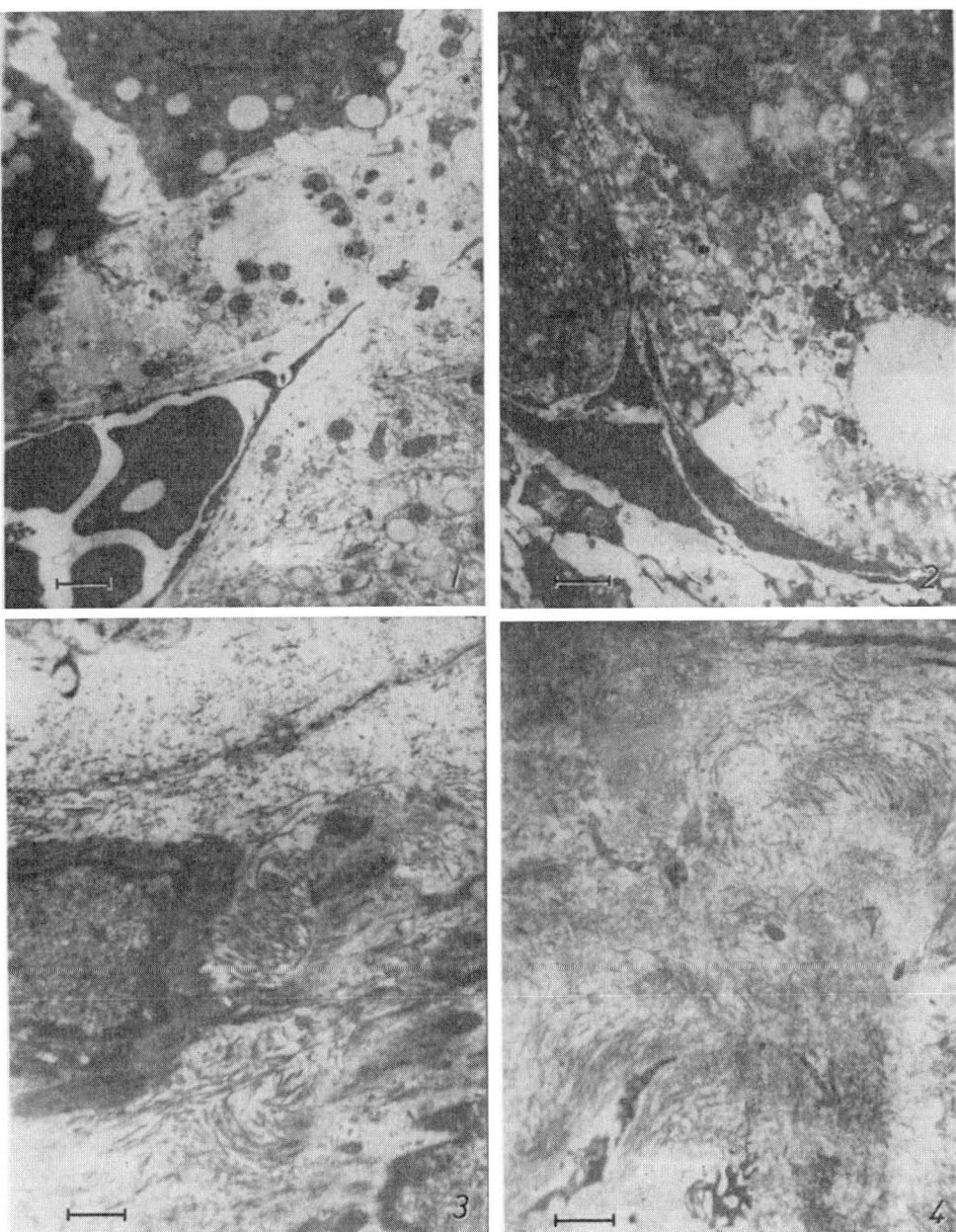

Fig. 77C. Age changes in the ultrastructure of the ovary and the uterus in rats of different ages. Scale: $2\,\mu$. *1* ovary of a young rat. Compactly arranged light and dark cells whose cytoplasm contains many mitochondria and secretory granules, and a moderately developed endoplasmic reticulum. *2* ovary of an old rat. Lipid and vacuole degeneration of the secretory cell of the ovary. *3* smooth-muscle cell of the ovary of a young rat. *4* large masses of collagenic fibres in the wall of the uterus of an old rat adrenaline do not change. However, shifts occur differently in all these elements in the neuromuscular apparatus of the extremities. When the systemic principle is used, the similarity of the structural disturbances in *Substantia nigra* and the striopallidal system as well as in *Locus ceruleus* and the hypothalamus becomes clear.

In our laboratory, Bezrukov (1979) determined the electric activity and excitability of several nuclei of the hypothalamus as well as their sensitivity to humoral factors. As we have seen, the physiological properties of these nuclei change not only differently, but also in different directions with age. This is due to their participation in both the regulation of definite functional systems of the organism and the realization of definite behavioural acts. For instance, some nuclei of the anterior hypothalamus are connected with the regulation of the basal level of gonadotropins, temperature control, the regulation of sleep, and so on, the posterior hypothalamus is connected with the realization of stress reactions, the regulation of endocrine glands, and so forth, and the lateral hypothalamus is connected with the formation of positive emotions, the appetite, etc.

The definite harmony of the dynamics of the age changes in various cellular structures of some functional systems is due to the primary and secondary shifts which occur with age. For instance, the sequence of the aging of the cells is determined by the level of their differentiation, mitotic activity, regulatory specifics and their relation to a certain system.

It has been established that 90 per cent of all the cells in the organism are postmitotic. They include neurons. The structural, metabolic and functional changes in such cells are especially significant during aging. The postmitotic cells die and their number diminishes as a result of the gross irreversible age changes. Table 1 presents data on the death of neurons in various structures of the central nervous system (Frolkis, Bezrukov, 1979). The number of neurons in various parts of the brain decreases sharply, though to a different extent. It has been shown that the death of neurons in the brain of a mouse can be described by the Gompertz curve, which characterizes the animal's extent of survival.

Ever since the work of Minot (1908), Metalnikov (1917) and Cowdry (1939), researchers have been studying the link between the specialization and differentiation of the cells, on the one hand, and their ability to divide and age, on the other. The great extent of differentiation is believed to reduce the ability of the cells to undergo division. Cells cannot become substantially renewed when they lose their ability to undergo division. Consequently, conditions are created for their aging. Evans (1979) draws our attention to the fact that the age changes in the late passages of the human fibroblasts *in vitro* are similar to the shifts which occur in the postmitotic cells. To analyze the aging of the dividing and postmitotic cells, it is important to study the cells which undergo facultative division, e. g. the hepatic cells. It has been discovered that they begin to divide actively under definite conditions (partial hepatectomy, etc.). There are certain distinctions in the regeneration of the liver of adult and old animals after hepatectomy. However, many age differences are levelled out when hepatectomy is repeated. Hence, aging is largely revealed during the cell's postmitotic state.

The role which the aging of the postmitotic nerve cells plays is clearly seen when the life cycle of the giant neurons of the pond snail is studied. A link has been established between the aging of this snail, on the one hand, and the structural and functional changes in its neurons, on the other. Is has been discovered that the final stage of the animal's life coincides with both the clear-cut changes in the morphology of its nerve cells and the disturbance of the state of their organoids. There is a great difference between the function and structure of the pond snail's neural ganglia, on the one hand, and the cerebral activity of mammals, including man, on the other. However, they have common evolutionary features of their neuron's aging. They share many structural and ultrastructural phenomena of the aging of their nerve cells. Interestingly, the correlation between age and the neuron's state is expressed to a far greater extent than between age and the structural changes in other cells in the pond snail. Hence, the changes in the postmitotic nerve cells are the pacemakers of the pond snail's aging.

The postmitotic cells are characterized by a high level of vitauct. These cells become capable of maintaining a high level of viability for many decades even if disturbances may not only originate, but also accumulate in them during this time. The dividing cells are liberated from many disturbances during mitosis. It may seem that damages should not accumulate in them. However, great age changes occur in their protein biosynthesis and their energy processes as a result of both the inevitable "errors" in metabolism and the effect of the regulatory factors. The human nerve cells can exist and function properly for a hundred years and even more. Prolonged viability and a high level of vitauct are maintained in the nerve cells due not to the stability and inertness of the metabolic proccesses, but to the high level and reliability of the adaptive regulatory processes.

Functional protein biosynthesis, or "export" biosynthesis, is expressed especially clearly in the hepatic and secretory cells. However, it occurs to a definite extent also in the nerve cells. This applies not only to the neurosecretory cells, but also to many neurons. What we have in mind is the axoplasmic flow with which proteins, RNA, transmitters and individual organoids move. This is probably an important mechanism ot the neuron's structural renewal that protects it from the accumulation of damaging factors. When the axoplasmic flow weakens, it not only affects the tissues being innervated, but also changes the neuron's trophism, thus promoting its aging.

Hence, we see that, on the one hand, the specialization of the cells grows, being accompanied by the perfection of several aspects of their metabolism and function as well as a high level of vitauct, while, on the other, the ability of the cells to divide diminishes and is even lost. Such are the inner contradictory tendencies which increase the life span of individual cells, but which eventually limit the life span of the whole organism.

Mechnikov (1907) was among the first to try to establish the regularities of the age changes in the tissues. He wrote: "In senile atrophy, we always see the same picture: the atrophy of the 'noble' cells of tissues and their replacement with the hypertrophied connective tissue. The nerve cells, i. e. those which are used for the highest activity, namely, mental and sensual activity, movement controlling activity, and so forth, disappear so as to give their place to the lower cells known as *neuroglia,* which is the connective tissue of the nerve centres. In the liver, connective tissue forces out hepatic cells, which play a significant role in the organism's nutrition. Such tissue swamps the kidneys and tightens the canals which are needed for ridding us of many soluble substances." Mechnikov associated these disturbances of the intercellular relationships with the growing self-poisoning of the organism with age.

Bogomolets (1940) had constantly noted the change in the relationships between the connective-tissue cells and specific cells. However, he assessed the age changes in the connective tissue in a different way. He wrote: "My point of view of the significance of the activity of the physiological system of connective tissue with respect to longevity is directly opposite to Mechnikov's viewpoint. I believe that the organism begins to age from connective tissue."

Bogomolets deserves great credit, because he regarded connective tissue not only as the organism's supporting skeleton, but also as its active participant and the regulator of metabolism as well as the trophism of cells and tissues. The changes in the connective-tissue cells disturb the barrier functions in the organism and cause both the disturbance of the organism's trophism and the development of hypoxia. Connective tissue has a trophic or "donor" function, whose disturbance limits the possibilities of the plasmic cells.

The collagen is an extremely important connective-tissue element. It constitutes 25–30 per cent of all the proteins in an adult human organism. In their monograph, Nikitin and others (1977) have thoroughly described the age changes in the basic properties of the collagen. According to Verzar (1968), the primary mechanisms of aging are connected with the change in the collagen and the appearance of crosslinks in them. However, it should be taken into account that the changes in the collagen correlate more with chronological age than with the aging rate. The molecular mechanisms of aging of various cells are not universal. The molecular mechanisms of some cells cannot be explained by the data which were obtained when another type of cells was being studied. The sequence of changes at the molecular level in the cells of one type cannot be regarded as a general regularity of aging. Indeed, the sequences of the age changes in the primarily aging neuron and, for instance, in the muscle cell after the destruction of the nerve ending which reaches it greatly differ from one another.

In some cells, primary changes occur in genome regulation, while in others, they occur in the membrane processes in energy metabolism. Secondary changes then occur in the genome with the subsequent disturbances in all the links of the vital activity of the cells.

A set of structural and metabolic disturbances can ultimately cause the death of the cells. The death of neurons in various structures of the brain in old age has already been mentioned. Tauchi and Hashigawa (1977) have described the great loss of cells in the myocardium, *Musculus gastrocnemius,* the liver and other organs.

A decrease in the number of cells in old age has a different effect on the level of various organ's activity. When an organ's activity is not intensive and is on the ordinary level, a part of its cells may not participate in its work (e. g. capillaries which are "on duty," *Alveoli pulmonis,* the neuromotor units in the muscles, and the nephrons in the kidneys). The reserve of the intensification of the organ's work is limited in old age due to the death of many cells. Moreover, the same work of an organ is done by a different number of cellular elements during various age periods owing to a diminution of the function of a part of the cells. According to Yankovskaya and Podrushnyak (1979), a larger number of neuromotor units are activated in an old person than in an adult when the same amount of work is performed. In old age, a definite level of antibody formation is maintained with the participation of many immunocompetent cells, while in young animals, it is maintained due to the high level of the activity of every immunocompetent cell and to the great possibilities of protein synthesis in them (Yekhneva, 1976).

A decrease in the number of cells affects the activity of various organs to a different extent. In most organs (the skeletal muscles, the kidney, the liver, etc.), the activity of all the cells has a common aim, which is to produce a single functional effect, namely, the contraction of the skeletal muscle, urination, cholopoiesis, and so forth. However, the relationships between the cells of the central nervous system are somewhat different. In this respect, individual groups in the growing mass of cells form specific nerve centres, which control definite aspects of the organism's metabolism and function. A decrease in the relatively small amount of the nerve cells can strongly affect the activity of the nerve centre and the peripheral tissues which are controlled by the centre. Therefore, the structural changes and the death of the nerve cells strongly affect the whole organism's aging.

Discussions are still being held on the possible active nature of the death of cells with age. In this respect, it is expedient to cite data which show that the post-denervation shifts that cause the death of the cells are active at a definite stage of their development. For instance, the agents blocking transcription retard the rate of the structural changes in the skeletal muscle after denervation (Frolkis, 1975). In our laboratory, Pakhlevanyan showed that the long administration of olivomycin, a blocker of the DNA-dependent synthesis of RNA, retards the rate of change in excitability, in the resistance of the cell membrane, and in the ionic composition of *Musculus gastrocnemius* after the sciatic nerve section. According to Orlova and Khromyak (1972), the long administration of RNAase reduces post-denervation osteoporosis.

After denervation, the synthesis of RNA and protein is at first activated, and then it is suppressed. This is due to a decrease in the supracellular control of protein biosynthesis and the disturbance of intercellular control. Under these conditions of the disturbance of genome regulation, it could be that the genes which were "silent" earlier are activated, new proteins appear, and the metabolism of the cell is disturbed. The inhibitors of protein biosynthesis, while retarding this process, help to maintain the structure of the cell somewhat. The unique gene is probably repressed, and this could result in the death of the cell. In this respect, we should recall our data which show that the inhibitors of protein biosynthesis inscrease the average and maximum life spans (Frolkis *et al.*, 1976b).

Membranogenetic Mechanisms of Cellular Aging

The primary mechanisms of aging are connected with a change in genome regulation. This is the basis on which a set of age changes occurs in the metabolism, function and structure of the cell. The membranogenetic mechanisms of aging are especially significant in this respect. As a result of the age changes in genome regulation, the synthesis of the membrane proteins is disturbed and the synthesis of a special factor which regulates the state of the membrane processes (the hyperpolarizing factor) changes. Not only do the changes in protein biosynthesis influence the state of the cell membrane, but also the shifts in the membrane processes affect genome regulation during aging.

Thus, we maintain that there are two types of relationships between the activity of the genetic apparatus of the cell and the membrane state: (a) the plastic type (the synthesis of the membrane proteins) and (b) the regulatory type (the synthesis of the peptides which regulate the membrane state and thus change the cellular function). The latter includes the cellular functions which are conjugated with protein biosynthesis (we have been described these functions during the last few years) and the hyperpolarizing factor which has been discovered recently (Frolkis, 1980).

The disturbances of the membranogenetic mechanisms during aging result in a change in (a) the number of receptors of the cell and its reaction to regulatory effects, (b) the mechanisms of the active transport of substances across the membrane, (c) the number of special membrane canals, and (d) the main electric properties of the membrane that determine the functional parameters of the cell.

The plasma membrane is an extremely important link in the regulation of cellular metabolism. Its state determines the intercellular relationships, the reaction of the cell to neurohumoral effects and its trophism, and the controlled transfer of substances into the cell and from it into the external environment. The molecular composition of the cell membrane and its basic physicochemical properties change with age. The cholesterol-phospholipid ratio grows in old age. Apparently, this affects the elasticity, or mobility, of the cell membrane, which becomes more rigid. This growth has been shown on the basis of the cell membranes of the liver and the skeletal muscles of rats (Carlson et al., 1968) as well as their fibroblasts (Grinna, Barber, 1976). Moreover, an increase in lipid viscosity affects the physicochemical properties of the membrane (Borochov et al., 1976). Functionally important enzymes, receptors, ionic canals, and so forth, are included in the membrane structure. The protein composition of the membrane changes with age, and this affects its function decisively. Suffice it to say that the amount of some hormonal receptors in the cells can decrease by 50 per cent and even more (Roth, 1979). The activity of several membranous enzymes, i. e. K^+- and Na^+-ATPase, 5-nucleotidase, and alkaline phosphatase, also changes in old age.

Structural changes in the cell membrane occur with age. Indurations, enlargements, microruptures of varicose inclusions, pockets, oil droplets, and so forth, originate in it (Stupina, 1978; Kelley et al., 1979). The plication of the membrane, the growth of its surface, the invagination into the cytoplasm, and so forth, can be of definite compensatory significance. It is believed that the cell membrane is relatively stable during aging (Artyukhina, 1979). But no account is taken of the fact that the gross shifts and the great ruptures in the cell membrane cause the death of cells, which are then eliminated from the population.

The neurohumoral regulation of the metabolism and function of the cells alters with age, because changes occur in (1) the neural and hormonal influences on the cell and (2) the state of a special apparatus which perceives these influences: the cellular receptors.

In the previous chapters, we have seen that the thresholds of the neural influences on many organs, tissues and cells grow with age. According to I. V. Frolkis (1973), shifts in the membrane potential of the cells of the skeletal muscle are more pronounced in mature rats than in old ones when the force of stimulation of the sympathetic chain is the same. Faizulin (1979) has shown that the shifts in the polarization of the membrane of acinar cells of the parotid gland are less stable in old animals than in mature ones when the sympathetic nerve is stimulated. Shevchuk has discovered that the stellate ganglion must be stimulated by a stronger current in old rats than in mature ones in order to change the membrane potential of the myocardial fibres. Thus, neural control of cellular activity diminishes with age. As we have seen, this is due to the attenuation of the synthesis of the mediators in the nerve endings, a decrease in their uptake by the terminals, and the weakening of the axoplasmic flow which carries the vesicles with the mediator to the nerve endings.

The given changes in the synaptic transfer in old age have a morphological basis. Great structural disturbances and a diminution of the number of nerve endings in the heart, the skeletal muscles, the stomach and various parts of the brain have been observed. The number of axospinose synapses as well as the synapses on the body of the nerve cells is reduced sharply in old rats. In these animals, endings with a small number of synaptic vesicles occur and the area of the "active" synaptic zones as well as the width of the dense postsynaptic membranous layer diminishes. According to Timchenko (1972), the number of synapses from which miniature potentials can be recorded decreases in their skeletal muscles.

All these shifts in the neural regulation of the cells are among of the causes of the gross disturbance of their structure and functions. According to Fudel-Osipova (1968), the disturbances of the neural apparatus of the skeletal muscles of rats occur earlier than the gross disturbances of the skeletal muscle fibres. The latter are largely the outcome of the former. The destruction of the neural apparatus together with atrophy and the degradation of the cells being innervated has been discovered in other organs, too.

Cellular activity is regulated due not only to neurohumoral control, but also to intercellular contacts. For instance, the intercellular nexus contacts are known to play an important role in the function of the smooth muscle cells of the vascular walls. They help to transfer the stimulus from one cell to another and probably promote plastic exchange between them. Accor ingito I. V. Frolkis (1978), the number of nexus in the smooth muscle wall of the portal vein decreases in old age. This number comes to 10–12 over an area of 2,500 μm² in rats 8–10 months old and only 4–6 over the same area in rats 24–26 months old. Nexus of the "lock" type are found in old rats (Fig. 78). Such nexus are more stable and can be a manifestation of vitauct when the total number of intercellular contacts decreases.

A change in cellular reception is one of the most important mechanisms of cellular aging. A decrease in the number of receptors not only affects a cell's reaction to neural and hormonal influences, but also changes the extent of trophic effects, which are constantly realized through these pathways of the information which goes to the cell. As the number of receptors diminishes, the cell not only gets out of the organism's control, but also loses the forms of metabolic stimulation without which it cannot normally exist.

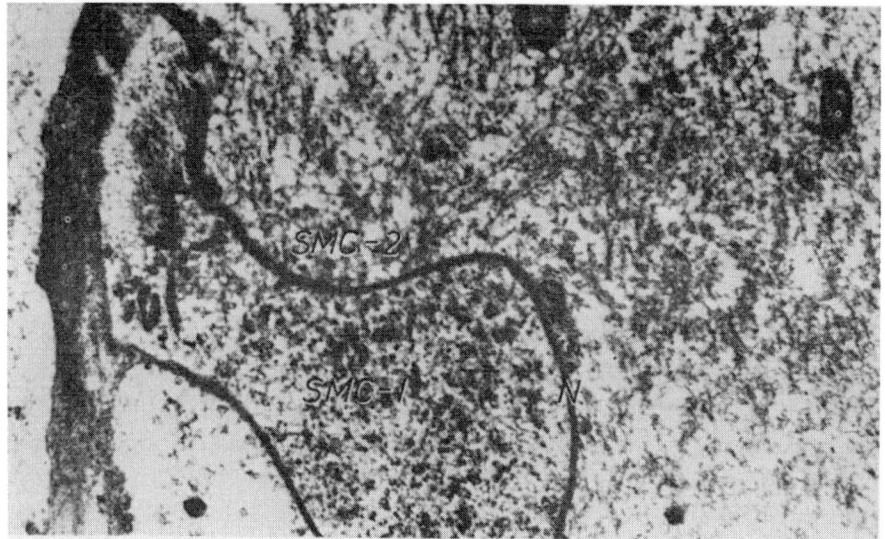

Fig. 78. Nexus (N) between the smooth-muscle cell of the longitudinal layer (SMC-1) and the smooth-muscle cell of the circular layer (SMC-2) of the portal vein of an old rat (28 months). 59,400 ×

Data are now available on a change in cellular reception in old age. They had been obtained when the effects of hormones and mediators on the brain, the liver, the heart, the skeletal muscles, adipose tissue, fibroblasts and erythrocytes were being studied. At the same time, it has been established that the ability of the receptors to become bound with a hormone does not change or, according to some data, even grows. After analyzing the literature as well as his own data, Roth (1979) noted several variants of a change in the number of receptors in ontogeny: (a) the concentration of the receptors decreases only in old age; (b) the concentration of the receptors in early mature age decreases and later does not change; (c) the concentration of the receptors does not change throughout life, and (d) the concentration of the receptors grows with age. However, most researchers note that the concentration of the receptors decreases in old age. A parallel can be drawn between a decrease in the number of receptors and a change in the hormonal effect. For instance, the ability of corticosteroids to suppress the oxidation of glucose in the hepatocytes and the incorporation of uridine into lymphocytes decreases as the number of gluco-corticoid receptors diminish in rats (Roth, Livingston, 1976).

In the previous chapters, our data have shown that the number of cholinoreceptors and beta adrenoreceptors decreases in the heart and the brain, while the number of alpha adrenoreceptors does not change in the cardiovascular system with age. Thus, cellular "dereception," so to say, probably occurs with age, limiting the ability of the cells to react to neurohormonal influences. A decrease in neurohumoral control is known to change the state of the cell substantially, while denervation can cause the atrophy of several cells. When cellular dereception grows, it limits the range of neurohormonal control and can become an extremely important mechanism of cellular aging.

The number as well as the state of cellular receptors changes with age. The reaction of a cell is known to depend on the affinity of the receptors for hormones, the duration of their interaction, and so forth. The calculated and experimental data given in the previous chapters show that the affinity of the receptors for physiologically active substances changes with age. Consequently, the reaction of the cells to the humoral factors changes in old age. This has been shown in the experiments carried out *in vivo* and *in vitro* with the cells of various organs, i. e. the neurons of various parts of the rat brain, the ganglia of the pond snail, hepatocytes, cardiocytes, skeletal muscle fibres, and the cells of the parotid gland, the adrenal cortex and the thyroid gland. A study has been made of the reactions to various substances with a mediatory effect and hormones, namely, catecholamines, acetylcholine, cholinergic and adrenergic blocking agents, insulin, hydrocortisone, estradiol dipropionate, the somatotropic hormone, and corticotropin. In most cases, the reaction of the cell was determined by a change in the electric properties of its membrane and by ionic shifts.

A study of the neurohumoral effects has shown that the reactions of different cells to the same substance as well as the reactions of the same cells to different substances are quantitatively and qualitatively diverse in old age. This diversity of the response engenders contradictory concepts of the age specifics of regulation.

The sensitivity of the cells to many hormones increases, while their reactivity decreases in old age. Fig. 79, which has been drawn up on the basis of the works by Frolkis and orthers (1972, 1976), Korotonozhkin (1973), Martynenko (1977, 1980) and Turaeva (1979), shows that the doses of insulin, adrenaline and estradiol dipropionate that cause the growth of the membrane potential of the cell are smaller for old animals than for mature ones. According to I. V. Frolkis (1978), smaller doses of noradrenaline cause the spontaneous electric and contractile activity of the cells of the portal vein in old animals. Gorban (1979) has shown that the shifts in the membrane potential, especially during the second hyperpolarization phase, are more pronounced in old rats when small doses of the thyrotropic hormone (0.5 unit per 100 g of weight) are administered. According to Faizulin (1979), however, sensitivity to adrenaline and acetylcholine in the acinar cells of the parotid gland is higher in mature rats than in old ones. Moreover, the sensitivity of even the same cell to various

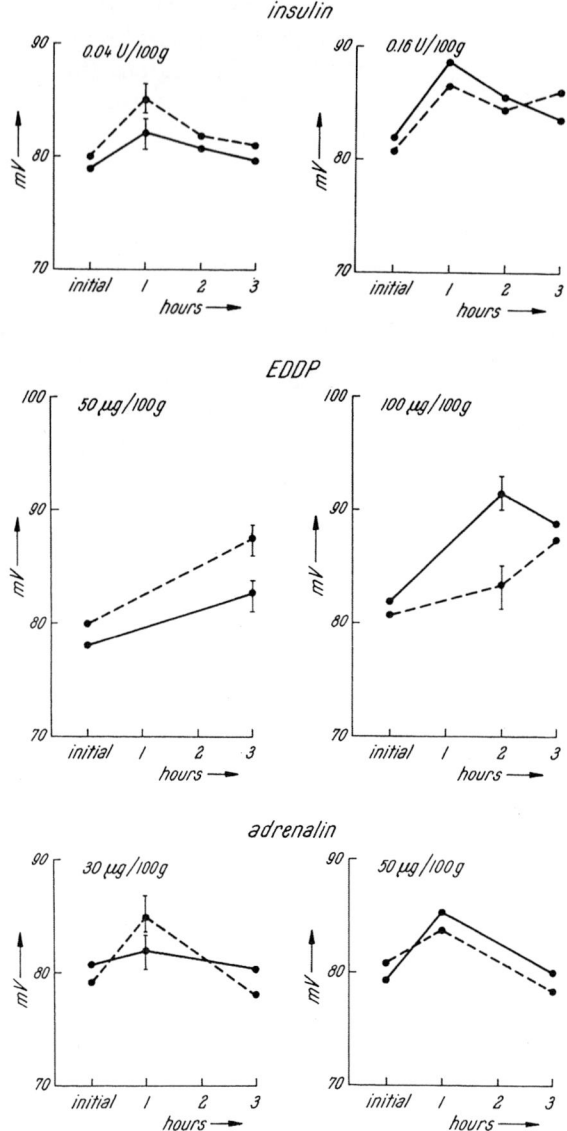

Fig. 79. Influence of various doses of insulin, estradiol dipropionate and adrenaline on the membrane potential of muscle fibers in mature and old rats. The dashed line stands for old rats, and the continuous line, for mature rats

substances can change differently in old age. According to Martynenko, for instance, the sensitivity of the neurons of the parietal ganglion of the pond snails which are 2.5 years old does not change with respect to insulin, but increases with respect to adrenaline. The range of the reactions, just as the reactivity to the action of several physiologically active substances, diminishes with age. A decrease in the number of receptors in one cell and in the number of cells in an organ is probably ʻhat reduces the range of the response and the reactivity of the cells and organs. A change in the state of cellular receptors affects the sensitivity of the cells. We do not know the nature of these changes. However, it is clear that they increase cellular sensitivity in some cases and reduce it in others.

In this respect, it is necessary to take a few examples from our laboratory's works which prove that the state of the receptors changes with age. Tanin (1977) has shown that the reaction of the neurons of the spinal cord to insulin and estradiol dipropionate virtually disappears in old age. This is due not to the disappearance of the respective receptors, but to a change in their state. The

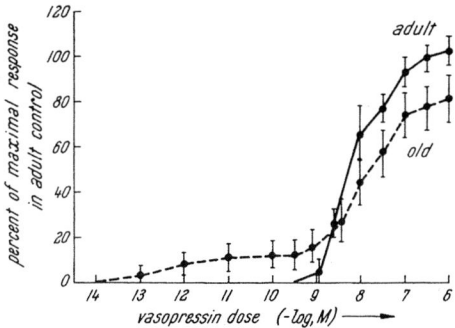

Fig. 80. Cumulative curve of the dose effect of the contraction of an isolated aortic strip of mature and old rats with respect to the growing concentrations of arginine vasopressin; percentage of maximum contraction in mature animals

reaction to hormones is restored after the administration of Ionol, which is an antioxidant. A change in the state of the lipid layer of the membrane and the accumulation of free radicals, lipid peroxides, and so forth, can probably so affect the state of the receptors that they no longer interact with the hormones.

The shifts in both the cholesterol-phospholipid relationship and the lipid state can cause conformation changes in the protein receptors of the membrane and disturb the molecular mobility of the receptors on the cellular surface in old age, thus affecting the ability of the cell to respond to stimulation.

We have shown earlier than the donator of the sulfhydryl groups, i. e. unithiol, increases sharply the lability of the neuromuscular synapse in old rats, thus apparently affecting the state of the cholinoreceptors of the postsynaptic membrane.

Fig. 80 presents Golovchenko's data on the effect of various concentrations of vasopressin on the contractility of the strips of the abdominal aorta of rats of different age. Old animals have a group of changed receptors which react to very low hormone concentrations. Thus, not only the quantity, but also the state of the receptors change with age, as a result of which the specifics of the cellular reactions are affected in old age.

When the number of receptors decreases, an increase in the sensitivity of the cells to several mediators and hormones is probably of adaptive regulatory significance.

Cellular receptors are proteins. Hence, their change is most probably due to the shifts in the protein-synthesizing system. The selectivity of definite receptors and the extent of diminution of their content can be explained from the standpoint of the genoregulatory hypothesis of aging. This may involve the selective age change in the regulation of definite genetic loci, which limit the synthesis of definite receptor proteins.

There is probably another mechanism of a change in the quantity of the receptor proteins of the cell. The genetic induction of receptor proteins exists just as the genetic induction of enzymes. This is evident from the data on the determination of the relationship between an increase or decrease in the concentration of the blood hormones and the number of receptors which perceive their action. It has been shown with the aid of enzymic induction that the long administration of a substrate or a hormone inductor can gradually reduce the synthesis of the appropriate protein (Salganik, 1972; Frolkis, 1970, 1975). This peculiar suppression of the inductive response is expressed differently when different enzymes are synthesized. For instance, it was discovered that the synthesis of tyrosine aminotransferase is easily exhausted when hormones act on it for a long time, while that of microsomal enzymes is virtually inexhaustible under experimental conditions.

Experiments carried out to study the age specifics of a change in sensitivity during pharmacological denervation are a definite confirmation of a link between aging and receptor synthesis. When reserpine is administered, the cells become more sensitive to catecholamines because the number of adrenoreceptors increases. However, sensitivity to adrenaline does not grow when actinomycin D (50 μg per 100 g of weight), which blocks RNA synthesis, is administered prior to reserpine. This is apparently because new adrenoreceptors cannot be synthesized. Interestingly, chemical denervation does not enhance sensitivity to catecholamines in old animals. The receptor proteins are probably inadequately synthesized in this case, too. The results of these experiments indirectly confirm the concept of the link between cellular dereception in old age and the shifts in protein biosynthesis.

The action of many physiologically active substances is known to occur due to the activation of adenylate cyclase and the synthesis of cyclic nucleotides, which are a second messenger, as it were, in the influence of many substances on the cell. Catecholamines, glucagon, vasopressin, and so forth, exert their influence through this system. According to some researchers, adenylate cyclase is a receptor subunit situated on the inner side of the membrane. The basal level of cyclic AMP and cyclic GMP does not change in most organs with age. However, as Kulchitsky and I. V. Frolkis have shown, small doses of catecholamines and acetylcholine increase the content of cyclic AMP and cyclic GMP to a greater extent in old animals than in mature ones (see Figs. 44, 45). Sensitivity to hormones and mediators grows in old age probably often due to the shifts in the properties of the adenylate cyclase system. This is evident also from the fact that sodium fluoride, which is a specific activator of adenylate cyclase, causes greater shifts in old rats.

Thus, a peculiar vicious circle may originate with age: constant neurohumoral stimulation promotes the age changes in the receptors, while the changes in the receptors largely limit the adaptive neurohumoral influences on the cell. The cell undergoes age degradation more rapidly if the amount of its receptors to various hormones is reduced and its neurohumoral "support" is changed.

Shifts in cellular functions accompanied by protein biosynthesis are very important in cellular aging. There is enough proof to maintain that a special peptide factor, which controls the state of the cell membrane, is synthesized when the genetic apparatus is activated. We called it the hyperpolarizing factor, since it causes the growth of the membrane potential of the cell, and the link between protein biosynthesis in the cell and the state of its membrane is realized with its participation. An important fact is that many hormones act on the cell through this regulatory mechanism. There are grounds to believe that this control of the genetic apparatus over the cell membrane change substantially with age.

Earlier, we formulated the concept of the cellular function which are conjugated with protein biosynthesis, having in mind the shifts which occur in the state of the cell membrane when the genetic apparatus of the cell is activated (Frolkis *et al.*, 1970–1980). There is now evidence of such a link, e. g. (a) the factors which activate protein biosynthesis (such hormones as insulin, the sex hormones, the somatotropic hormone and hydrocortisone, and also regeneration, loss of blood, etc.) cause the hyperpolarization of various cells (neurons, hepatocytes, muscle fibres, etc.) (see Fig. 79); (b) under the action of hormones, hyperpolarization precedes the activation of protein biosynthesis; (c) the inhibitors of protein biosynthesis (actinomycin D, olivomycin, puromycin, cycloheximide, etc.) prevent hyperpolarization (Fig. 81).

In the last series of studies, we have clearly shown that all those facts can be ascribed to one cause, i. e. a special hyperpolarizing factor is synthesized when protein biosynthesis is activated in the cell. This is how we found the factor:

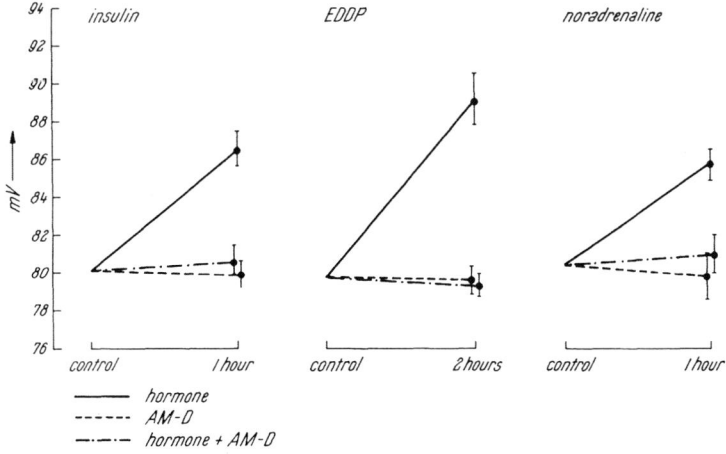

Fig. 81. Influence of actinomycin D (10 μg/kg) on the development of the hyperpolarization of the muscle fibres due to insulin (1.6 U/kg), estradiol dipropionate (1 mg/kg) and noradrenaline (300 μg/kg)

protein biosynthesis was activated in the liver of the donor animals by hydrocortisone administration, blood-letting or hepatectomy. Consequently, hyperpolarization originated. At the peak of polarization, the liver was homogenized
and filtered off. Afterwards, the recipient's liver was subjected to filtrate action
(application or perfusion).

The hyperpolarization effect is transferable, i. e. the membrane potential
grows in the recipients. The homogenate of the liver of intact animals does not
cause such changes.

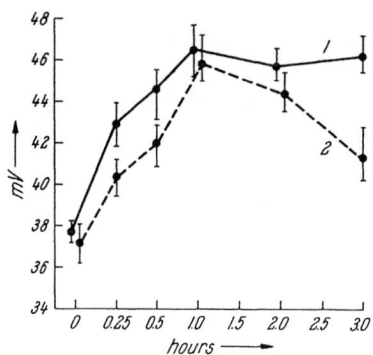

Fig. 82. Influence of the hyperpolarizing factor separated from the liver of rats 8–10 months old *(1)*
and rats 26–28 months old *(2)* on the membrane potential of the hepatocytes of the recipient

The inhibitors of protein biosynthesis (actinomycin D and cycloheximide)
were administered to rat donors in a special series of experiments. In this case,
the hormones did not cause the hyperpolarization of the cell membranes, while
the homogenate did not change the membrane potential in the recipient. Hence,
the given hyperpolarizing factor originates during protein biosynthesis. The
factor which we discovered is probably a simple peptide.

The growth of the membrane potential, being caused by the effect of the
hyperpolarizing factor, greatly influences trophism and the restorative processes
in the cell. Cellular excitability diminishes when hyperpolarization develops.
Protein biosynthesis is known to require great energy expenditures, while the
diminution of excitability stops the cell from participation in other processes and
thus creates the best conditions for restorative processes. Hence, this diminution
is of adaptive regulatory significance. Hyperpolarization deforms the membrane
and increases its permeability with respect to several substances (Zierler, 1960).
The "laminar" structure of its lipoprotein acquires a micellar, or globular
configuration. In this case, pores which can be penetrated by many
water-soluble substances are formed, and the configuration of ionic canals
changes. Thus, the activation of the genetic apparatus includes the mechanism of
a change in the state of the cell membrane. According to the data obtained by
our laboratory (Paramonova, 1977), prolonged hyperpolarization reduces the
intensity of protein biosynthesis in the cell.

This extremely important mechanism of intracellular regulation changes in
old age. Fig. 82 shows that the hyperpolarizing effect of the homogenate of the

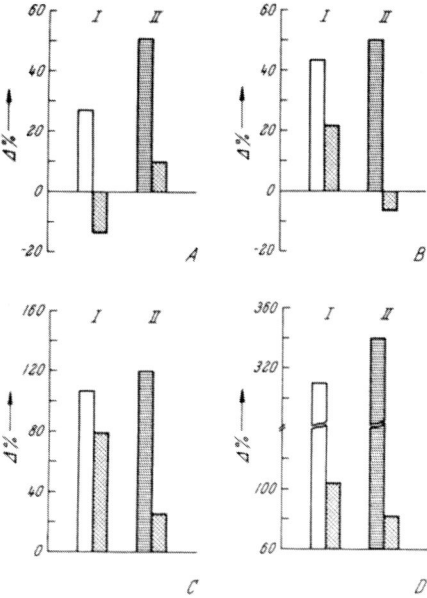

Fig. 83. Influence of the hyperpolarization of the plasma membrane on the inductive synthesis of hepatic enzymes when hydrocortisone is administered to mature rats (I) and old rats (II). A gluco-se-6-phosphatase; B fructose-1,6-diphosphatase; C tyrosine aminotransferase; D tryptophan pyrrolase. First column in each pair–hydrocortisone effect, second column–effect of hydro-cortisone + hyperpolarization

hepatic tissue is lower in old rats than in mature ones. A smaller amount of the hyperpolarizing factor is probably formed in old animals when all the other conditions are equal. In other words, the genetic apparatus of the cell weakens its control of the state of the cell membrane, and the conjugation of protein biosynthesis and the cellular function change in old age. This probably affects the optimum restorative processes.

According to our data, the hyperpolarization of the cells can be caused by a smaller amount of a hormone in old animals, but it does not take as long time as in mature ones. During hyperpolarization, ionic shifts develop (in some cases, intracellular potassium accumulates) and substrates accumulate. Consequently, protein biosynthesis may be suppressed. Fig. 83A, B, C, D shows that when the anode hyperpolarization of the cell membranes is the same in mature and old rats, its inhibiting effect on the genetic induction of several enzymes is more pronounced in the latter.

The adaptive trophic and restorative effect of hyperpolarization decreases when the process begins to exert less influence on protein biosynthesis. Many structures and processes are restored in the cell due to the activation of protein biosynthesis. However, the temporary suppression of the intensity of protein biosynthesis plays an important role in restoring cellular potentialities. A change in the relationship between hyperpolarization and protein biosynthesis is an extremely important mechanism of a change in cellular trophism in old age.

Thus, the cell has a self-regulatory system which conjugates the activity of the genetic apparatus and the cellular function by means of bilateral bonds. The age changes in the chain linking the genetic apparatus, the synthesis of the hyperpolarizing factor, the growth of the membrane potential, ionic shifts and the activity of the genetic apparatus are an important molecular functional mechanism of cellular aging.

Electric Properties of Cells During Aging

The membrane potential changes differently in various cellular populations in old age. It virtually does not change in the muscle fibres, hepatocytes, motoneurons of the spinal cord, and the neurons of the sensorimotor region of the cortex, while it grows somewhat in cardiocytes, the smooth muscle cells of vessels, the acinar cells of the parotid gland, and so forth (Martynenko, 1967; Tanin, 1976; Faizulin, 1979; Turaeva, 1979, and others). These data have been obtained from rats 24 and 25 months old, which are usually considered to be old. However, the membrane potential sharply diminishes in very old animals, i. e. in those 36–38 months old. It changes differently in the same cellular population. Cells with a low membrane potential are found more frequently in old animals. In most cases, these cells are structurally changed.

Definite distinctions can be seen in adult and old animals when the thresholds of the direct stimulation of individual muscle fibres are measured. In adult rats, the average value of the threshold current is $6.3 \pm 0.14 \times 10^{-8}$A. In old rats, the threshold response of the muscle fibre to electric stimulation originates most frequently when the force of the current is $8.9 \pm 0.14 \times 10^{-8}$A (Martynenko, 1971). The action potential originates when depolarization is at a critical level, i. e. 49.3 mV, in adult rats and 33.4 mV in old rats. The higher the critical level of depolarization, the smaller is the force of the stimulating current which causes the necessary shift in the potential, and the higher is excitability. The threshold shift in the potential is at 30.9 ± 1.0 mV in adult animals and at 46.7 ± 0.6 mV in old ones. An increase in the threshold of critical depolarization in old rats also shows that the membrane should be depolarized to a greater extent in them so as to allow the spreading action potential to originate in them. Such a direction of the changes in excitability is characteristic of not all the cells. According to Tanin (1976), the excitability of the interneurons and motor neurons of the spinal cord grows in old age. A calculation of the input resistance of the muscle fibre, specific membrane resistance, and membrane resistance per unit length of the fibre in white rats showed that these parameters have definite distinctions in conformity with an animal's age. The input resistance of the muscle fibres of adult rats averages 390 ± 8 kilo-ohms, while it is 270 ± 17 kilo-ohms in old ones. The specific membrane resistance in old rats is almost one-half of that in adult rats. Membrane resistance per unit length of the fibre also decreases substantially in old animals.

The action potential of the muscle fibres changes with age: the amplitude decreases, while the duration increases (Solomatin, 1970; Frolkis et al., 1976c). In adult dogs, the amplitude of the action potential of the muscle fibres is

116.9 ±1.8 mV, while it is 72.5 ± 3.2 mV in old dogs. It is 113.6 ± 2.4 mV and 91.2 ± 2.3 mV, respectively, in adult and old rats.

The fact that the excitation process changes in old age is evident from the changes in the duration of the absolute and relative refractory phases. The cell is completely unexcitable during the absolute refractory phase, which coincides with the excitation process. Cellular excitability is restored during the relative refractory phase, which coincides with the repolarization of the cell membrane. The duration of the absolute relative refractory phases increases substantially in old animals. For instance, the relative refractory phase is 5–5.6 milliseconds in rats 2–6 and 20–24 months old, while it is 7.5–10 milliseconds in rats 30–36 months old.

To characterize the functional state of the nerve cells, it is important to determine the rate at which a stimulus is propagated. Most researchers note that the stimulus is propagated more slowly along the peripheral nerves in elderly persons. This change is expressed differently in various nerve trunks. The stimulus is propagated at a rate of 70.57 ± 0.76 meters per second in the ulnar nerve of young persons and 50.38 ± 0.84 meters per second in that of old persons, 53.92 ± 0.99 and 42.9 ± 0.9 meters per second in the fibular nerve of young and old persons, respectively, and 47.7 ± 0.67 and 37.56 ±1.03 meters per second in the tibial nerve of young and old persons, respectively (Timko, 1971).

The latent period of the arbitrary inclusion of the motor unit into activity is longer in elderly persons. It is 0.1–0.5 seconds in young persons and 0.6–3.0 seconds in elderly persons (Fudel-Osipova, 1968; Yankovskaya, Podrushnyak, 1979). The electromyogram of old persons has many low-amplitude potentials (below 400 microvolts). In young persons, the amplitude reaches 900–1,200 microvolts. The frequency of the action potentials of the motor unit of the biceps muscle is 11–13 Hz in young persons and 6–8 Hz in elderly persons. Long polyphasic currents occur more frequently in elderly persons than in young persons.

To ascertain the age changes in the cellular function, it is important to study the active and passive transport of ions through the cell membrane. This process is known to not only determine the level of membrane polarization, but also regulate the activity of many intracellular enzymes and the intensity of protein biosynthesis (Malenkov, 1976). The potassium permeability of the membranes of the muscle fibres of the skeletal muscles and the heart diminishes with age (Martynenko, 1971). According to Kuprash (1974), the intracellular content of potassium in the fibres of the myocardium, the liver, the kidneys and the skeletal muscles decreases greatly, while the concentration of sodium and chlorine does not change very much in old age. According to Novikova (1964), the intracellular concentration of potassium is maintained on the same level in the muscles of rats from the day they are born until they are 3 months old. However, it diminishes greatly in animals 12 and 24 months old. The concentration of sodium ions remains relatively stable when the animals are between 1 and 12 months old, but it increases by the time they are 24 months old. The content of intracellular potassium decreases and that of chlorine increases in old age. Novikova (1978) and Turaeva (1979) have observed that intracellular sodium accumulates, while the content of potassium diminishes in the hepatocytes. Zs.-Nagy (1979), however, has presented opposite data. He determined the activity of potassium ions inside the cells and found that they accumulate in the cell in old age.

An important fact is that not only the content of ions, but also the neurohumoral regulation of their transport changes with age. In our laboratory, Korotonozhkin (1973), Martynenko (1977, 1980) and Turaeva (1979) studied the dynamics of the ionic asymmetry in the cells of the skeletal muscles and the liver under the influence of insulin, estradiol dipropionate, hydrocortisone and adrenaline in animals of different age. Small doses of hormones caused ionic shifts of greater intensity in old rats. Another important fact is that ionic transport changes differently under the effect of hormones in old age. Consequently, shifts may occur in the intracellular ionic content, changing the metabolic state of the cell. It is believed that ionic shifts can become a cause of the age changes in the biosynthesis of the protein (Zs.-Nagy, 1979).

A description of the age changes in the electric activity of the cell membranes gives a definite idea of the change in ionic transport. Membranous permeability is known to increase sharply as a result of stimulation. This permeability is 20 times higher for Na^+ than for K^+. The inflow of Na^+ into the cell surpasses the outflow of K^+, thus causing depolarization. Then, sodium conductivity is inactivated and the outflow of K^+ from the cell intensifies. Consequently, the membrane is repolarized with possible trace hyperpolarization. According to Martynenko (1977, 1980), repolarization takes longer and less trace hyper-polarization is found in the parietal ganglion of old pond snails. This relates to the action potential elements which are connected with the potassium outflow. It should be recalled that repolarization takes longer also in the muscle fibres and motoneurons of the spinal cord of old rats, thus confirming the concept that the potassium permeability of the membrane diminishes in old age. The data presented by Turaeva (1979) are interesting in this respect. She showed that adrenaline hyperpolarization is connected largely with the accumulation of intracellular potassium in adult animals and with the diminution of the sodium content in old ones. Various components of the ionic current probably change differently with age.

The synthesis of ionic canals is known to be coded by definite genes. Great changes occur in genome regulation and protein biosynthesis with age. These shifts probably affect the regulatory system, which determines the formation of the potassium and sodium canals. This may reduce the number of ionic canals in the membrane of an old cell and change the duration of the action potential. Tetrodotoxin is known to block selectively the sodium canals of the membrane. Tanin (1976) has shown that the application of tetrodotoxin causes the growth of the membrane potential of the neurons of the spinal cord by 4–5 mV in adult animals, but does not change it in old ones. This may indicate that the state of the sodium canals is changed in old age. Consequently, they do not interact with tetrodotoxin, or the number of these canals diminishes in old age. The synthesis of the proteins of the plasma membrane is activated in response to the administration of insulin. In adult animals, activity reaches its peak three hours after the administration of the hormone (two units per 100 g of weight), while in old animals it does so only five hours later.

The active transmembranous transport mechanism is ensured by the energy of the macroergic phosphorus compounds. ATP is hydrolyzed by a specialized enzymic membranous Na^+-K^+-ATPase system, whose work is vectorial: the sodium ions are pumped out constantly, while potassium accumulates in the cell.

Recent investigations have shown that the mechanism of the active transfer of ions through the membrane can function in two ways. One of them is the exchange of the intracellular ions for extracellular ones on an electroneutral basis ("charge for charge") and does not affect the membrane potential directly. The other is the active transfer of ions on an electrogenous basis, when the amount of charges transferred in one direction is not compensated by the amount of ions transferred in another direction, i. e. the transport mechanism can separate the charges and thus create directly the difference of potentials on the membrane.

A change in the work of this mechanism is an extremely important factor of the age changes in the cells. This is evident from the following:

1. There is clear evidence that the activity of the K^+-Na^+-ATPase of the membrane of several cells decreases with age (Novikova, Malysheva, 1975; Sousa, Baskin, 1977), although some authors did not find any changes in the activity of the enzyme. A description has been given of even the growth of the activity of the K^+-Na^+-ATPase of the membranes of the hepatocytes in old age.

According to our data, the energy provision of the cell diminishes, oxidative phosphorylation becomes less intense, and the content of ATP, creatine phosphate and other substances decreases in old age (Frolkis, 1970).

2. The membranous K^+-Na^+-ATPase is known to be blocked by ouabain. The role which the electrogenous transport of ions plays in maintaining the value of the membrane potential can be seen by measuring the potential under the effect of ouabain. According to Gorban (1979), ouabain reduces the membrane potential of the muscle fibres of the diaphragm by 14.6 ± 0.75 mV in mature rats and by 8.2 ± 0.86 mV in old ones. According to Tanin (1976), it does not reduce the membrane potential of the neurons of the spinal cord in old rats, while it reduces this potential by 9./ mV in mature rats. However, ouabain causes greater hyperpolarization in the cells of the liver and the parotid gland of old rats than of mature ones. The different nature of the given shifts is apparently due to the different ionic mechanisms of maintaining the membrane potential in various cells.

3. The work of the sodium pump in the electrogenous mode can be simulated by various methods. The reversible suppression of the sodium pump's functioning by cooling the preparations down to 0–5 °C for a definite length of time leads to the accumulation of large amounts of sodium ions in the cell. When a preparation is later put into a solution with room or elevated temperature, the membranous K^+-Na^+-ATPase is activated sharply and the excessive amounts of the accumulated sodium ions are pumped out. In this case, the sodium pump begins to operate in the electrogenous mode and the so-called temperature hyperpolarization develops on the membrane, while the membrane potential is much higher than the calculated potassium equilibrium potential.

Gorban (1979), our fellow worker, studied the temperature relationship between the repolarization of the membranes of the cells of the adrenal glands and the repolarization of those of the diaphragm. He discovered that great age differences in repolarization originate in old age, while the value of the membrane potential of the cells of those organs remains unchanged. In this respect, the Q_{10} of the process and the E_{act} of the reactions, which determine the growth of the membrane potential of the cells of the adrenal cortex in the temperature range of 7–17 °C and the growth of the membrane potential of the muscle cells in the temperature range of 10–20 °C after they are cooled at first to 0 °C in a potassium-free solution, are twice as high in old animals as in young ones (Q_{10} is 1.4 and 2.7 for the cells of the adrenal cortex and 1.5 and 3.8 for the muscle cells of mature and old rats, respectively). Hence, the role of the non-enzymic reactions probably increases in the overall balance of the processes which determine the repolarization of the cell membrane in old animals.

Thus, the activity of the ionic pump and the energy provision of ionic transfer decrease greatly with age, causing substantial changes in the cellular function. The state of the membrane and of its lipids and lipid peroxides as well as free-radical reactions play apparently an important role in the changing activity of ATPase which is built into the membrane. Gorban showed that the addition of the antioxidant Ionol (2,6-di-tert-butyl-4-methylphenol) levels out the age differences during temperature hyperpolarization and reduces both the temperature coefficient and the energy of activation of reactions. Apparently, the activity of the membranous K^+-Na^+-ATPase in old age is determined largely by its lipid micro-environment, which changes in old age.

Hence, not only the phospholipid composition, but also the lipid state changes with age. This can change the physicochemical properties of the membrane and its fluidity substantially and can influence the basic properties of the membrane properties, their mobility and accessibility, and consequently the basic properties of the membrane.

Aging is characterized by the redistribution of the pathways of the metabolic ensurance of the function. The mechanisms of intracellular self-regulation make it possible to maintain the same level of the cellular function when irregular changes occur in various metabolic cycles. The energy expenditures on various needs in the cell as well as various ways of energy generation change with age. The results obtained (Korotonozhkin, 1973) suggest that, with age, the relationship between glycolytic and oxidative phosphorylations changes in the mechanisms of the formation of the ionic asymmetry and in the mechanisms of the maintenance of the membrane potential. For instance, shifts in the membrane potential are more pronounced in old rats than in mature ones when sodium fluoride is administered, but they are more pronounced in the latter than in the former when 2,4-dinitrophenol is administered.

Thus, when the intracellular mechanisms of aging are analyzed from the standpoint of the adaptive regulatory theory, it becomes evident that irregular changes occur in various links of the metabolic ensurance of the function (a change in the relationships between glycolysis and oxidative phosphorylation, enzymic and non-enzymic reactions, the active and passive transfers of ions, the processes of protein biosynthesis, etc.). The adaptive mechanisms make it possible to maintain the cellular function for a long time in spite of the growing age changes. The above-mentioned data suggest that the membrane disturbances play the leading role in the mechanism of aging at the cellular level. They change the transfer of substances, the excitability of the cell and its reaction to the incoming information, upset the active transport of ions and the intercellular relationships, weaken the general membranous mechanisms of the regulation of cellular metabolism, and so forth. It should be borne in mind that the most important metabolic cycles, including protein biosynthesis, are controlled with the participation of the membranous mechanisms (cyclic adenyl nucleotides) which regulate ionic shifts.

13. Neurohumoral Regulation of the Cardiovascular System

Hemodynamics and Age

As far back as in 1883, Pavlov showed in his classical work *Centrifugal Nerves of the Heart* that extracardial nerves can change only the current activity of the heart, but also regulate the trophism of the myocardium. In 1965, Randall, a prominent specialist in blood circulation, wrote that the heart needed nerves only for love. Thus, the study of the blood circulation function is characterized by both constant vacillation and a search for a reasonable measure in the correlation between mechanical work and the central regulation of the heart.

Researchers have been interested in the age changes in blood circulation for several centuries now. Even Laurenz (1597) said that the representatives of the Alexandrian School of Philosophy associated aging with changes in the activity of the heart, which gained two drams annually until the age of 50, and then lost weight. Casalis' well-known, though clearly exaggerated, aphorism that a "person's age is determined by the age of his vessels" is the best expression of the importance which was attached to the age changes in the cardiovascular system.

However, the role of physiological (age changes in the cardiovascular system) and its pathological (especially atherosclerotic lesions) are still disputed in gerontology generally and also when the age changes in blood circulation are being studied. Are these processes interconnected, or are they completely identical? This dispute occasionally flares up as new concepts of the essence of aging appear. Its settlement is of general biological significance, as it relates to the essence of the aging process itself.

The bulk of factual material on the changes in the functions of the cardiovascular system was obtained clinically. This is very important, because the state of this system in a person can be determined directly. However, it is difficult to understand the deep-seated mechanisms of the changes in blood circulation, as the experimental analysis of these changes is lagging behind obviously.

The cardiovascular system is self-regulatory. Its age changes are due to the interaction between two contours of self-regulation; intrasystemic regulation and neurohumoral regulation. Each of these contours is modified during vitauct and aging. Arterial pressure is one of the main parameters of the system that is being regulated. The dynamics of the changes in arterial pressure has been described in many works. In spite of clear-cut sex, population and ecological distinctions, most researchers note the growth of mainly systolic arterial pressure.

Age norms have been the subject of a long heated dispute. What group of persons should be used to determine the age norms of various functional indices? According to some researchers, virtually all healthy persons should be used, while others maintain that a cross section of entire population should be used, since healthy persons are rarely found and the norm will be unrealistic for a given age group or a given population in which most persons are suffering from some diseases. Both of these variants should be corrected. Age norms should be determined on the basis of a group of persons who are not suffering from the diseases of a given system being studied. In this respect, objective data on age dynamics can be obtained without relying only on unique cases of ideal health. Indeed, the regulation of the central nervous system or the cardiovascular system can remain on a high level in a person who lost a leg or an eye or is suffering from osteochondrosis, and so forth, and he may live to very old age. For instance, Lasser and Master (1959) reported in their first work that the levels of systolic and diastolic pressures were 180–190 and 100–110 mm Hg, respectively, at the age of 55–60. According to them, such a shift should not be regarded as a pathological one. However, such arterial pressure is good grounds for diagnosing "arterial hypertension." In their next work, they excluded persons with arterial hypertension from the population. A thorough examination of 5,757 persons has shown that systolic and diastolic pressures were 145 ± 22 and 82 ± 10 mm Hg, respectively, in men aged 65 and 156 ± 28 and 84 ±/ 15 mm Hg, respectively, in women of the same age.

In assessing the age changes in arterial pressure, attention should be paid more to their possible stability than to their age dynamics, which is not very significant. It can be assumed that the ability to preserve the optimum level of arterial pressure is an exhibition of vitauct. A group of workers of the Institute of Gerontology of the USSR Academy of Medical Sciences (Muravov, Shchegoleva, Derkach, 1965) analyzed the changes in the level of arterial pressure in 24,824 persons over 80 and came to the conclusion that this pressure was somewhat lower in them than in persons of the preceding age groups. According to Sichinava (1963), arterial pressure in the inhabitants of Abkhazia who are over 100 years old is within the following limits: systolic pressure is 110–170 mm Hg and diastolic pressure is 60–90 mm Hg. It would be correct to assume that persons with clearly expressed vitauct processes, i. e. persons in which the age changes in blood circulation did not cause the development of gross pathology, live to such an old age. Age changes in arterial pressure in animals indicate the significance of the vitauct processes. Interestingly, the level of systemic arterial pressure does not change in rats and rabbits as they become older, but it reliably grows in dogs, which have a longer life span, and man. In other words, there is a definite link between the life span of a species and hemodynamic shifts. Perhaps shifts in arterial pressure "have no time" to originate in rats and rabbits owing to the vitauct processes and to their small life span.

The age dynamics of arterial pressure, its invariability, is maintained for a certain length of time owing to diversely oriented changes in various links of the regulation of the cardiovascular system. Table 13 gives data, which we obtained together with Shevchuk, on the direction of hemodynamic shifts in animals in old age. These data show that the disturbed level of arterial pressure in rats and rabbits is maintained due to the divergent shifts in cardiac output and total peripheral resistance. Many researchers have noted the drop in cardiac output and the stroke volume in people. For instance, Strandell (1964) indicated that cardiac output and the stroke volume dropped by 24 and 23 per cent, respectively, in old persons. However, David and others (1963) did not observe any changes in the stroke volume, while Modestov and others (1966) noted an increase in the stroke volume. Many contradictions are due to the selection of groups of those being examined and to the degree of expression of their pathology.

There is a certain relationship between cardiac output and oxygen consumption, or basal metabolism. This relationship is determined by several regulatory mechanisms which are aimed at maintaining tissue metabolism. This gave rise to assumption that the decrease in cardiac output in old age is of certain adaptive significance. However, this decrease was more pronounced than that in oxygen consumption. For instance, Strandell (1964) observed that oxygen consumption decreases by 11 per cent, while cardial output decreases by 24 per cent as a person grew older. According to Tokar (1977), cardiac output decreases to a greater extent than basal metabolism in persons over 65.

In assessing these very complex relationships, it should be noted that tissues do not receive the necessary amount of oxygen and, what is more, they cannot fully use it at a definite stage of the organism's aging. This is connected with a change in the oxidative processes, shifts in the respiratory chain, and change in the amount and state of mitochondria, etc. (Frolkis, 1970; Korkushko, 1976; Korkushko, Ivanov, 1980). Even Strazhesko (1939) emphasized that arterial hypertension may be a peculiar compensatory reaction to progressing hypoxia. Tokar (1977) drew attention to the fact that arterial hypertension occurred in the form of "hypertension of cardiac output" in elderly and old persons. He regarded it as a compensatory reaction aimed at restoring the oxidative balance in old age. Apparently, the developing shifts in arterial pressure can be of different significance to the aging organism. The combination of the growth of arterial pressure and a greater or even normal arteriovenous difference is undoubtedly important adaptively under the conditions of a changed hemato-parenchymatous barrier and tissue hypoxia. However, if tissues can no longer utilize oxygen at the next stage of the development of hypoxia, a peculiar vicious circle originates, i. e. hypoxia causes the growth of arterial pressure. However, owing to the changes in oxidative metabolism, the tissues do not respond with a corresponding increase in oxygen consumption. Hypoxia remains, thus promoting the process of arterial hypertension. Hence, an adaptive increase in arterial pressure and its disregulatory growth can occur with age.

Cardiac output diminishes because of a decrease in the contractile capacity of the myocardium. This is evident from the clinical and experimental data on the state of various indices of the contractile capacity of the myocardium (Table 13). In old animals, the maximal rates of both the rise of left ventricular pressure and the shortening of the myocardial fibres as well as the index of contractility and

Table 13. *Parameters of the hemodynamics and contractile function of the myocardium in rats of different ages* $(M \pm m)$

	Rats			Rabbits			Dogs		
	adult		old	adult		old	adult		old
Systemic arterial pressure, mm Hg	78.2±1.6	p>0.05	84.2±2.6	93.8±2.2	p>0.1	96.5±1.6	123.8±2.6	p<0.01	139.0±3.1
Heart rate, beats/min	349±21.0	p>0.05	335±10.6	270.7±6.2	p>0.2	258.2±6.0	200.7±4.29	p<0.05	172.0±4.3
Cardiac output, ml/min	92.6±3.0	p<0.05	76.2±2.4	304.0±7.0	p<0.02	254.0±11.7	2097±40.0	p<0.001	1591±57.2
Stroke volume, ml	0.26±0.02	p<0.05	0.22±0.02	1.2±0.06	p<0.02	0.85±0.04	10.9±0.43	p<0.01	9.03±0.31
Cardiac index, lit/min/m²	1.890±0.02	p<0.05	1.342±0.06	2.000±0.08	p<0.01	0.993±0.05	2.317±0.06	p<0.001	1.821±0.07
Working index of the left ventricle, kgm/min	2.016±0.18	p<0.02	1.533±0.037	2.500±0.08	p<0.01	1.280±0.07	4.188±0.13	p<0.001	3.423±0.16
Total peripheral resistance of vessels, dyne/sec/cm⁻⁵	70360±3319	p<0.05	90757±8512	22663±851	p<0.02	31519±1492	4886±127	p<0.02	7057±135
Systolic pressure in the left ventricle of the heart, mm Hg	89.7±3.1	p>0.05	92.0±3.0	113.4±4.2	p>0.05	103.5±3.7	157.0±1.33	p<0.05	147.3±1.48
Maximum rate of growth of intraventricular pressure, mm Hg/sec	3378±250	p<0.02	2650±189	3375±273	p<0.05	2480±196	2736±31.9	p<0.02	2207±43.5
Maximum rate of shortening myocardial fibres, muscle length/sec	2.35±0.02	p<0.05	1.80±0.02	1.86±0.03	p<0.05	1.30±0.02	1.08±0.008	p<0.05	0.93±0.02
Contractile index, relative units	60.0±2.3	p<0.05	47.4±3.9	73.7±5.0	p<0.05	61.2±2.8	34.6±2.57	p<0.01	23.3±0.54

the intensity of the functioning of the myocardial structures decrease and the phase structure of the systole changes. It should be noted that these changes in the contractile capacity of the myocardium correlate well with the structural and metabolic changes which occur in the heart in old age, and they have a definite cellular basis. Total peripheral resistance increases in old age. Functional and morphological data show that the state of various vascular regions changes differently in old age. For instance, the relative preservation of the share of the cerebral and coronary blood flows in the general hemodynamic shifts in old age is of certain adaptive regulatory significance.

The slowing down of the blood flow, which occurs in this respect, may also be very important adaptively, since it is conducive to the greater extraction of oxygen from the blood. Indeed, according to Drozdova (1969), the arterio-venous difference grows in elderly persons.

The mechanisms of the interrelation between the age changes of cardiac output and peripheral resistance are very important areas whose functionings are still not clear. What is the explanation of their diversely oriented shifts which determine natural changes in arterial pressure? Are they parallel age processes or interconnected shifts in different links of the system of self-regulation?

Arterial pressure could be calculated providing cardiac output decreases while total peripheral resistance remains unchanged in old age. It would be 53.6 mm Hg in rats, 57.5 mm Hg in rabbits, 77.7 mm Hg in dogs, and 45.7 mm Hg in people. In other words, sharp shifts would occur in arterial pressure if there were no diversely oriented shifts in both cardiac output and total peripheral resistance. Of course, vascular sclerosis, which occurs in aging, inevitably increases the total peripheral resistance of the vessels. However, it should be admitted that the growth of this resistance in old age is connected in many respects with the myogenic, functional change in the vascular tone. This is evident from the fact that many vasodilating agents with different sites of their action cause a substantial decrease in the total peripheral resistance of vessels both in people and test animals.

Consequently, the growth of total peripheral resistance in old age is largely of a regulatory nature. It is connected with a change in the function of the smooth muscle fibres of the vascular wall and their reaction to regulatory neurohumoral influences. This is evident from the data presented by I. V. Frolkis (1978) on a change in the electric activity and contractility of the smooth muscle cells of vessels. According to Folkow (1960) and Osadchy (1975), a decrease in the contractility of the myocardium reflexively causes an increase in the vascular tone.

In accordance with the principal of heterometric regulation and the Frank-Sterling law, the systolic contraction of the myocardium is determined by the diastolic dilatation of the myocardial fibres and the venous inflow. The possibilities of diastolic dilatation are limited in aging owing to the substantial structural changes in the cardiac muscle, shifts in the state of the connective-tissue skeleton of the heart, a decrease in its elasticity, the appearance of atrophied and hypertrophied fibres, and a change in the actomyosin complex. This affects the adaptive increase of cardiac output. According to our data, the index of relaxation is among the first to drop in aging. If it is taken as 100 per cent in dogs 2 and 3 years old it is 41 per cent in dogs 12–15 years old. Moreover, the duration of diastole tends to decrease in old age. It should be recalled that the volume of residual blood in the cavities of the heart increases in elderly and old persons (Tokar, 1977). However, it should be noted that the decrease of heterometric regulation is one of the main mechanisms of the limitation of the adaptive capacities of the myocardium.

Long ago, the opinion that latent physiological insufficiency of the heart develops in old age was expressed (Strazhesko, 1939; Bürger, 1960). Regardless of whether this is true or not, the limitation of the adaptive cacpacities of the cardiovascular system is exhibited especially clearly under different loads. Clinicians have long known that cardiac insufficiency develops more frequently and more rapidly in old people, and we have shown this experimentally (Frolkis *et al.*, 1976d, 1977). In mature and old animals, a greater load on the heart was attained by aortic coarctation. In the first 5 days of aortic coarctation, 48 per cent of old rats died from acute cardiac insufficiency, while only 12 per cent of mature rats died from it. Fig. 84 A, B, C shows that shifts in the hemodynamics

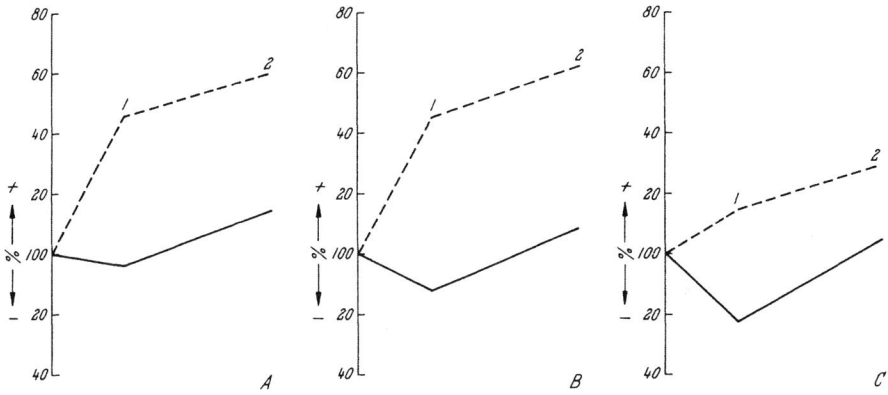

Fig. 84. Influence of the aorta coarctation on the contractile function of the left ventricle in rats of different ages with the experimental hyperfunction of the myocardium. *A* systolic pressure in the left ventricle; *B* maximum rate of growth of intraventricular pressure; *C* myocardial contractility index. *1* emergency stage; *2* stage of stable hyperfunction. The dashed line stands for mature rats, and the continuous line for old rats

and contractility of the myocardium are more pronounced in old animals than in mature ones at the so-called emergency stage (4–6 days after coarctation) and the stage of stable hyperfunction (13–15 days after coarctation). This is due to the fact that, in old animals, the content of ATP, creatine phosphate and glycogen decreases to a greater extent, a larger amount of lactic acid accumulates, and the activation of protein biosynthesis is less pronounced.

But it is important to remember that old animals do not represent a homogenous population. The hypertrophy and hyperfunction of the myocardium in some old animals did not differ from those in mature rats.

Hemodynamic Centre in Aging

In 1959, we proposed the concept of the hemodynamic centre as the totality of central neurons which ensure the regulation of the optimum level of the most important integral function of blood circulation. This was important because physiologists dealt mainly with the description of individual groups of neurons whose stimulation caused chiefly pressor and depressor responses in a certain vascular region. The matter in question is the "hemodynamic" centre and not the "centre of the cardiovascular system," since the object of regulation is the final adaptive effect (hemodynamics, respiration, alimentary behaviour), and not simply the structures which constitute it.

There is now enough factual material on a change in the function of the hemodynamic centre in aging. Two groups of facts testify to this: (a) a change in reflex reactions which are ultimately realized with the participation of the hemodynamic centre, and (b) a change in hemodynamic effects in the direct stimulation of the central nervous structures.

The conditioned reflex effects on the cardiovascular system weaken in old age. Working out conditioned reflexes in old people requires more stimuli presentations (Parchon, 1959). Examinations of elderly and old persons have revealed the inertness of vascular reactions, their long latent period, and the origination of prolonged changes in the vascular tone under the action of temperature, tactile and other irritants (Mankovsky, Mints, 1972). According to Collins and others (1981), cardiovascular reactions are weakened in old persons in an orthostatic test, on cooling and under the action of negative pressure on the lower part of the body.

Owing to the central programmes, the nerve centres function according to the principle of "forward fit control." They allow the organism to adapt itself to current as well as future activity. In aging, it becomes difficult to realize this form of central programmes in blood circulation reactions. This is expressed in the retarded engagement of the cardiovascular system in current activity. The peculiarities of the cardiovascular reactions during muscular work are also connected largely with the changes in the central mechanisms of regulation. In elderly persons, changes in the function of the cardiovascular system after a load become more prolonged (Fig. 5). Contradictions exist in the assessment of shifts in blood circulation under loads also because account is not taken duly of the "law of force relations." It has been discovered that the amplitude of shifts is expressed more in elderly persons under small loads and more in young persons under great loads (Frolkis, 1975). Moreover, it has been shown experimentally that considerable loads and a strong pain stimulus, while causing an optimum reaction in adult animals, lead to gross disturbances of hemodynamics in old animals and even to their death. The changes in the state of the hemodynamic centre are important in the genesis of these disturbances. Moreover, a definite level of the trained state of the cardiovascular system can be attained in old age. For instance, Kotelnikov and Fedorovich (1981) studied the influence of the training loads of the same duration and intensity (swimming every other day for 3 months) on the specifics of the development of the adaptive reactions of the organism of mature and old rats. It has been discovered that the level of the trained state, being expressed in the hypertrophy of the myocardium, an increase in the mass of the body, a decrease in the heart rate, the growth of cardiac output and stroke volume, and less expenditure on the work of the left ventricle with the simultaneous increase in the velocity of blood output and the duration of total diastole, is expressed more strongly in old rats under the adequate loads. It can be assumed from the results of the investigation that the alternation of a physical load with periods of rest corresponds largely to the possibilities of the organism of old rats. This should be taken into account when the physiological norms of work loads are being determined.

Reflex effects on the cardiovascular system are often prolonged. A change in the function during the prolonged action of a stimulus has become known as the "adaptation of reflexes," which has been thoroughly studied on the basis of the cardiovascular system (Chernigovsky, 1960; Frolkis, 1959). Cardiovascular reflexes become adapted more quickly in old animals when the receptive fields and sensory nerves are stimulated for a long time. For instance, when the receptors of the rectum are stimulated for a long time, the adaptation of the pressor reflex takes 10.5 ± 2.1 minutes in mature rabbits and 4.5 ±1.3 minutes in old animals. Adaptation of reflexes from the receptors of the carotid sinus (depressor reflex) takes 20–55 minutes in young rabbits and 5–25 minutes in old ones.

The hemodynamic centre is a complex hierarchy of neurons which are arranged at different levels of the brain. They are of diverse significance in hemodynamic regulation. Some of them are involved mainly when reflexes to the cardiovascular system originate, while others determine the basal level of the reflex regulation of blood circulation. The bulbar level of hemodynamic regulation plays a special role in the integration of hemodynamics. The phylogenetic development of nerve control so occurred that not only the mechanisms of the regulation of a certain function of the organism (different behavioural reactions, emotions, etc.), but also the mechanisms of their autonomic, particularly hemodynamic, ensurance were consolidated in definite structures of the brain. For instance, the structures of the mesencephalon coordinate the changes in the hemodynamics and motor manifestations of behavioural reactions, the structures of the limbic system control the relationship between blood circulation and emotional behavioural acts, etc. It has been shown that bulbar neurons are involved in the realization of the hemodynamic effects from the subcortical structures of the brain.

In work carried out together with Bezrukov and Duplenko, we determined the hemodynamic effects when different structures of the brain were stimulated. The experiments involved adult and old rabbits. Interestingly, the thresholds of current intensity, while causing changes in arterial pressure when various structures of the brain are stimulated, vary within a wide range. According to our data, their excitability ranges from 20 to 400 μA. It turned out to be the maximum when the central amygdaloid nucleus and the piriform region of the cortex were stimulated and the minimum when the tegmental reticular nucleus and the oblongate medulla were stimulated (Fig. 21). In many structures, which are characterized by great excitability in mature rabbits, the thresholds grow in old rabbits (the sensorimotor region of the cortex, the lateral hypothalamus, the medial amygdaloid nucleus). This smoothing out of differences in the excitability of various structures of the brain which participate in the regulation of hemodynamics can have serious functional consequences. The distinctions in excitability apparently promote the differentiation, specificity of hemodynamic shifts in various complex reactions. The smoothing out of this differentiation can lead to a generalized type of reactions of the cardiovascular system. It is known that with an involvement of the hemodynamic centre there may occur both local vascular shifts (which do not involve general hemodynamics in a reaction) and systemic cardiovascular reactions. As a result of the shifts in the central systems of regulation, these gradational peculiarities are smoothed out in old age. This reduces the adequacy of the correlations between a change in metabolism and its hemodynamic ensurance and promotes the development of pathologic processes.

Interestingly, the electric excitability of the bulbar level of the hemodynamic centre decreases substantially. It should be taken into account that the effects of the higher levels of the central nervous system on blood circulation can be realized through the above-mentioned structures. Therefore, the decrease in the excitability of the bulbar structures with age affects the general regulatory influences of the brain on blood circulation substantially. Particular attention is now being given to the hypothalamic mechanisms of the regulation of the cardiovascular system. According to Bezrukov, the excitability of various sections of the hypothalamus changes differently: that of the lateral one decreases and that of the posterior one increases, while that of the anterior one does not change virtually (Fig. 21). The realization of various reactions of the organism, whose hemodynamic ensurance changes differently in old age, is connected with those structures. It is important to note that hemodynamic shifts change qualitatively in old age when hypothalamic structures are stimulated: the same type of reactions (pressor or depressor ones) is maintained owing to other relationships between cardiac output and total peripheral resistance (Frolkis, 1970). In old rabbits, hypothalamic reactions occur more frequently with the clearly expressed growth of cardiac output. It is assumed that the autonomic nervous regulation of cardiac output is realized largely through a change in pressure in the right auricle, which determines the venous return to the heart. We have already mentioned our laboratory data concerning the fact that the reliability of the hypothalamic mechanisms which regulate blood circulation decreases and they are disturbed more easily when the organism ages. Rushkevich (1980) has shown that arterial hypertension and myocardial necroses (Fig. 36) occur more frequently in old rabbits when the hypothalamus is electrically stimulated daily. An important fact is that the correlation between the ways of realizing central influences on the periphery changes in connection with the shifts in adrenergic and cholinergic relation and in hypothalamic effects: the humoral link of regulation becomes important in old age; this promotes the origination of prolonged pathologic reactions.

Efferent Neurohumoral Regulation of the Cardiovascular System

The regulatory effects of the hemodynamic centre on the cardiovascular system are realized through the adrenergic and cholinergic neural pathways. It is known that the extracardial nerves influence not only all the aspects of the work of the myocardium, but also its metabolism, producing a trophic effect.

In our laboratory, the peculiarities of the adrenergic and cholinergic control of the cardiovascular system were thoroughly studied (Shevchuk, 1973; Frolkis et al., 1977; Lakiza, 1979). The work was carried out in the following way: the initial values of the hemodynamics and contractile capacity of the myocardium of rats, rabbits and dogs of different age were recorded. Then, the thresholds of the stimulation of the stellate ganglion and the cervical sympathetic nerve or the vagus nerve were determined and acetylcholine or catecholamines were administered in various doses. Such experiments have allowed us to compare the dynamics of the age changes in the reactions of the cardiovascular system ranging from threshold to maximum values.

The stimulation of stellate ganglia enhances systolic pressure in the auricles and the ventricles of the heart, reduces the refractory period of the ventricles, increases the frequency and force of cardiac contractions, and dilates the coronary vessels. Fig. 39 shows Shevchuk's data on a change in the parameters of the hemodynamics and contractile capacity of the myocardium when the cervical sympathetic nerve is stimulated by a current whose power grows. It turned out that the threshold value of stimulation of this nerve is 1.2 ± 0.2 V in adult rabbits and 2.4 ± 0.3 V in old rabbits. Such a regularity has been observed also when the stellate ganglion was stimulated. It has been shown in Lakiza's experiments on rabbits that the hemodynamic effects, i. e. greater arterial pressure, the growth of cardiac output, a higher cardiac index, a larger left ventricular work index, greater left ventricular pressure, an increase in the maximum rate of the shortening of the myocardial fibres, a higher contractility index, and so forth, develop in mature rats when the current which stimulates their stellate ganglion is weaker than that which stimulates it in old rats. Shifts in the hemodynamics and contractile capacity of the myocardium grew as the power of the stimulating current increased. However, the functional changes in the cardiovascular system grew far more rapidly in mature animals than in old ones. Thus, the sympathetic neural effects on the heart attenuate and sympathetic stimulation causes less pronounced inotropic shifts when the organism ages. These effects on the cardiovascular system attenuate because neurons are destroyed in the sympathetic ganglia and sympathetic terminals, noradrenaline synthesis becomes less active in these endings, and the transport of vesicles with catecholamines along sympathetic axons decreases. This is confirmed by our data on a change in hemodynamics in pharmacological desympathization caused by reserpine. Fig. 85 A, B shows that reserpine causes more pronounced changes in hemodynamics in old rats 4 hours after its administration. In these animals, the period of half-removal of noradrenaline from neuronal depots is twice as short and the ability of the adrenergic granules to retain and absorb catecholamines is reduced in comparison with mature rats (Limas, 1975). Reserpine exhausts greatly the reserves of catecholamines in the sympathetic terminals of old animals and thus causes more pronounced effects. These data on the specifics of the influence of reserpine in old age should be taken into account to the extensive use of the preparations of Rauwolfia in clinics.

Thus, sympathetic neural control of the activity of the cardiovascular system weakens when the organism ages. This is revealed when the sympathetic nerves are stimulated without involving the nerve centres. Consequently, the disturbances of sympathetic autonomic ganglia, sympathetic terminals and postsynaptic membranes can limit the realization of the central programme of regulating blood circulation. Indeed, as we have seen, substantial changes in the nerve centres and in the hemodynamic centre are sometimes not realized by the appropriate effects at the periphery. This attenuation of the sympathetic neural effects is apparently among the causes of the "inertness" of blood circulation reactions under different loads in old age.

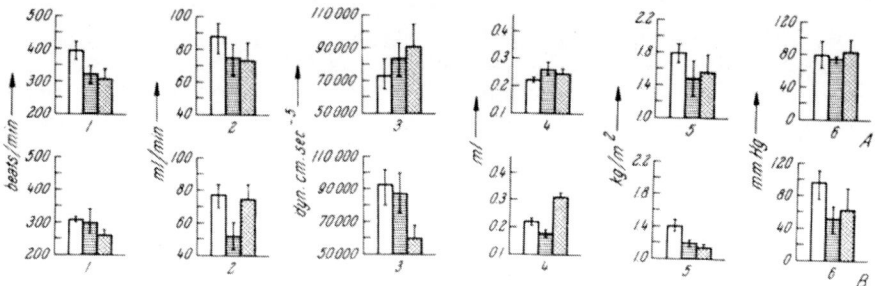

Fig. 85. Influence of reserpin on the hemodynamics in mature rats *(A)* and old rats *(B)*. *1* rhythm; *2* cardiac output; *3* total peripheral resistance; *4* stroke volume; *5* working index of the left ventricle; *6* arterial pressure. Light columns stand for control, shaded columns, for reserpin (5 mg/kg), 4 hours, and dotted columns, for reserpin, 24 hours

The attenuation of the sympathetic neural effects on the myocardium is among the causes of its reduced contractile capacity. It is known that homeometric regulation, direct inotropism and enhanced cardiac contractions without a preliminary increase in diastolic filling are connected with sympathetic neural effects. This important type of adaptive regulation of the myocardium is affected in old age. Moreover, adrenergic effects synchronize the contraction of myocardial fibres, thus intensifying cardiac contractions. This attenuation of the positive inotropic sympathetic effects is especially important owing to a change in the mechanisms of heterometric regulation

The summation of the changes in homeometric and heterometric regulations is the main cause of the reduced contractility of the myocardium in old age.

Sympathetic effects on the cardiovascular system are realized through noradrenaline. This agent causes diverse hemodynamic effects, which are occasionally the opposite of one another, depending on the functional state of the heart and the vessels and on the dose of the transmitter. Moreover, catecholamines can influence the contractile ability of the heart as well as the vascular tone, changing the venous inflow to the heart and thus indirectly influencing the cardiac function. For instance, Almazov and others (1976) have noted that, under the influence of noradrenaline, cardiac output increases in one group of animals, while it diminishes in another group. Abe and others (1973) have described the growth of the stroke volume under the action of noradrenaline, while Gurevich and Kondratovich (1969) have described its diminution. Some researchers have observed an increase, while others, a decrease in the rhythm of cardiac activity (Gurevich, Kondratovich, 1969; Nuzhny et al., 1977). Most researchers have now concluded that noradrenaline increases the contractility of the myocardium (Kanmann, 1977; Martinez, McNeil, 1977).

Noteworthy is the fact that many researchers use not the physiological doses of catecholamines, but the pharmacological ones, and therefore they overlook the physiologically significant threshold concentrations of substances and the reactions of the cardiovascular system. Data on a change in the reaction of the cardiovascular system to the action of catecholamines in old age is contradictory (Tuttle, 1966; Hruza, Zweifach, 1967). In our laboratory, Shevchuk and Lakiza had studied the age specifics of the changes in the hemodynamics and contractile capacity of the myocardium when noradrenaline, adrenaline and isadrine were used in varying doses. Hemodynamic changes occurred in mature and old rabbits when the same dose of noradrenaline (0.05 μg/kg) was administered. However, the shifts occurred in different directions: cardiac output decreased and total peripheral resistance increased in mature animals, while cardiac output increased and total peripheral resistance decreased in old animals. Such shifts were also observed when the stroke volume, the cardiac index, the left ventricular work index and the heart rate were being determined. At the same time, the same dose of noradrenaline induced similar changes in the myocardium contractility indices in mature and old animals. When large doses of the transmitter are administered to mature and old rabbits, shifts occur in the same direction, but they are more pronounced in mature rabbits. When large doses of noradrenaline are administered, changes in the contractility of the myocardium occur in two phases. The indices of the contractility of the myocardium grow and then diminish during the first few minutes after the transmitter is administered.

Largely similar results were obtained in experiments on rats. In old rats, the doses of noradrenaline which caused hemodynamic shifts were smaller (0.025 μg/100 g) than those in mature ones (0.05 μg/100 g). Just as in rabbits, shifts occurred in different directions in them when small doses of the transmitter were administered.

This phenomenon of higher sensitivity to noradrenaline was shown in experiments not only *in vivo*, but also *in vitro*, in which the relationships are simplified greatly. Fig. 40 shows Lakiza's data on the age specifics of the reaction of the aorta abdominalis strips of rats of different age to noradrenaline. It can be seen that the sensitivity of the strips is higher in old animals than in mature ones. Interestingly, noradrenaline in a concentration of 1×10^{-17}M causes the relaxation of the strips in old rats. When the concentrations are 1×10^{-16} to 1×10^{-14}M, the contraction of strips is more pronounced in old animals than in mature ones. At the same time, when the noradrenaline concentration grows further, the amplitude of the growth of the contractile response of the strips is less in old animals than in mature ones (reactivity diminishes). I. V. Frolkis (1978) has shown that the sensitivity of the smooth muscle cells of the portal vein to the action of noradrenaline grows in old age.

The reaction of the cardiovascular system not only to the transmitter, noradrenaline, but also to the hormone, adrenaline, changes when the organism grows old. Adrenaline can produce opposite hemodynamic effects, depending on its dose (Almazov et al., 1976). It turned out that the doses of adrenaline that cause the rise of arterial pressure are smaller for old rabbits (33.8 ± 3.0 ng/kg) than for mature ones (183.0 ± 23.6 ng/kg) (Bezrukov, 1969). At the same time, adrenaline bradycardia is less pronounced in old rabbits than in mature ones (Frolkis, 1978). This bradycardia has parasympathetic genesis and is realized through the vagus nerve. Apparently, bradycardia is less pronounced in old age because this extracardial neural control of cardiac activity weakens. In their experiments on rabbits and rats of different age, Shevchuk and Lakiza thoroughly described the changes in the hemodynamics and contractility of the myocardium when adrenaline was administered in doses varying from 0.01 to 10.0 µg/kg. Old rabbits turned out to be more sensitive than mature ones: a dose of 0.05 µg/kg did not change the hemodynamic parameters in mature animals and caused substantial shifts in old ones. The threshold dose was 0.15 µg/kg for mature rabbits. Interestingly, a qualitatively different reaction occurs when large doses of adrenaline (5.0–10.0 µg/kg) are administered, i. e. cardiac output, the stroke volume and the cardiac index decrease, while total peripheral resistance increases. Higher sensitivity of the cardiovascular system to adrenaline was revealed in experiments on rats. According to Dillon and others (1981), small doses of adrenaline and noradrenaline cause a more pronounced increase in arterial pressure and cardiac output and a decrease in total peripheral resistance in old persons. Verkhratsky (1962) has shown that the spasm of the capillaries of the nailbed and skin occurred under the action of adrenaline in a concentration of 1×10^{-9} M in old persons and 1×10^{-6} M in young persons.

Each of the hemodynamic parameters which have been studied is a summary one. For instance, different changes in the vascular tone of many regions lie behind the shifts in total peripheral resistance. According to our data, the reactivity of various vascular regions changes differently when the organism ages. Consequently, an increase in arterial pressure may be due to different topographies of a change in the vascular tone. In old rats, the thresholds of stimulation of the sympathetic chain grow (causing a change in the tone of the hind limb vessels), the thresholds of the sympathetic effects on the tone of the vessels of the small intestine decrease, while the thresholds of these effects on the vessels of kidneys do not change. In old animals, the sensitivity of the hind limb vessels to adrenaline increases, while the sensitivity of the vessels of the kidneys and the intestine to it does not change (Frolkis et al., 1967).

Systemic reactions and their regulation are ultimately determined by the specifics of the response of individual cells and largely by a change in their electric properties. We have data which testify to a change in the adrenergic regulation of individual cells of the heart and vessels. For instance, I. V. Frolkis (1978) has shown that the doses of noradrenaline which cause changes in the electric activity of the smooth muscle fibres of the portal vein are smaller in old rats than in mature ones.

Catecholamines in the cells of the conducting system increase the rate of spontaneous diastolic depolarization and the value of the membrane potential, while they reduce the threshold of cell excitability and promote the appearance of spontaneous activity. In myocardial fibres, catecholamines increase the amplitude and duration of the action potential and cause both the growth of the membrane potential and the prolongation of the slow repolarization phase. In our laboratory, Shevchuk studied the effect of adrenaline and noradrenaline (whose concentrations ranged from 1×10^{-12} to 2.5×10^{-5}M) on the electric properties of the cells of the right auricle in experiments *in vitro*. Noradrenaline in small doses causes a more pronounced increase in the membrane potential of the myocardial fibres, an increase in the amplitude and duration of the action potential, and a change in the excitation frequency in the cells of the auricles of old rats. An opposite effect occurs when the concentration of noradrenaline is raised: the value of the membrane potential as well as the duration and amplitude of the action potential decrease. It has been observed that individual myocardial cells become more sensitive to adrenaline in old age. Electric potentials of the myocardial cells of the heart were recorded *in situ* by "floating" electrodes in a special series of experiments. It turned out that catecholamines influence also the electric properties of the left auricle when they are administered in doses which change substantially its contractility. An important fact is that these shifts occur under the action of adrenaline whose amount is smaller in old animals (0.05 μg/100 g) than in mature animals (0.15 μg/100 g). The values of the membrane potential and the action potential diminish progressively when considerable doses of adrenaline are administered. Thus, we have shown that the cellular and systemic responses to adrenergic stimulation are correlated clearly. In old age, the weakening of the sympathetic neural effects on the heart and vessels is combined with greater sensitivity and decreased reactivity to the action of catecholamines. This direction of the shifts is of certain adaptive significance, since the sensitivity of the cell to noradrenaline can compensate for the insufficient secretion of the neurotransmitter and promote the maintenance of synaptic transmission.

Extremely important adaptive reactions of the cardiovascular system are started along the sympathetic nerves, and they also occur due to the release of adrenaline into the blood and the diffusion of noradrenaline from the synaptic clefts. Catecholamines cause substantial metabolic changes in the myocardium, leading to structural disturbances and often necroses. The metabolic nature of many necroses, even myocardial infarction, is widely known in different stress situations. The limited reactivity of the cardiovascular system to the action of catecholamines in old age under the conditions of the existing metabolic and structural shifts is also of definite adaptive significance. If a substantial amount of catecholamines is have caused released into the blood of old persons in stress situations, this would cause gross changes in the heart under the conditions of greater cellular reactivity and pre-existing hypoxia.

Interestingly, as the organism ages, not only quantitative, but also qualitative changes occur in reactions of the cardiovascular system to adrenergic stimulation. For instance, small doses of noradrenaline cause an increase in total peripheral resistance and a decrease in cardiac output in mature animals, while they cause a decrease in this resistance and an increase in cardiac output in old animals. Noradrenaline stimulates both the β_1-adrenoreceptors of the myocardium and the α-adrenoreceptors of the vessels. It can be assumed that the reaction of the α-adrenoreceptors of the vessels is more pronounced in mature animals; consequently, the vascular tone increases and the venous return decreases, as a result of which cardiac output diminishes. The β_1-adreno-receptors react more in old animals, and this stimulates the contractile function of the myocardium. The experimental data obtained by Shevchuk and Lakiza show clearly that the sensitivity of the β-adrenoreceptors grows in old age. These data have been given in the preceding chapters. It should be recalled that general hemodynamics and cardiodynamics change in old rats and rabbits when the doses of Obzidan administered to them are less than those administered in mature ones. Smaller doses of this β-adrenergic blocking substance reduce the effects of catecholamines. Age distinctions in the action of the α-adrenergic blocking agents were not observed. It can be assumed that the number of α- and β-adrenoreceptors in the cardiovascular system changes differently in old age.

Definite relationships exist between different types of adrenoreceptors. Fig. 86 A, B gives data on a change in the contractile reaction of aortic strips of

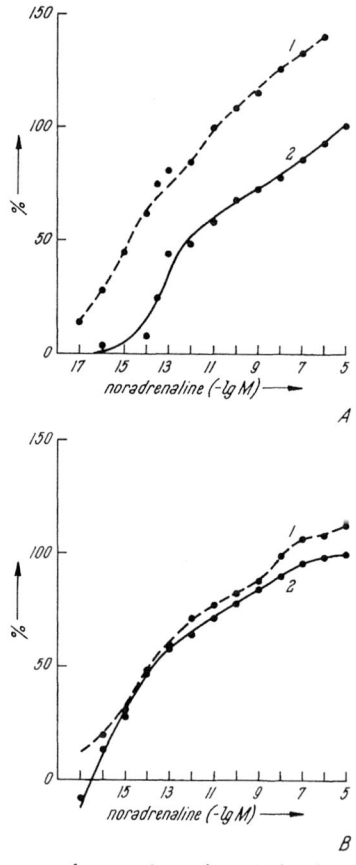

Fig. 86. Influence of Obzidan on the reaction of an isolated aortic strip under the action of noradrenaline in mature rats (A) and old rats (B). 1 control experiment; 2 action of noradrenaline against the background of Obzidan

mature and old animals under the action of noradrenaline against the background of a blockade of β-adrenoreceptors (introduction of Obzidan). The treatment leads to an increased contractile reaction in mature animals: it appears when the dose of noradrenaline is less and the amplitude of the reaction is greater. In other words, more pronounced effects develop in the case of a blockade of the β_2-adrenoreceptors, being connected with the stimulation of the α-adrenoreceptor. It can be assumed with great caution that the partial blockade of the β_2-adrenoreceptors by Obzidan somewhat simulates the shifts (greater sensitivity to noradrenaline) which occur in old age. Such a pronounced shift in the reaction is not observed when Obzidan acts on the aortic strips of old rats. It can be assumed that owing to a decrease in the amount of β-adrenoreceptors in old animals, their blockade does not cause such great prevalence of the α-adrenergic reactions in a blockade of β-adrenoreceptors.

Thus, substantial changes in the adrenergic control of the cardiovascular system occur when the organism ages. They are due to the attenuation of the sympathetic neural effects on both the heart and several vascular regions, a decrease in their reactivity and a reduction of the overall content of catecholamines. Under these conditions, the greater sensitivity of some structures to catecholamines plays a definite, though limited, adaptive role. The shifts in adrenergic control not only change the reactions of the cardiovascular system, but also become one of the main causes of its metabolic and functional disturbances. To confirm this, it is enough to recall the role of the adrenergic effects in the regulation of cardiac contractility, in chronotropic influences, in the ability of the cardiovascular system to rapidly adapt itself and pass over from one process to another, and in the regulation of energy exchange. It is these aspects of cardiac activity which change substantially in old age. The role of adrenaline increases when neural control is limited and the content of noradrenaline diminishes considerably. Consequently, local "economical" reactions are replaced more often by general hemodynamic ones. All these shifts, which have already been ascertained in the initial state, become especially significant in intensive activity and often promote the development of pathology.

The cardiovascular system is regulated cholinergically by the parasympathetic section of the autonomic nervous system. It is assumed that the fibres of the vagus nerve spread to all the sections of the heart. This determines the possibility of its influencing the rhythmic activity as well as the contractility of the heart.

Age changes in the metabolism of acetylcholine and the structural disturbances of the nervous system of the heart affect different links of cholinergic regulation.

Data on the attenuation of the negative chronotropic effects of the vagus nerve on the heart have already been given in Chapter 4. This is a general biological phenomenon to a certain extent, as it has been observed in old animals of different species: rats, rabbits, cats and dogs. The heart is constantly under the tonic influence of the vagus nerve; this is expressed differently in animals of different species. The tonic influence of the vagus nerve on the heart attenuates in old age. For instance, Dukhovichny (1974) has shown that the heart rate increases by 37.6 ± 3.6 per cent in young persons and only by 13.7 ±1.9 per cent (p < 0.001) in old subjects when one milligram of atropine is administered.

A link is known to exist between the extent of the tonic excitation of the centre of the vagus nerve and the intensity of the cardiac reflexes. The reflex response is expressed clearly in rats and rabbits when the tone of the centres of the vagus nerve is low: the stimulation of the respiratory tracts, pain stimulation, and so forth, cause severe bradycardia and brief cardiac arrest (Frolkis, 1959). This reflex bradycardia is less severe in old animals, owing to which the heart and hemodynamics as a whole are protected somewhat from great changes.

It is known that the heart slips away from the action of the vagus nerve when the nerve is stimulated for a long time: the heart rate increases in spite of continuing stimulation. There are various hypotheses of the mechanism of this phenomenon: the reserves of the transmitter are exhausted, ion redistribution occurs on the postsynaptic membrane, the sympathetic neural effects are reflexively activated, and the activation of protein biosynthesis lessens. In our laboratory, Pugach compared the age distinctions in the development of the phenomenon and discovered that when the vagus nerve is stimulated for a long time, the heart rate begins to accelerate earlier in old animals than in mature ones.

Complex relationships exist between the nodes of automatism in the heart: the sinoatrial node suppresses the underlying sources of automatism, but it can activate them at a definite frequency. The origination of the heterotopic sources of automatism and extrasystoles depends on the excitability of the local foci and on the inhibitory influence of the sinoatrial node. Apparently, a change in these mechanisms promotes the appearance of arrhythmias more frequently in old age. Extrasystoles originate more frequently in old animals than in mature ones when bradycardia is the same. Moreover, when the vagus nerve is stimulated, bradycardia develops more frequently in the former than in the latter due to the incomplete atrioventricular blockade.

Shevchuk has shown in our laboratory that the thresholds of the influence of the vagus nerve on the hemodynamics and contractile capacity of the myocardium grow as the organism ages (Fig. 39). Interestingly, the shifts in the contractility of the myocardium can originate when bradycardia is inconsiderable or even absent. This makes it possible to link them with the direct influence of the vagus nerve on the contractile elements of the myocardium.

The influence of the vagus nerve on the heart is realized through acetylcholine. Bezrukov (1969) has shown that the doses of acetylcholine which cause changes in arterial pressure are less in old rabbits (1.4 ± 0.5 ng/kg) than in mature ones (9.4 ± 2.7 ng/kg). This conclusion was confirmed to a certain extent in investigations involving people (Chebotarev, Korkushko, 1966; Korkushko, Ivanov, 1980). In subjects 20–29 years old, arterial pressure, cardiac output and the power of contraction of the left ventricle decreased and the heart rate slowed down when 75 mg of acetylcholine was administered, while in subjects 60–69 years old, that occurred when only 25 mg of acetylcholine was administered.

Shevchuk (1973) studied the change in the hemodynamics and contractility of the myocardium in animals of different age when the transmitter was administered in varying doses (from 0.001 to 5 μg/g). It was discovered that the effect was more pronounced when small doses of acetylcholine (from 0.01 to 0.15 μg/kg) were administered to old rabbits and large doses (from 2.0 to 5.0 μg/kg) were administered to mature ones.

Such a correlation between the changes, i. e. the attenuation of the cholinergic neural effects, an increase in sensitivity to small doses of the transmitter and a decrease in the reactive capacity may indicate some mechanisms of age shifts in cholinergic regulation. When the organism ages, neurons in the parasympathetic ganglia of the heart are destroyed, the parasympathetic nerve endings die, and the transmitter synthesis becomes less intensive in both ganglia and the presynaptic nerve endings. The origination of two limiting links in the ganglion itself and the peripheral synapse weakens the parasympathetic neural effects on the heart. Owing to these changes in the centrifugal pathways of information, the central cholinergic effects may not be realized at the periphery in certain cases. In mature animals, excitation in a convulsive seizure involving the centre of the vagus nerve causes bradycardia and brief cardiac arrest. In old animals, convulsions are simulated, but bradycardia is not pronounced. As the synthesis of the transmitter decreases, its hydrolysis becomes less intensive, thus preserving acetylcholine for a longer time in the sphere of its action and prolonging its effects.

A change in the cholinergic effects on the heart is connected with the shifts in the state and amount of the receptors. We have already shown in Chapter 4 that smaller doses of atropine block the cholinergic effects in old animals.

The above-mentioned changes in the cholinergic effects on the heart have a definite cellular basis. Acetylcholine is known to change the electric activity of the myocardial cells. Under the action of acetylcholine, the form of the action potential changes, its duration, the repolarization rate and amplitude diminish and, according to some researchers, the value of the membrane potential grows. It is assumed that acetylcholine can change the electric properties of the myocardial fibres of not only the supraventricular sections of the heart, but also the ventricles.

In our laboratory, the influence of acetylcholine on the myocardial fibres of the right auricle was studied *in vitro*. The amplitude of the action potential tended to decrease (by 3.2 ± 0.6 mV, $p > 0.05$) and the value of the rest potential tended to increase (by 4.9 ± 0.3 mV, $p < 0.05$) in old animals under the influence of acetylcholine whose concentration was 1×10^{-8} M. Shifts occurred in the cells of the auricles of mature animals when the concentration of acetylcholine was 1×10^{-7} M. Thus, there is a definite relationship between the specifics of cellular reactions and those of systemic reactions in response to the action of acetylcholine.

In view of the rapid cholinesterase-induced hydrolysis of acetylcholine in blood and the closed type of the cholinergic synapse, the cholinergic effects on the cardiovascular system are more local then the adrenergic ones. Therefore, substantial changes may occur in the myocardium when the cholinergic neural control of the heart is weakened. This confirms the data on the role of the cholinergic mechanisms in supporting the energy and plastic metabolisms of the myocardium.

When changes occur in hormonal regulation, the disturbances of blood circulation are exhibited in the "thyrotoxic heart," "diabetic angiopathy," "vasopressin coronary insufficiency," "corticoid necroses," etc. However, not so much is known about the role of the hormonal effects in regulating the physiological reactions of the cardiovascular system and maintaining the basal level of metabolism as well as the functions of the heart and vessels.

It can be asserted that, in aging, many metabolic changes of the heart and vessels are often secondary with respect to the age shifts in hormonal regulation. We have already seen how vasopressin, thyroxine, adrenaline and insulin influence hemodynamics. As the organism ages, the possible range of changes in hemodynamics in response to the action of these hormones decreases, but sensitivity to them increases. The hormonal regulation of the metabolism and functions of the heart becomes more important when neural extracardial control is limited. At the same time, gross pathological disturbances of cardiac activity occur more easily in old age under the influence of the growing concentrations of hormones against the background of disturbed myocardial metabolism. For instance, coronary insufficiency and arterial hypertension develop in old animals when the doses of vasopressin administered to them are smaller than those administered to mature animals (Pugach, 1970; Frolkis et al., 1976d; Golovchenko, 1976). In hyperthyroidism, changes in cardiac contractility occur and cardiac insufficiency develops earlier in old animals than in mature ones, under the action of adrenaline, polytopical extrasystoles and ventricular fibrillation occur earlier as well (Frolkis et al., 1978). Higher sensitivity of the cardiovascular system in old age has also been observed with respect to the action of some other physiologically active substances. According to Oginara and others (1981), the infusion of angiotensin II (600 μg/kg/min) causes a more pronounced shift in arterial pressure in old persons than in middle-aged persons. According to Pugach, angiotensin II which is administered intravenously in a dose of 10 μg/kg causes the growth of arterial pressure in old rabbits. In mature animals, changes in arterial pressure occur when angiotensin is administered in a dose of 100 μg/kg.

Reflexes of the Cardiovascular System

The reflex effects of the cardiovascular system ensure the adaptation of blood circulation, the correspondence of the shifts in this system to the changes in the current state of the organism, and the specification of the central programme of autonomic reactions in the course of its fulfilment. It is assumed that the blood circulation system is regulated not only by the deviation principle. If the "baroceptive" reflexes act only in a stabilizing way in any circumstances, they would obstruct the changes in blood circulation during muscular activity as well as during the orientational or defense reactions (Khayutin et al., 1977). It is assumed that complex relationship may originate between the central mechanisms of regulation and the baroreceptors. The realization of the programme of the hemodynamic centre can influence the receptors of the cardiovascular system not only by changing its activity, but also by engaging special mechanisms of their activation and attenuation (Korner, 1971).

Age-related changes in the cardiovascular reflexes began to be analyzed seriously in our laboratory more than 15 years ago (Frolkis, 1962; Shchegoleva, 1962; Frolkis, Shchegoleva, 1963). At the first stage, we concentrated our attention on the characteristics of the reflexes of the baroreceptors and chemoreceptors of the vessels (aortic arch, carotid sinus, intestinal vessels). The results of these studies, which were thoroughly analyzed elsewhere (Frolkis, 1970, 1975), include:

1. The reflexes of the mechanoreceptors of vessels weaken in old rabbits (carotid sinus, aortic arch). Depressor reflexes occur when intravascular pressure grows in them more and the value of the pressor reflexes of the carotid sinus in them is less than in mature rabbits. The reflex shifts in hemodynamics are weaker also when the aortic nerve is stimulated. For instance, the threshold of the depressor reaction is 0.45 ± 0.01 V in mature rabbits and 0.85 ± 0.02 V in old ones when the aortic nerve is stimulated. The attenuation of the sinocarotid reflex of old persons has also been described (Chebotarev, Korkushko, 1966; Lindblad, 1977). The baroreceptors in rats 10 weeks old are more sensitive than those of the animals 20 weeks old (Brown, 1979). The sensitivity of the baroreceptors is less in rats with hypertension.

The reflexes of the vascular baroreceptors are aimed at restoring arterial pressure when the position of the body changes orthostatically. According to Dukhovichny (1974), arterial pressure decreases 3.3 times more often in old persons than in young persons when an orthostatic test is carried out.

2. The chemoreceptors of the carotid sinus and the intestinal vessels become more sensitive to hypoxic effects when the organism ages (Fig. 87 A, B). Extremely important is the fact that the reaction of the receptors to hormones, which are constantly secreted into the blood during intensive activity, changes with age. For instance, according to Anokhin (1952) and Navakatikyan (1967),

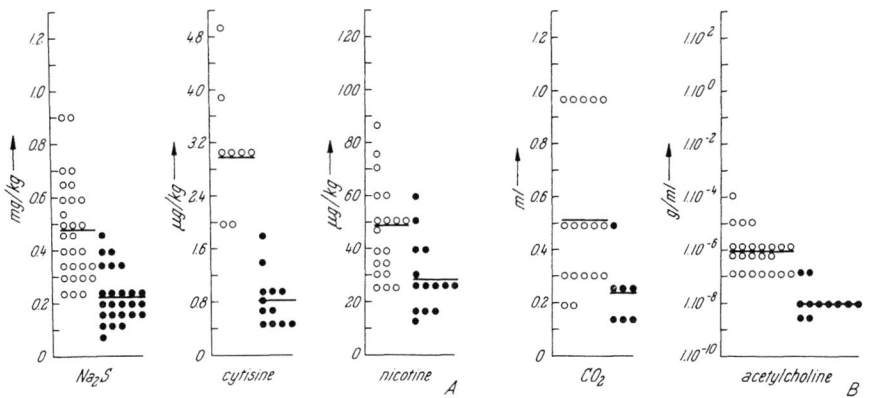

Fig. 87. Threshold doses of various substances which cause reflexes from the chemoreceptors of the carotid sinus in rabbits *(A)* and the chemoreceptors of the intestine vessels in cats *(B)*. Light circles stand for mature animals, and dark circles, for old animals

the nature of the potentials in the aortic nerve changes when adrenaline is administered owing not only to greater arterial pressure, but also to the direct action of adrenaline on the receptors. When adrenaline is administered (3 μg/kg), the volley impulse becomes a continuous one in 70 per cent of the cases involving old rabbits and only in 14.2 per cent of the cases involving young ones. In this study, we did not observe any differences in blood pressure changes. Consequently, the matter in question is the direct action of adrenaline on the afferent nerve endings, on their sensitivity to shifts in arterial pressure. Under these conditions, adrenaline activates the mechanisms of the adaptation of the cardiovascular system when it gets into the blood.

3. Recently, great attention has been paid to the experimental study of cardiac reflexes (Shevchuk, 1979). The mechanism of cardiogenic reflexes has been discussed in detail in several reviews and monographs (Kositsky, 1975; Tkachenko et al., 1975; Udelnov, 1975; Moibenko, 1979). We showed as early as 1952 that the reflex effects of the rhythmically contracting heart are of definite significance in maintaining the optimum excitability of several nerve centres.

The reflexes of the receptors of the pericardium, epicardium, myocardium and endocardium have already been described and structural evidence of the existence of afferent nerve fibres in the heart parts has been obtained. Reflexes from the mechanoreceptors and chemoreceptors of the heart cause a change in its rhythm and in the level of arterial pressure and hemodynamics. Shevchuk (1979) has shown that the epicardial chemoreceptors are more sensitive in old rabbits than in mature ones. Hemodynamic and cardiodynamic changes occur in old rabbits when the concentration of nicotine, veratrine and acetylcholine which act on the epicardium are smaller than those in mature rabbits. The threshold doses of veratrine and acetylcholine which cause hemodynamic shifts when applied to the epicardium were 1×10^{-7}M and 1×10^{-5}M, respectively, in mature rabbits and 1×10^{-9}M and 1×10^{-8}, respectively, in old rabbits. At the same time, quantitative differences in blood circulation reactions as well as qualitative hemodynamic changes were discovered. When the epicardial chemoreceptors are stimulated, arterial pressure and total peripheral resistance change more in mature rabbits, while cardiac output and intracardiac pressure change more in old rabbits (Fig. 88). In other words, the reflexes from the heart

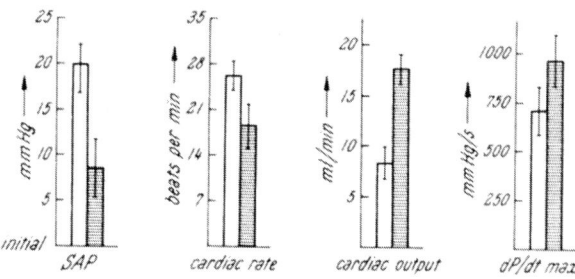

Fig. 88. Change in the hemodynamics and cardiodynamics of rabbits of different ages when the cardiac chemoreceptors are stimulated. *SAP* systemic arterial pressure; *dP/dt max* maximum rate of growth of intraventricular pressure. Light columns stand for mature rabbits, and shaded columns, for old rabbits

to the heart are more pronounced in old rabbits, while the reflexes of the heart to the vessels are more pronounced in mature ones. When the concentration of nicotine applied to the epicardium was increased substantially (1×10^{-3} M), hemodynamic shifts became so great that 35 per cent of the old animals died. Experiments involving the section of the vagosympathetic trunks and the application of Novocain to the site of action of chemical stimulants were a control test which proved the reflex nature of the shifts which originate when chemoreceptors are stimulated. Under these conditions, the reflexes of the heart weaken in old animals, while the depressor reflex does not originate, but arterial pressure and total peripheral resistance grow in mature animals.

The reflexes of the mechanoreceptors of the heart and especially of the auricles are important in the mechanisms of the self-regulation of blood circulation. These reflexes promote the regulation of the load on the myocardium and the establishment of the optimum relationships between a change in the rhythmic and contractile activity of the heart and the vascular tone and regulate the correlation between the inflow and outflow of blood and the work of the heart. The distension of the auricles decelerates the heart rate, reduces systemic arterial pressure, and increases the maximum rate of growth of intraventricular pressure, the index of contractility, and systolic pressure in the left ventricle. According to Shevchuk, the reflex effects on the heart of old rats were weaker than those on the heart of mature ones when pressure in the right auricle increased to the same extent (this was done by introducing an extra amount of liquid with regard to the initial volume of the auricles of animals of different age). Afferent impulses from the right auricle pass along the fibres of the vagus nerves (Udelnov, Yasinovskaya, 1969). The nature of these impulses in the right vagus nerve of animals of different age was studied in a special series of experiments. In old age, the amplitude and frequency of the impulses in the vagus nerve are reduced even in the initial state. When the auricle is distended by saline, the frequency and amplitude of the impulses in the peripheral section of the vagus nerve grow more in mature animals than in old ones. This also attests to the fact that the reflex of the mechanoreceptors of the heart weaken in old age.

Thus, the reflexes of the mechanoreceptors and chemoreceptors of the heart and vessels change greatly in the aging process. This is due to the metabolic age changes in the nerve endings. Shifts in providing reception with energy are of definite significance. It was shown earlier (Frolkis, 1975) that the energy processes in chemoreceptors change as the organism ages. For instance, when chemoreceptors are stimulated for a long time, the reflex reaction weakens and the reflex becomes adapted sooner in old animals. Under these conditions, the intensity of the reflex is restored rather rapidly by the effect of some substances participating in energy metabolism (ATP, sodium succinate, pyruvic acid) on the nerve endings. This restoration is more pronounced in old animals. Two important conclusions are drawn in this respect: (a) in old age, shifts in chemoreception are connected with a change in the energy processes in the nerve endings, and (b) in old animals, shifts in the receptors, and in young ones, shifts in the centres are more significant in the attenuation of the reflexes during long stimulation.

The baroreceptors of the vessels and auricles are stimulated when they are distended. The rate of growth of pressure is of great significance in stimulating the receptors; if blood pressure grows suddenly, an impulse characterizing a high degree of tension of the aortic wall can originate at values which are far below the optimum ones. It can be assumed that the decrease in the elasticity of the vascular wall and the tissues of the auricles is of great significance in the attenuation of the reflexes from the vascular baroreceptors in old age. In other words, greater distension is needed to attain the threshold of baroreceptor stimulations. It can be assumed that the attenuation of the reflexes of vascular baroreceptors is one of the reasons why prolonged changes in arterial pressure and hypertensive reactions occur in old age. The role of the baroreceptive zones in the genesis of arterial hypertension has long been disputed. Anokhin (1952) assumed that a prolonged rise in the level of arterial pressure caused by a certain factor will inevitably lead to the adaptation of baroreceptors, the attenuation of the reflexes of these regions, and stable arterial hypertension. We have shown that the depressor reflexes of the aortic nerve is adapted, or "disengaged," far more rapidly in arterial hypertension (Frolkis, 1959). When the organism ages, this mechanism of the attenuation of the depressor reflexes becomes especially significant in the genesis of arterial hypertension. This is evident from the fact that the adaptation of baroreceptors during a prolonged increase in pressure develops and the reflexes of these reflexogenic zones weaken more rapidly in old animals. Even the "virtually indefatigable" depressor reflex weakens sooner in old animals when the aortic nerve is stimulated for a long time (Frolkis, 1962). Moreover, the greater sensitivity of the vascular wall, i. e. its receptors, to the hormonal factors also changes the perception of the shifts in arterial pressure by baroreceptors. When the myocardium is working intensively, the attenuation of the heart reflexes limits the mobilization of many adaptive mechanisms.

We believe that there is another point which is hardly taken into account in works on vascular reception. In many cases, researchers quite justifiably use the isolated stimulation of certain vascular regions to describe the receptors of the vessels. However, vascular mechanoreceptors ensure feed-back in the system of regulating blood circulation in most cases under natural conditions, i. e. they are stimulated againgst the background of the changed function of the cardio-vascular system. Therefore, unlike in model experiments, the ultimate effect of the stimulation of vascular receptors will depend on the coordination of the information which comes from them to the centre and the current integration of the neural processes in the hemodynamic centre as well as the programme of autonomic shifts, the afferent image, and the "acceptor of action" according to Anokhin (1952). In other words, the intracentral mechanisms differ greatly from one another when vascular mechanoreceptors are stimulated separately for the first time and are drawn into a reaction under natural conditions. It can be assumed that the growing disparity between the afferent image and the neurodynamic prediction of a possible reaction in the centre, on the one hand, and the back information which enters the centre from vascular receptors, on the other, is of definite significance in the mechanism of the age changes in the reflexes of vascular receptors, i. e. the hemodynamic centre is misinformed about the events at the periphery. This is evident from a comparison of the data on a change in the reflexes of vascular mechanoreceptors when they are stimulated separately and are drawn into the natural reactions of the organism (a change in the position of the body in space, pain stimulation, etc.). The attenuation of the reflexes of the mechanoreceptors in old animals was expressed more in the latter case than when separate receptor zones were stimulated. This is seen in the prolonged restoration of arterial pressure after physical loads are applied, in pain stimulation, and in a substantial difference of thresholds, which cause shifts in arterial pressure when the position of the body is changed in space.

Regulation of Coronary Blood Circulation in Old Age

A truly paradoxical situation has arisen. It is well known that the disturbances of coronary blood circulation develop mostly in elderly and old subjects. However, the age changes in the coronary blood flow have still not been studied experimentally. Important mechanisms of the neurohumoral regulation of the coronary vessels have been ascertained recently (Sakai et al., 1980). It turned out that most regulatory factors dilate coronary vessels and only some of them constrict the vessels of the heart (vasopressin, angiotensin). The intensity as well as the direction of the reactions of the coronary vessels to the action of the regulatory factors can change in old age.

The specifics of the regulation of the coronary blood flow were studied in experiments on dogs of two age groups (1–2 years and 10–12 years). These experiments were carried out together with Shevchuk and Golovchenko (Frolkis, 1980). The experiments involving catheterization and the extracorporal perfusion of the coronary vessels were carried out on animals with a closed thorax. At the same time, systemic arterial pressure, perfusion pressure in the femoral artery, systolic pressure in the left ventricle and its first derivative were recorded and an electrocardiogram was taken. The stimulation of the vagus nerve and the subclavian loop of the sympathetic nerve caused a decrease in perfusion pressure in the coronary vessels. Neural control of the coronary vessels weakens in old animals. In old age, we see a rise of the thresholds of the vagus nerve effects on the coronary vessels (from 0.4 ± 0.02 V in mature dogs to 0.9 ± 0.03 V in old dogs) and those of the sympathetic nerve (from 0.55 ± 0.03 V in mature dogs to 1.2 ± 0.02 V in old dogs). This weakening of neural control limits the adaptive possibilities of ensuring the hemodynamics of the heart in old age, i. e. it promotes the development of coronary insufficiency. Metabolism and the contractile function of the heart intensify substantially under the conditions of various reactions which are realized through the sympathoadrenal system. The dilation of the coronary vessels, while being part and parcel of such a reaction, is an extremely important mechanism of maintaining a high level of cardiac activity. In the above-mentioned work, a study was made of the reactions of the coronary vessels as well as the hemodynamics and cardiodynamics with respect to the intracoronary administration of adrenaline, noradrenaline and acetylcholine in varying doses (from 0.001 to 15.0 μg in a volume of 0.05 ml). It turned out that the threshold doses of adrenaline and acetylcholine, which cause the reaction of the coronary vessels, decrease in old age (the adrenaline dose is $0.015 \pm 0.003 \mu g$ in mature animals and $0.007 \pm 0.001 \mu g$ in old animals; the acetylcholine dose is $0.01 \pm 0.002 \mu g$ and $0.005 \pm 0.001 \mu g$, respectively). There were no age-related changes in the threshold doses of noradrenaline. The vasodilating effect increases to a greater extent in mature dogs as the doses of catecholamines and acetylcholine grow. It is important to note that qualitative changes in the reactions of the coronary vessels also occur in old animals. For instance, the intracoronary administration of $0.1 \mu g$ of adrenaline caused an increase, and not a decrease, in perfusion pressure in the coronary vessels of 6 out of the 13 dogs which were over 13 years old (Fig. 89 A, B). At the same time, the maximum rate of growth of intraventricular pressure, the maximum rate of shortening of myocardial fibres and the index of contractility decreased. Such a paradoxical reaction occurred in three cases when noradrenaline was administered.

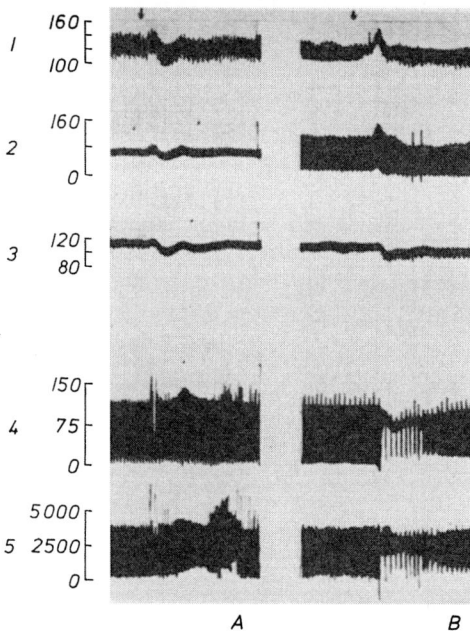

Fig. 89. Effect of the intracoronary administration of epinephrine $(0.1 \mu g)$ on the tone of the coronary vessels and the hemodynamic indices in dogs of different ages. *1* perfusion pressure in the coronary artery; *2* systemic arterial blood pressure; *3* perfusion pressure in the femoral artery; *4* left ventricular pressure; *5* maximal rate of increase in intraventricular pressure. *A* adult dogs (2 years); *B* old dogs (15 years). Arrows indicate hormone administration

These data are very important in understanding the mechanism of the disturbance of coronary blood circulation in old age. Indeed, the substantial activation of the sympathoadrenal system in stress situations is accompanied by the stimulation of cardiac activity, or cardiac contractility, which requires a greater coronary inflow. Under these conditions, ischemic lesions inevitably occur when the tension of the metabolism and functions of the myocardium is accompanied by a spasm of the coronary vessels. Consequently, the changes in the coronary blood flow and the specifics of the reactions of the coronary vessels to the regulatory effects are among the factors which limit the functional possibilities of the heart. Noteworthy is the fact that these regularities have been established by us in studying of dogs which were not affected by spontaneous atherosclerosis.

Coronary blood circulation is also disturbed in old age due to the change in the reactions to vasopressin (which is released into the blood in large amounts during intensive activity) and stress. The spasm of the coronary vessels is expressed more clearly in old animals when small doses of the hormone are administered (Fig. 31). This correlates with the data given in Chapter 3 on the more clearly expressed changes in the electrocardiograms of rats and rabbits when small doses of vasopressin are administered. Thus, substantial changes occur in coronary blood circulation when the organism ages. These changes are an extremely important cause of the disturbances of the activity of the cardio-vascular system.

Thus, the relationships between vitauct and aging determine the age dynamics of the cardiovascular system, its adaptive possibilities. A decrease in the lability of sinus automatism and an increase in the neurogenic control of cardiac activity at the early stages of ontogeny were an extremely important exhibition of vitauct. The energetically most economical form of cardiac activity, a form of maintaining cardiac output by an infrequent rhythm while the stroke volume is large, had originated owing to those factors. This type of cardiac activity is characteristic of many types of animals with long life spans. The trophic neural and humoral effects on the heart, the neural regulation of inotropism, the optimum tonicity of the vessels, and so forth, are important in achieving the optimum level of blood circulation. The lability of sinus automatism, its initial level and regulation decrease until very old age, thus protecting the myocardium from the "energetically" unbearable tachycardias. However, the progressive weakening of neural control accompanied by shifts in myocardiocyte genome regulation may cause the progressive disturbance of the structure and functions of the heart with its latent insufficiency which easily becomes a clearly expressed one.

We have traced the age dynamics of all the links of the neurohumoral regulation of blood circulation: the intracentral relationships, direct neural and hormonal links, and the feed-back of the vessels and the heart. It was discovered that the "hemodynamic programme" of ensuring various reactions of the organism, its realization at the periphery, and information on the course of its fulfilment change differently in the aging process. This is what engenders the different level of hemodynamics and largely becomes a cause of the discrepancy between the hemodynamic requirement and its satisfaction.

14. Experimental Life Prolongation*

The mean life span of the Romans was 22 years. By the end of the last century, i. e. in approximately two thousand years, the human life span increased by 20–30 years. In the last 70–80 years, it grew by another 20–30 years in the developed countries. In other words, the rate of human life prolongation increased almost 30-fold in one century. In the Soviet Union, the mean life span almost doubled in comparison with the level which existed before the Great October Revolution. Such a sharp growth of the life span became the basis of many optimistic predictions, which were often made by quite competent scientific organizations. At the end of the 1960's, for instance, the U.S. scientific corporation Rand predicted that the life span will increase by another 50 years by the year 2020, while Smith Kline & French Laboratories predicted such a growth by the 1990's. Experts of both corporations were of the same opinion that the main mechanisms of aging will be revealed and control over them will be established with the subsequent sharp growth of the life span by the middle of the next century (Bender *et al.*, 1970). However, the presently high growth of the life span is obviously connected not with a change in the aging rate and not with the shifts in the life span of a species, but with both a sharp decrease in infant mortality and the elimination of some infectious diseases. In recent years, the life span growth rate dropped sharply in the highly developed countries. According to demographers, this rate will drop even more in the future. The human life span will grow only by 8–10 years even when malignant tumours and cardiovascular diseases can be treated successfully.

Two tasks, one tactical and one strategic, must be tackled in order to increase the life span (Frolkis, 1979b). The tactical task is to increase the life span right up to the highest limit allowed by a species, while the strategic task is to increase the life span of a species itself. Until now, the life span was increased by successfully solving tactical problems. In the future, it can be increased mainly by successfully solving more complicated strategic problems.

Therefore, most gerontologists are not very optimistic about the further growth of the life span. There are grounds for such pessimism, especially if researches involving life prolongation will be continued at the same pace. To assess this situation, it is enough to read Shock's well-known gerontological bibliography, which includes the main researches into aging, beginning with ancient civilizations. This bibliography, which is naturally not quite complete, now includes more than 100,000 researches, of which less than 1 per cent

---

* This chapter has been written together with Kh. K. Muradian.

involves the solution of the main problem of gerontology: life prolongation. Many researchers believe that life can be prolonged only after the mechanisms of aging are completely revealed and control is established over them. Although there is some logic in this, it should be taken into account that much is known about aging. Firstly, several definite mechanisms of aging and the key links which limit the organism's life have already been revealed. The tactical as well as the strategic task of gerontology can be successfully tackled by influencing these links. Secondly, the general biological concept of the essence of aging and the processes which determine the life span has greatly changed. According to the adaptive regulatory theory (Frolkis, 1970), vitauct processes, which serve the purpose of increasing the organism's viability and life, had originated together with the aging processes during evolution. Hence, the means which influence the aging processes as well as those which activate opposite tendencies in the organism can be used to increase the life span. Thirdly, there are many examples in the history of natural science and especially biology and medicine which show that very difficult problems were solved long before the necessary mechanisms were understood. Fourthly, the ways of increasing the life span must be studied experimentally in order to reveal the mechanisms of aging. Only the model experiments in prolonging the life span can be an adequate criterion of the truth of certain hypotheses of aging.

Criteria of the Life Span

The main criteria of the life span are the values of the mean and maximum lifetime. In spite of the seeming simplicity of these criteria, they are still interpreted in different ways. In experimental gerontology, for instance, the average life span implies the mean arithmetic life span of all the animals of the selected group, while in demographic investigations, it implies the mean future life span. In some investigations, the life span is studied not from the moment of birth, but from a later period of ontogeny, and the mean life span is determined. The age at which the observations began is automatically added without taking account of the mortality at the previous stages, and this naturally produces exaggerated results. The criteria of the maximum life span are even more diverse. Some authors take the life span of the longest living specimen of a selected group as the maximum life span, while others propose that the mean life span of 1, 5 or 10 per cent of the longest living specimens of the population under consideration should be taken as the maximum life span.

Besides the mean and maximum life spans, wide use is made of such indices as the time of 50 per cent of mortality that corresponds to the moment of death of one-half of the specimens which are under observation. The times of 20, 40, 70 and 80 per cent of mortality are also often used.

An important fact is that the experiments involving the study of the life span take a very long time (except those when short-living species are concerned). Therefore, it is very difficult to take account of all the factors which can influence the ultimate result. No wonder the repeated determinations of the life span of biological subjects differ greatly from one another even when they are carried out by the same researchers under the same conditions. These differences are even greater when a comparison is made of the data obtained by various authors from the same inbred strain of animals, i. e. from the same genetic material. After analyzing the mean life span of mice that were obtained by various authors in 12 series of experiments in 1948–1975, Goodrick (1975) gave the following data on four inbred strains:

No.	Strain	Females			Males		
		minimum	maximum	increment, %	minimum	maximum	increment, %
1	A/J	405 ± 7	688 ± 22	70	488 ± 11	662 ± 20	36
2	Balb/cJ	462 ± 7	816 ± 32	77	460 ± 14	648 ± 21	41
3	C57BL/6J	561 ± 8	874 ± 14	56	519 ± 7	870 ± 5	68
4	DBA/rJ	407 ± 6	683 ± 26	68	407 ± 9	722 ± 30	77

Even greater differences (up to 300–400 per cent) are observed when a comparison is made of the data presented by various authors on the mean life span of laboratory insects, e. g. fruit flies. Apparently, such sharp differences in the life span are mostly due not to genetic distinctions, but to the different conditions of maintenance. This is especially clear when a comparison is made of the animal life span which are determined during different periods. For instance, according to the data given in the forties and the fifties, the life span of the C57BL/6J mice was rarely longer than 500–600 days, while the figure increased to 800–900 days in the sixties and the seventies (Kunstyr, Leuenberger, 1975). An interesting fact is that the difference between the females and the males decreases as the life span increases, while the males live longer than the females in the longest-living populations. Kunstyr and Leuenberger (1975) have estimated that the difference between the life spans of the females and the males of the C57BL/6J mice decreased by 8.2 days per year in the last three decades. They attributed this to the genetic instability of the given strain, which is widely used. However, a more convincing explanation was offered by Deerberg and his associates (1980), in whose experiments the average life span of the females of the Han-Wistar rats reached 30–33 months, while that of the males, 33–36 months. It is interesting to note that the longest-living specimens of this population lived 48 months. An analysis of the causes of mortality under such apparently almost "ideal" conditions of maintaining laboratory rodents shows that it is mainly due to malignant tumours in several organs, especially in the organs of neuroendocrinal origin (hypophysis, adrenal gland, the tissues of the genital system). In this respect, a large number of the females die of cancer of either the uterus or the mammary gland. Naturally, this does not occur in the males. Therefore, as the maintenance conditions are improved and mortality due to such diseases as pneumonia and infections is reduced, cancer of the mammary gland and the uterus becomes an important factor in determining the life span of females.

The duality of the factors which determine the values of the life span of biological subjects, i. e. the genetic and stochastic factors, is clearly revealed also when the mortality curves are being analyzed. Thus, the curve of the survival of the heterogenous population of animals which are maintained under "ideal" conditions of the external environment should be like a trapezium (Fig. 90 A).

As for the population which is maintained under the conditions that are unfavourable for longevity, where the main cause of death is not aging, but casual damaging factors, the curve of survival is shaped like that of the rates of the first-order chemical reactions (Fig. 90 B). In this respect, the maximum life

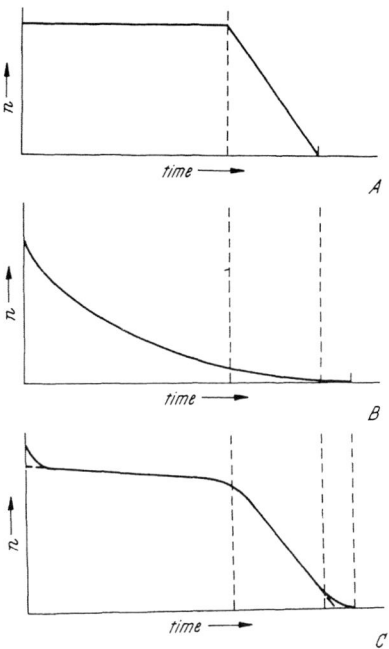

Fig. 90. Comparison of the curves of survival of the populations maintained under conditions which are "ideal" (A) or extremely unfavourable (B) for longevity with a similar curve obtained under real conditions (C)

span may be increased somewhat, since individual unfavourable factors can be transformed into factors of life prolongation due, for instance, to the "super-stimulation" of the restoration processes. The real mortality curve, which is usually obtained in the life span experiments, is a hybrid of the curves represented in Figs. 90 A and 90 B (Fig. 90 C). Obviously, this is an exponential curve except for the small sections at the very beginning and the end of postnatal ontogeny. Gompertz was the first to draw attention to this as early as in 1825. He proposed the following well-known dependence of mortality (R_t) on age (t):

$$R_t = R_0 e^{\alpha t} \tag{1}$$

where R_0 — constant obtained by extrapolating mortality by the moment t = 0;

   e   — base of the natural logarithm;

   α — constant of a given biological species.

The significance of the constante R_0 and α is seen especially clearly when the Gompertz equation is linearized (Fig. 91). R_0 is hypothetical mortality at the moment $t = 0$, while it is easy to find α from Equation (1), $\alpha = \dfrac{\ln R_t / R_0}{t}$. Since the life span can be increased by reducing both R_0 and α, it is proposed (Dubina, Razumovich, 1975) that a distinction should be made between the concept of "retarded" aging (decrease in α) and "postponed" aging (decrease in R_0). Mortality can differ greatly from the Gompertz relationship under real

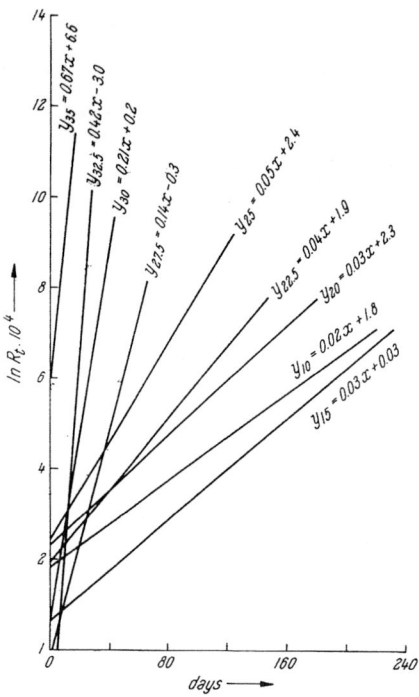

Fig. 91. Linearized curves of the survival of the imago of the fruit flies of the D-18 strain which were kept at nine different temperatures ranging from 10 to 35 °C. The regression equations were obtained by the method of least squares

conditions of animal maintenance, especially at the initial stages of life, when aging still does not play a significant role. Therefore, Makeham proposed that constant A, which takes account of the background mortality due to chance causes, should be introduced into Equation (1). The Gompertz-Makeham equation is now written as:

$$R_t = R_0 e^{\alpha t} + A \tag{2}$$

Attempts to modify this equation were often made and will apparently continue to be made. Endeavours to linearize Equation (1) were especially fruitful. Taking its natural logarithm, we obtain:

$$\ln R_t = \ln R_0 + \alpha t \tag{3}$$

In other words, the relationship between $\ln R_t$ and t is shaped like a line whose slope tangent (α) and the point of intersection of the ordinate axis ($\ln R_0$) determine mortality at any age. The term $\ln R_0$ in Equation (3), which Sacher calls the vulnerability index, is determined by mortality at the initial stages of life that are not connected with aging. The link between the expected life span (L) and the constants of the Gompertz equation is determined by the following equation (Sacher, 1977):

$$L = -\alpha^{-1} \times \ln(1.76 R_0 \alpha^{-1}) \tag{4}$$

Thus, the aging of the population can be described quite correctly by the vulnerability indices R_0 and the growth of mortality with age (α). For instance, the 30-fold increase in the life span of man as a species in comparison with the mouse is due to a 500-fold decrease in vulnerability and only by a 15-fold decrease in α. It is convenient to express the aging rate of the populations also by the period of the duplication of mortality (T_d), which, as Equation (3) shows, is

$$T_d = \alpha^{-1}\ln 2 \tag{5}$$

For instance, in mice and man, T_d is equal to 220 days and 8.5 years, respectively (Sacher, 1977).

The existing methods make it possible to linearize not only the Gompertz equation, but also the Gompertz-Makeham equation. To this end, Gavrilov (1980), for instance, proposes to use not the values of mortality, but those of its increment. Since constant A and its increment are equal to zero, we obtain the following from Equation (2):

$$\ln \Delta R_t = \ln(R_{t+\Delta t} - R_t) = \alpha t + \ln(R_0 e^{\alpha \Delta t} - 1) \tag{6}$$

In other words, when Δt is constant, $\ln \Delta R_t$ is a linear function of t. This was shown experimentally by analyzing the mortality of 86 human populations (in the 25–85 age bracket when $\Delta t = 5$ years) and 20 populations of inbred mice (Gavrilov et al., 1978). In replacing the relationship between R_0 and α that has been shown by Strehler and Mildvane ($\ln R_0 = M - B\alpha$, where M and B are the constants of a given biological species) in the Gompertz-Makeham equation, we obtained the following in logarithmic form:

$$\ln(R_t - A) = M + (t - B)\alpha \tag{7}$$

An interesting conclusion which is drawn from this equation is that when t = B, then $\ln(R_t - A) = M$, i. e. the mortality curves in the coordinates $\ln(R_t - A)$ and t should have one point of intersection with the coordinates M and B regardless of the conditions under which all the populations of a given species exist. It turned out that such a point corresponds to the age of 90–95 years for human populations and 55–60 days for the fruit flies (Gavrilov, 1980). After determing the values of the constants α and R_0 for the age period from t_1 to t_2 by means of Equation (5), we can estimate constant A by the following equation:

$$A = \frac{\sum_{t_1}^{t_2}(R_t - R_0 e^{\alpha t})}{t_1 - t_2} \tag{8}$$

An analysis of the statistical data of the mortality of men in Sweden from 1911 to 1975 has shown that the value A of the 45–75 age bracket, which was about 0.5 per cent in 1910, had gradually diminished and virtually became nil between 1945 and 1950. Mortality due to age ($R_0 e^{at}$) did not change during the given period, averaging 0.32 per cent annually. Since the level of background mortality (A) approximated the zero level in the developed countries (as was the case with Sweden), Gavrilov and Gavrilova (1979) came to the conclusion that a decrease in mortality due to age alone would be the main way to prolong life in the developed countries.

While discussing the possible mechanisms of prolonging life in direct experiments and predicting the possible methods of prolonging it on the basis of indirect results, mention should be made of another interesting direction of researches in this respect. Many attempts are now being made to determine the nature of the link between the life span of a species and various anatomical and physiological parameters of the organism. The investigations which Rubner and Friedenthal started in this respect at the end of the last century and the beginning of this century were renewed only in the last decades due largely to interesting researches carried out by Sacher and Cutler. Sacher (1978), for instance, obtained the following relationship between the life span (L) and the mass of the body (m_b) or the brain (m_r) for 63 mammalian species:

$$L = 2.95 \, m_b^{0.197} \tag{9}$$
$$L = 4.83 \, m_{br}^{0.325} \tag{10}$$

Approximately the same relationship was obtained by Economos (1980a) for 40 mammalian species:

$$L = 2.61 \, m_b^{0.20} \tag{11}$$
$$L = 5.20 \, m_{br}^{0.313} \tag{12}$$
$$L = 9.39 \, (m_{br}/m_b)^{-0.53} \tag{13}$$

It follows from Equation (13) and from a comparison of Equations (9) and (10) that the relationship between the life span and the relative mass of the brain (m_{br}/m_b) is not positive, as could have been expected from Friedenthal's rule, but negative. Moreover, according to the data presented by Economos (1980a), the mass of the body or the brain is not the only morphological index which correlates with the life span of a species. The correlation ratios of the mass of the liver (m_1) or the adrenal gland (m_a) can be used just as m_b and m_{br} for determing the potential life span of a species. The appropriate equations of the dependence of the life span of the mass of the liver or the adrenal gland are written in the following way:

$$L = 4.44 \, m_1^{0.24} \tag{14}$$
$$L = 14.2 \, m_a^{0.27} \tag{15}$$

Using the method of multiple correlation for 253 mammalian species, Sacher (1978) obtained the following relationship between the life span of a species, the cephalization coefficient (K), the intensity of metabolism (M) and the body temperature (T):

$$L = 8 K^{0.6} \times M^{-0.5} \times 10^{0.025 T} \tag{16}$$

Since the body temperature of most mammals is about 37 °C, we obtain:

$$L = \frac{67.3\,K^{0.6} \times M^{-0.5}}{37°} \qquad (17)$$

In other words, the different life span of a mammalian species is determined by two independent parameters: K and M. The author worked out two hypotheses of aging (those of the genes of aging and the genes of longevity) and concluded that only the hypothesis of the genes of longevity was correct.

After collecting the data given by several authors, Economos (1980b) obtained the following relationship between the life span and the mass of the body for 170 species of mammals:

$$L = 10.4\,m_b^{0.172} \qquad (18)$$

When the animals were divided into orders, it turned out that there were clear-cut distinctions in the nature of the relationship between the life span and the mass of the body even within a single class. For instance, this relationship is written in the following way for rodents:

$$L = 8.8\,m_b^{0.252} \qquad (19)$$

for ungulates:

$$L = 7\,m_b^{0.217} \qquad (20)$$

for carnivores:

$$L = 10\,m_b^{0.193} \qquad (21)$$

for primates:

$$L = 15.7\,m_b^{0.236} \qquad (22)$$

for other mammalian species:

$$L = 6.8\,m_b^{0.260} \qquad (23)$$

It follows from these data that the dependence of the life span on the mass of the body virtually does not differ in rodents and carnivores. In ungulates, the life span is about 30 per cent lower than the carnivorous species of the same mass, while in primates, it is higher. Among other species, *monotrem* and *chiroptera* are interesting. Their life span is apparently three or four times higher than the level suggested by the mass of the body. For instance, the fruit bat weighs 0.7 kg and lives 18 years, while the echidna weighs 4 kg (its body temperature is 30–33 °C) and lives more than 50 years.

Several authors have tried to establish a link between the life span and the ontogenetic changes in individual morphological and physiological indices. By making several allowances, Beier (1980) obtained the following relationship between the life span (T), the level of aging (μ), the level of growth (K), the mass at the time of birth (m_0) and the mass when weight became stable (M):

$$T = \frac{1}{\mu} - \frac{\ln (m_0/M)}{K}$$

Zotin and others (1978) believe that the life span of man and other mammalian species can be determined by using the dynamics of growth and the mass of the body as well as the intensity of basal metabolism that diminishes with age. According to them, this diminution is mainly what determines the limits of the mammalian life span since, regardless of the species, all mammals have a minimum of basal metabolism that is 20 cal/kg per day. This minimum is attained with age by the moment of death.

Thus, we can now draw several conclusions which are important in analyzing the subsequent material of life prolongation. For instance, when the possible mechanisms of the prolonging effect are being considered, it may be expedient to determine the constants α and R_0 by Equation (3), since they can be used to quantitatively differentiate mortality due to chance damaging causes and mortality due to aging. The values of Makeham's constants A, which approximate zero, show clearly once more that the further prospects of the growth of the human life span should be associated with a decrease in the constants R_0 and α. An analysis of the nature of the link between the life span of a species and the anatomical physiological indices shows that a purposeful search for the possible prolonging factors can be carried out by using the evolutionary "experience."

Influence of Physical, Chemical and Biological Factors on the Life Span

Much data on the influence of various factors on the life span has accumulated since the first scientific attempts to increase the life span were made about a century ago. For the reader's convenience, we tried to divide these data into three groups according to the nature of the life prolonging factor: physical, chemical and biological. Of course, such a division is nominal to a certain extent, since the "application" of many factors of diverse nature and the definite mechanisms of their life prolonging action can have much more in common than various factors of the same nature.

Influence of Physical Factors on the Life Span

Many physical factors, such as temperature, radiation, light and sound of different frequencies, and electric and magnetic fields, can strongly influence the life span. Most of the physical factors which have been studied have a clearly defined optimum range of effects outside whose limits the life span decreases sharply. In this respect, the nature of the dose-effect curve can differ not only quantitatively, but also qualitatively in accordance with the nature of the subject being studied. This is evident when an examination is made of the influence of the temperature of the external environment on the life span of the cold-blooded animals as well as the heterothermal and homoiothermal warm-blooded animals.

Temperature

The first to study the influence of temperature on the life span was apparently Loeb, who published data on the influence of the incubation temperature on the duration of development (Loeb, 1908) and somewhat later presented data together with Northrop (Loeb, Northrop, 1917) on the duration of all the life stages (larval, pupal and imaginal stages) of the fruit fly. In all the cases, maintenance at high temperatures reduced the life span, while it increased the life span at low temperatures. Using the temperature dependence of the rate of the processes that has been discovered by Arrhenius, these authors showed that the energy of activation of the aging processes in flies is about 20 kcal/mole, i. e. it reaches a value that is characteristic of most chemical reactions. Hence, they proposed the "chemical hypothesis" of aging, according to which "duration of life is determined by the production of the substance leading to old age and natural death, or by the destruction of a substance or substances which normally prevent old age and natural death." Later, a similar relationship between the life span and the temperature of the external environment was shown by many authors on the basis of various strains of the fruit fly (Alpatov, Pearl, 1929; Smith, 1958; Strehler, 1961; Shaw, Bercaw, 1962; Sondhi, 1967; Hollingsworth, 1969; Cohet, 1975; Parsons, 1977), paramecia (Smith-Sonneborn, Reed, 1976), wasps (Clark, Kidwell, 1967), seed beetles (Sharma *et al.*, 1979), nematodes (Suzuki *et al.*, 1978), aphides (Reggi, 1975), rotifers (Meadow, Barrows, 1971), daphnids (Ewer, Ewer, 1942), silk moths (Osanai, 1978), house flies (Sacher, 1977), sea ascidians (Nomaguchi, 1974), prawns (Suyama, Iwasaki, 1976), and cold-blooded vertebrates (Bourlière, 1958; Liu, Walford, 1972, 1975; Sacher, 1977). Apparently, the inverse dependence of the life span of poikilotherms on the habitation temperature is so great that the given fundamental property of living organisms is defined clearly in spite of the different subjects of research, different conditions under which experiments are carried out, and so forth.

However, the authors' unanimous assessment of the effect of temperature on the life span of poikilotherms does not mean that the problem is not debated. The possible mechanisms of the temperature effect have engendered especially long and heated debates. After Loeb and Northrop, Pearl and his co-workers (Pearl, 1928; Alpatov, Perl, 1929) had shown the inverse dependence of the life span of the fruit flies on the incubation temperature and proposed their well-known hypothesis of aging known as the "rate of living." Seeing that the "total activity" of flies grows with an elevation of incubation temperature and vice versa, Pearl concluded that the "shorter duration of imaginal life is primarily simply because it is more active at those temperatures or, in other words, has a higher 'rate of living' and consequently shorter absolute duration of life." After correctly observing that the causes of aging of the fruit flies at extremely high incubation temperatures (higher than 30 °C) have little in common with the mechanisms of aging at temperatures which approximate optimum values (20–25 °C), Smith (1958) has shown by several fine experiments that the diminution of the life span, while being connected with an elevation of temperature, is observed from a certain moment, and that the rate of aging does not depend on the "rate of living" before that age. The author divided the life of the fruit flies into two stages: aging and extinction. He maintained that the rate of aging does not depend on the incubation temperature, and that the extinction phase, which depends on temperature, sets in only after the age disturbances reach a certain "threshold" value.

Shaw and Bercaw (1962) tried to combine the "chemical" hypothesis proposed by Loeb and Northrop and the "rate of living" hypothesis proposed by Pearl, maintaining that, just as the rate of chemical reactions, the "rate at which vital substances or substances which determine longevity are lost" is higher at elevated temperatures. However, such an explanation is hardly enough for understanding why, for instance, the values of the life span are often higher than those calculated by the "rate of living" hypothesis when animals are transferred from high temperatures to low ones. A similar pattern is observed when a study is made of the influence of the incubation temperature which, according to the sinusoidal rule, is not constant, but variable, on the duration of the development and imaginal life of the fruit flies and rotifers (Halbach, 1973). Reggi's investigations shed light on some of the possible mechanisms of that phenomenon. He used aphids to show that, just as in the research carried out by Shaw and Bercaw (1962), the dependence of the life span (L) on temperature is determined by the line of regression, i. e. $\ln L = \frac{4509}{T} - 12.2$ (where $\ln L$ is the natural logarithm of L, while T is absolute temperature on the Kelvin scale), and that the energy of activation of this dependence is 9.2 kcal/mole. If the insects are exposed to X-rays in a dose of 30 kR at the beginning of the experiment, the energy of activation (11.7 kcal/mole) and the inclination of direct regression, $\ln L = \frac{5839}{T} - 17.1$, will increase. The author believes that such an additive effect of the elevation of temperature and radiation occurs because the "weak point" of aging is apparently the reparation of macromolecules and subcellular structures that are damaged constantly (Reggi, 1975). This is evident also from much data on either a substantial decrease in the survival of the cellular cultures of mammals which were subjected once to moderate hyperthermia and radiation (Rubachev, 1978) or an increase in radioresistance during hibernation (Lui, Walford, 1972).

According to Strehler (1961), the decrease in the rate of aging of poikilotherms with a drop in the temperature of habitation may be due to both the retardation of all the biological processes and the manifestation of the evolutionarily acquired protective feature, which makes it possible to survive the low-temperature periods that are usually accompanied by a reduction of the sources of nutrition. Morrison and Milkman (1978) have presented interesting data in this respect. They showed that the selection inside the isofemales of the fruit flies produces great differences in an increase or decrease in heat resistance already after ten generations. In this respect, heat resistance decreases more than it increases. On the chromosome level, this is caused mainly by a single locus with a recessive effect, while the additive polygenous effects constitute only 10 per cent. Investigations involving 20 natural populations of the fruit flies caught in various regions of Australia have shown that the insects in the given regions have a temperature ratio of the aging rate which is almost as high as that of the insects after many laboratory-bred generations (Parsons, 1977).

The great shifts which occur in the life span of the poikilotherms as the temperature of habitation changes may be due largely to the changes in various subcellular structures, including the genetic apparatus. Genomic changes may occur under the influence of various external effects which are reversible, but which are maintained for a long time in the cells and even in sexual generations. For instance, the correlation of the DNA fractions changes at low temperature: the content of the satellite DNA increases, while the amount of the copies of the structural genes of histones, the packing of the nucleoprotein complex, and so forth, can change in accordance with the genotype.

It has already been mentioned that there is no work in which the authors failed to show the inverse relationship between the life span and the body temperature in spite of the diverse objects of investigation, whether they be dipteria or nematodes, rotifers or seed beetles, vertebrates or the silk moth (which does not feed on anything and is virtually a closed system), notwithstanding the diverse temperature ranges that have been studied and the conditions under which the experimental animals were kept. Extremely important is the fact that such a relationship exists not only for the poikilotherms, but also for the culture of their tissues (Shima et al., 1980) as well as the tissue culture of warm-blooded animals, including man. According to Shari and co-workers (1978), the viability of the cells of the HeLa and PK-13 cultures is preserved for 17–21 days under ordinary thermoecological conditions (37 °C), for 56 days under hypothermal conditions, and for 70 days during preliminary adaptation to hypothermia. When the cultures were returned from the hypothermal state to ordinary conditions, unadapted cultures began to grow again in 39 days, while adapted cultures, in 7 days. Approximately the same relationship, although with a somewhat smaller temperature ratio, is characteristic also of the aging rate of the cells of plant origin (Haber, 1971). These data show that an increase in the life span with a diminution of temperature is an inseparable property of the cell itself and is apparently due to the rather prolonged changes in the intracellular relationships, whose realization can be made less painful to the preliminarily adapted cells. Another important fact is that the effect of temperature on the life span of the biological objects is qualitatively and quantitatively the same in spite of the diversity of the objects of research and the conditions under which it is carried out. In virtually all the cases, the temperature ratio of the aging rate (Q_{10}) in the 20–30 °C range is 2–3 and grows by leaps in the high temperature range. Hence, the prolonging effect of low temperatures is probably due to the changes in the fundamental mechanisms which are the same for all cells.

In trying to establish the mechanisms which determine the long life span of the poikilotherms when the temperature drops, it is expedient to recall another significant achievement of experimental gerontology, i. e. Rubner's inverse relationship between the level of basal metabolism and the life span of several domestic mammals. Pearl (1928) was among the first to notice such a relationship also in the cold-blooded animals which were incubated at different temperatures. Somewhat later this was confirmed in experiments with various species of sea and land vertebrates and invertebrates (Prosser, 1977).

The genetic apparatus plays an important role in determining the life span of biological subjects. Hundreds of works deal with the age changes in various stages or replication, transcription and translation. However, there are only a few works whose authors studied the nature of the link between the life span and the main functional parameters of the genetic apparatus. The poikilotherm incubated at different temperatures are very convenient for solving that problem. Therefore, we studied and compared the temperature relationship of the life span, basal metabolism and the rate of synthesis of total RNA and protein in the fruit flies which were incubated at ten different temperatures in the 10–37.5 °C range. Fig. 9 shows that the mean and maximum life spans of flies increase clearly as the incubation temperature drops at least to 15 °C. The somewhat smaller life span of flies at 10 °C is probably due not to an increase in the aging rate, but to the substantial growth of initial mortality (Fig. 9) that is apparently connected with the difficulties of adaptation or other experimental errors. The incorporation of the labelled precursors into the intracellular pool and macromolecules shows that the rate of synthesis of RNA and protein (being determined by relative specific radioactivity, i. e. by the relationship between the specific radioactivity of macromolecules and the intracellular pool of precursors) was minimum at 10 °C, that it increased sharply in the 15–30 °C range (activation energy was about 10–20 kcal/mole), and that it dropped even more sharply at high incubation temperatures (Fig. 9). Approximately the same values of the activation energy were obtained when a study was made of the temperature relationship between the rate of elongation of the peptide chains which are being newly synthesized and the total synthesis of protein in the toad fish *Opsanus tau* (Mathews, Haschemeyer, 1978). The amount of carbon dioxide being released by the flies also increased until 30 °C was reached, then it decreased at 32.5 °C and, unlike in the RNA and protein synthesis, increased again at 35 °C. The inverse relationship between the life span and the intensity of transcription and translation is observed only in the 15–30 °C range. The relationship is positive outside this range. The relative specific radioactivity (RSR) of RNA and protein as well as the amount of carbon dioxide shows that the value of the product (life span multiplied by metabolism) has a faint maximum at 20–25 °C in all the cases, and that it decreases sharply beyond this range, especially at high temperatures.

The single type of course followed by the curves of the life span and the ratio of the RSR of protein and RNA (Fig. 9) are interesting. The last index indicates the efficiency of the genetic apparatus and shows how effectively the information taken from the genetic apparatus is used (it indicates, in relative units, the number of protein molecules which were synthesized per RNA molecule). The curve of the temperature relationship of that index almost fully coincides with the life span curve. Only at 35 °C and 37.5 °C, when the duration of preliminary adaptation is obviously not great (1 day and 15 minutes, respectively), the ratio of the RSR of protein and RNA again approaches the 25 °C level.

A sharp decrease in both the life span and the rate of synthesis of RNA and protein at incubation temperatures which are higher than 30 °C is apparently due to the growth of the damaging effect of the denaturation and degradation processes. This is evident also from the high energy of the activation of the processes which reduce the RSR of RNA or protein or the life span (about 200–300 kcal/mole). In this respect, there are interesting data which show that the rate of protein breakdown in the free-living nematodes at 30 °C is about one-tenth of that at 36 °C (Prasanna, Lane, 1979). Our data show that, in accordance with the curves of the aging rate in the coordinates of Arrheius' equation, the energy of activation of the aging processes is 15–20 kcal/mole up to 30–32.5 °C, while it is about 200 kcal/mole at 32.5–37.5 °C. According to Hollingsworth (1969), such a break in the curves of *D. subobscura,* which are known to have smaller heat resistance, occurs at lower temperature, i. e. at 28–29 °C.

Thus, the given literary material shows that an inverse relationship exists between the life span and the incubation temperature at least in the temperature range which is the optimum for a given species. Regardless of the diversity of the subjects of research and the experimental conditions, this relationship has manifested clearly itself in all cases, being of a single type not only qualitatively, but mostly also quantitatively. The main disagreements in this respect are connected with the possible explanations of the phenomenon being observed. The "chemical" hypothesis proposed by Loeb and Northrop, Pearl's "rate of living" hypothesis and Smith's "thresholds" cannot explain the whole experimental material which has accumulated. We believe that the main shortcoming of these hypotheses is the overestimation of the role of the damaging factors and the underestimation of the role of the restorative factors. The aging rate of the cell, which has rather effective mechanisms of restoration and reparation, is not always determined by the level of the damaging factors. In most cases, it is determined by the relationship between the damaging and restorative processes. By their nature, most restorative processes are enzymic ones ($Q_{10} = 1.5$), while the chance damaging processes are chemical ones ($Q_{10} = 2 \div 3$). Therefore, the difference in the rates of the damaging and restorative processes should decrease as the temperature rises, since these processes have smaller activation energy and the temperature ratio of the rate. In other words, the rate of most restorative processes should decrease by 50 per cent and that of the damaging processes by 100–200 per cent as the incubation temperature of the cold-blooded animals drops by 10 °C every time. Such a diminution of the relationship between the rates of the damaging and restorative processes can be one of the main reasons why the aging rate decreases and the life span increases. When various metabolic shifts are combined favourably in some cases, the difference in the rates of the damaging and restorative processes can become negative. In this interval, the organism may grow younger rather than age. In this respect, Lerman's (1978) hypothesis of aging is interesting. He believes that the rate of degradation of macromolecules is minimum and is almost nil in the dividing cells, while degradation occurs most intensively in the resting cells and its rate is the inner feature of every biological species. During the breakdown of macromolecules, the value of erroneous information can decrease substantially, and then the cell is rejuvenated. There is a definite share of resting cells which are capable of being rejuvenated in all the cellular populations.

Influence of Temperature on the Life Span of
Warm-Blooded Animals

Warm-blooded animals are divided into homoiotherms (the body temperature is maintained at a constant level by regulating heat production and heat loss) and heterotherms (whose body temperature is not constant and which are capable of alternating the periods of active life with torpor and hibernation) in accordance with the principle of thermal regulation. Naturally, the effect of the temperature of the external environment on the life span of these species differs owing to the different strategy of thermal regulation. In homoiotherms, a substantial decrease in the temperature of habitation additionally intensifies metabolism, which is intended to increase heat production, while in warm-blooded heterotherms, the mechanism of torpor or hibernation begins to operate and the level of metabolism decreases sharply. Therefore, a decrease in the temperature of the environment reduces the life span in the former case, but increases it the latter. As experiments with laboratory mice and rats (Kibler, Johnson, 1961, 1966) have shown, a drop in temperature below 10–15 °C increases the consumption of food and oxygen and reduces proportionally the life span. In warm-blooded heterotherms, however, a decrease in the temperature of the environment reduces the temperature of the body and increases proportionally the life span, while the specimens live less when this does not occur (Sacher, 1977). No wonder warm-blooded heterotherms live much longer than the species of approximately the same size which have evolved similarly and whose body temperature is fixed. Various strains of mice and rats live not more than 3 or 4 years, while bats and other hibernating rodents of roughly the same size live 15–20 years (Liu, Walford, 1972; Sacher, 1977). The lower the body temperature during hibernation and the longer its duration, the greater is the life span. Estimates based on these data show that the energy of activation of the processes which determine the value of the life span of the warm-blooded animals is 30–50 kcal/mole, which corresponds to the energies of activation of macromolecular denaturation.

The division of homoiotherms and warm-blooded heterotherms is somewhat nominal, because the mechanisms of thermal regulation maintain the body temperature far above the temperature of the environment even at the height of hibernation, while the body temperature of the species in which it is fixed varies by 1–3 °C daily or seasonally. There are great individual differences in the body temperature in any population of homoiotherms. It may seem that specimens with a low body temperature could have a longer life span. However, the nature of the link between the rectal temperature of rats and their life span differs during different age periods. On the whole, the life span of the animals with a lower body temperature was greater than that of the animals with a higher body temperature. The following relationship existed between the life span and temperature (t °C) in rats aged 85 days that were divided into two subgroups with high and low body temperatures: $L = 4,752 - 106\,t$ (Kibler, Johnson, 1966).

The negative effect of the "temperature" factor on the life span has been shown in other experimental models, too. For instance, the extrapolation of the

Arrhenius curve at 37 °C shows that more than 0.2 per cent of the cells disappear irreversibly every hour from the proliferating population of the cells of the Chinese hamster owing to thermal damages even by physiological temperatures (Johnson, Pavelec, 1972). Although the exact nature of these damages, which affects all the organisms even at normal body temperature, is unknown, they are most probably due to denaturation and the ruptures of the initial structure of proteins and nucleic acids (Johnson, Pavelec, 1972). Interestingly, the extent of damages to macromolecules increases and the effectiveness of the reparation processes decreases with a rise in temperature, although the rate of the reparation processes grows in absolute terms (Weniger et al., 1979).

It has often been emphasized in gerontological literature that one of the most promising and real ways of increasing the life span of the warm-blooded organisms, including man, is by reducing the body temperature. Unfortunately, it is still unknown how to reduce greatly the body temperature of homoiotherms for a long time or to increase the thermal stability of their vitally important macromolecules. In virtually all the known cases, however, an increase in the life span to a certain extent involves the effect of temperature. For instance, an increase in the life span is accompanied by a decrease in the body temperature when nutrition is limited, regardless and whether the animals' diet has enough calories and proteins or not. When the low-calorie diets, which increase the life span by 40–50 per cent, are fixed reasonably, the temperature drops by 1.5–2.5 °C, and when the models of low-protein diets are involved, the growth of the life span (by 25–30 per cent) and the diminution of the body temperature (by 0.2–1.2 °C) are proportionally less (Miller, Payne, 1968; Liu, Walford, 1972; Barrows, 1977; Arshavsky, 1979). The energy of activation of the processes which determine the life span values in the cases of limited nutrition is 30–50 kcal/mole, just as when the closely related heterothermal and homoiothermal mammals are compared. Since starvation as a model of life prolongation has virtually no influence on the cold-blooded organisms, it could be that the body temperature drop is the main reason why the life span increases in mammals which receive a low-calorie or a low-protein diet. In other words, limited nutrition in this case may be a more or less adequate physiological means of reducing the body temperature. A decrease in the body temperature and an increase in the heat resistance of macromolecules plays an important (and probably the leading) role in all the presently known methods of increasing the life span of the warm-blooded organisms. Hydrocortisone, for instance, is among the few hormones which can increase the mammalian life span (Bellamy, 1968; Everitt et al., 1980). At the same time, it is one of the most universal hypothermal factors of many species of mammals (Putthoff et al., 1977). Chronic exposure to small doses of ionizing radiation increases the life span by 10–20 per cent and causes noticeable hypothermia (Kalendo, 1972). Heterosis, which usually prolongs life by 10–30 per cent, is accompanied by a great increase in heat resistance, as can be easily seen from the smaller elongation of the metaphase chromosomes when the cells are heated (Vanyushin, Berdyshev, 1977, and others).

The possibility of greatly increasing the life span by reducing the body temperature can be attributed in the most general form to the relationship between aging and vitauct. There is good reason to believe that the vitauct processes, whose purpose is to increase the organisms's viability, are mainly connected with the enzymic reactions, whose activation energy is 4–12 kcal/mole. Chemical and denaturation reactions, whose activation energy reaches 50–60 kcal/mole and the Q_{10} of which is several times higher than that of the enzymic reactions, are important especially in the mechanisms of aging, which is destructive process. Therefore, the rate of vitauct may prevail over that of aging as the body temperature drops, thus increasing the life span.

Hence, it has been shown by means of tissue culture and by tens of species of cold-blooded vertebrates and invertebrates that there is a clear-cut inverse relationship between the life span and the body temperature. Temperature shifts can cause changes in the life span by more than ten times the normal level even in the temperature range which ensures the normal development and reproduction of a species. This inverse relationship obviously exists in the warm-blooded heterotherms, too. Virtually all the presently known methods of increasing the life span of the warm-blooded homoiotherms involve a decrease in the body temperature or an increase in the heat resistance of the vitally important macromolecules of the cell. Rough estimates have shown that the processes which determine the life span of the warm-blooded animals have an activation energy of 30–50 kcal/mole. Hence, their aging is probably mainly due to the denaturation of macromolecules, such as proteins and nucleic acids. Therefore, the life span can probably be increased mainly by reducing the rate of these processes and increasing the rate of the restorative processes.

Influence of Ionizing Radiation on the Life Span

Since many features of aging and those of the radiation injury are externally alike, gerontologists believed for a long time that ionizing radiation is a convenient method of both modelling accelerated aging and establishing the causes of aging. However, subsequent researches have shown that the mechanisms of aging and those of the radiation injury are different fundamentally.

When the organism is exposed once to radiation, the dependence of the extent of the reduction of the life span on the dose can be regarded as a linear one in a somewhat simplified form, at least if the dose is up to 1 krad (Yuhas, 1969). When small laboratory rodents are totally exposed once to radiation, their life span diminishes by 200–400 days/krad. The threshold dose in this case is apparently 50 krad. The negative effect of a single exposure to neutron radiation is two or three times greater than the exposure to X-rays and is characterized by a complicated dose-effect relationship (Darenskaya, 1978).

In the case of ionizing radiation, the extent of damages and their influence on the life span differs for different organs. For instance, in order to reduce the life span of mice approximately to the same extent (50 per cent), it is necessary to expose the whole body to a dose of 845 R and the abdomen area to a dose of 975 R, while subtotal exposure with the abdomen area being screened requires a dose of 1,885 R (Darenskaya, 1978). However, the life-span reducing effect of the exposure of the head of mice was almost 2.5 times higher than that of the exposure of the trunk with a similar dose and 4 times higher than that of the exposure of the pelvis, the extremities and the tail (Sato *et al.*, 1973).

An important fact is that the life-span reducing effect of radiation (as calculated per unit dose) differs hardly in various species of mammals (the mouse, the rat, the guinea pig and the dog) with a five- or six-fold difference in their life span, thus indicating that the extent of both the damages and their influence on the life span is approximately the same in various species of mammals (Sacher, 1977). In the cold-blooded animals, however, a drop in the temperature increases the life span and at the same time raises greatly the level of survival of the animals which were exposed to radiation (Kalendo, 1972).

Interestingly, in most cases, the females are affected less by the life-span reducing radiation than the males. The radiation reduced the life span of the male rats by 290 days/krad and that of the females by only 39 days/krad under equal conditions (Darenskaya, 1978). Gnotobiotic animals also turned out to be more sensitive to radiation, while the effects of the electric shock, parabiosis with an unexposed partner, and so forth, increased the life span of the exposed animals.

Exposure to radiation once in a small or medium dose does not reduce substantially, but occasionally even increases the life span of various species of insects and warm-blooded animals to 20–60 per cent (Yuhas, 1971; Ducoff, 1975). The prolonging effect of exposure to small doses is more pronounced in females than in males. Some authors attribute this to the sharper diminution of basal metabolism owing to the cessation or great reduction of the reproductive function. The higher level of the "resistance reserve" of the sex chromosomes, which are important to the life span, may play an important role in the greater radioresistance of the females. The data presented by Clark and Cole (1967) also indicate that the chromosome number may play a certain role in increasing radioresistance. They showed that the diploid females live 5–15 per cent longer in intact wasps, while the life span of the troploid females is 10–15 per cent greater than that of the diploid ones after exposure to radiation.

The influence of the fractionated doses of radiation, in which gerontologists take especially great interest, are more complicated and have been poorly studied. In this respect, the life-span reducing effect per unit dose decreases substantially even when the exposures are made at 40-second intervals. In the case of regular exposure to small doses, ionizing radiation more often increases the life span than reduces it. For instance, the life span of rats was reduced by 10, 20 and 30 per cent when they were exposed once to radiation in a dose of 120, 240 and 480 R, respectively. A dose of 120 R did not influence substantially the life span when it was divided into three fractions, while the life span increased by 10 per cent when the dose was divided into six fractions (Darenskaya, 1978).

When the animals are being exposed to radiation, it is important to know their age in order to determine the effect of radiation on their life span. According to several authors, a smaller number of exposed animals survive in old age. But according to Yuhas (1971), the exposure of the long-living

C57BL/6J mice of five age groups (120, 270, 450, 540 and 730 days old) to ten equal fractions of X-ray radiation in a total dose of 1,400 R reduced the life span of only the animals aged 120 and 270 days by 14.8 and 30 days, respectively, while it increased the life span by 53, 65 and 53 days, respectively, in the other age groups. In the older age groups, radiation has a great life-prolonging effect because it acts more therapeutically, e. g. it may suppress the foci of malignant tumours, infections, the reproduction of parasites, etc.

Thus, large doses of radiation can reduce substantially the life span, whose length is determined by the nature of radiation, the conditions, the extent of the influence of the dose, age, and the sexual and physiological state of the animal. In mammals, the specific effect of a decrease in the life span hardly depends on the value of the life span of a species, but it can be reduced if endogenous radioprotectors are worked out or exogenous ones are introduced.

The life span often increases under the action of small regular doses. This may be due to the possible suppression of the foci of tumours or infections or to the reduction of the level of the metabolic processes or the body temperature. The slight stimulation of the reparative mechanisms may be of definite importance in this respect. For instance, there is an optimum dose of radiation (400 R) for mice, and the reparation rate decreases when it is higher or lower (Darenskaya, 1978). In their experiments, Planel and Giess (1973) have shown that flies lived less when they were maintained under the conditions of low background radiation (10 per cent of the natural background) as compared with the ordinary conditions.

In considering the effect of radiation, it should be taken into account that the stereotype non-specific mechanisms of adaptation are switched on at the cellular level. These mechanisms are intended to increase the viability of the cell and are engendered by a decrease in most of the metabolic processes and temperature (Kalendo, 1972), probably being one of the main reasons why the life span increases when the animals are exposed to soft radiation.

Influence of the Electric and Magnetic Fields on the Life Span

The negative effect of the positive electric field and the positive effect of the negative electric field have apparently been studied most thoroughly with respect to the influence of the fields of different nature on the life span. In his experiments on laboratory mice, Molnar (1973) concluded that the positive charge acts as an electrochemical oxidant, which damages the macromolecules, while the negative field protects them in the same way as the cathodes are protected technically. Komarov (1978) observed that the life span of the house flies increases when electric and magnetic fields constantly act on them or when they are fed with magnetized products.

Influence of the Chemical Factors on the Life Span

There are many chemical agents which can influence strongly the life span. Among them, the most thorough study has been made of the salts of some metals and halogens, chelating agents, the precursors of free radicals and antioxidants, membrane stabilizers, the analogues of amino acids and nucleotides, lathyrogens, and some other agents.

Influence of Microelements and Chelating Agents on the Life Span

Schroeder and his associates (1963, 1971) thoroughly studied the influence of various microelements on the mammalian life span. They investigated the influence of the ions of chromium, nickel, cadmium, lead, titanium, germanium, yttrium, rhodium, palladium, tin, arsenic, selenium, tellurium, scandium, indium, zirconium, niobium, gallium, fluorine, antimony and vanadium of different valencies on the life span of mice and rats. Among all the elements which were studied, only three-valent chromium, yttrium and palladium increased substantially the life span. According to Priduba (1978a), manganese in a concentration of 5 μg/ml reduced the life span of the fruit flies, while it did not influence substantially this life span in a concentration of 1 μg/ml.

Among other metals, the influence of calcium on the life span has been studied most thoroughly. As early as 1942, Lansing showed that an inverse relationship existed between the life span of the rotifers and the concentration of calcium ions. This was confirmed in the experiments carried out by Sincock (1974). In these experiments involving radioactive calcium, he showed that calcium salts are deposited from a certain "threshold" age after the growth period is passed, and that the rate at which they are deposited is proportional to the calcium content of the medium. Moreover, it was learned that the life span of rotifers can be increased by 44–76 per cent (Sincock, 1975) and that the life of the fruit flies can be prolonged (Priduba, 1978b) by administering optimum concentrations of substances which bind calcium and some other polyvalent ions [citrate, tartrate, ethylene diamine tetraacetate, 1,2-di(2-aminoethoxy)-ethane of tetraacetic acid]. An increase in the life span by 20–25 per cent was detected when rats were fed EDTA (Dubina, Berlov, 1974). However, in the experiments on rotifers, whose life span decreased proportionally to the concentration of calcium or magnesium chlorides, the addition of such well-known chelating agents as sodium citrate, ethylene diamine tetraacetate or ethylene bis(hydroxy-ethylene nitrilo)-tetraacetate to the culture medium in different concentrations did not produce a prolonging effect, but caused a greater decrease in the life span (Enesco, Holtzman, 1980). Curtis and Tilley (1970) did not detect any correlation between the content of calcium in the blood and the life span of various strains of mice; the life span changed only slightly when calcium was excluded from food and water for 132 days. The authors then concluded that calcium has a limited effect on the aging processes.

Thus, some microelements can prolong the life span, while others can reduce it. In studying the influence of some elements on the life span, it is extremely important to establish to optimum concentrations of a chemical agent, since virtually all chemicals can reduce substantially the life span when they are administered in large doses. Unfortunately, only one or several doses are tried in most research works. Therefore, it can only be concluded preliminarily that the given chemical agents play a definite role in both aging and the determination of the life span.

Influence of Antioxidants on the Life Span

The free-radical nature of the action of many factors which reduce the life span (radiation, mutagens, carcinogens, etc.) suggested that the substances which stimulate the formation of free radicals can reduce the life span, while the inhibitors of the free-radical processes are potential geroprotectors. Indeed, it has been shown subsequently that the life span of the laboratory rodents and insects is markedly reduced when the free-radical processes are stimulated by increasing the partial pressure of oxygen or using such food additives as sodium hydrochloride, 2-amino-1,2,4-tyrosine and their combinations (Massie, Williams, 1980), hydroxylamine and hydrogen peroxides (Harman, 1968; Molnar, 1973), and fatty acids with a different degree of saturation (Driver, Cosopodiotis, 1979). However, the life span increased inconsiderably when use was made of most of the tested antioxidants of synthetic or biological origin, such as 2-ethy-6-methyl-3-hydroxypyridine (Emanuel, Obukhova, 1978 a, b), 2-mercaptoethylamine, 2,6-di-tert-butyl-4 methyl phenol and propyl gallate (Harman, 1968), ethoxyquinine (Comfort *et al.*, 1971), tocopherol-*p*-chloro-phenoxy acetate and thiazolidine carboxylate (Miquel, Johnson, 1975), 1,4-diazobicyclo-(2,2,2)-octane (Massie, Williams, 1980), tocopherol (Enesco, Verdone-Smith, 1980), and others.

Many aspects of the influence of the antioxidants on the life span are still unknown, although numerous works have been written in this respect. The opponents of the free-radical hypothesis of aging advance the following main arguments: (1) in most cases, the life-prolonging effect of the antioxidants is not great, being within the limits of the possible range of the life span of the intact populations; (2) the most successful attempts to increase the life span by antioxidants are connected with the experiments involving the short-living strains of rats which are predisposed to tumours (Harman, 1968), while the life-prolonging influence of the most effective antioxidants on the genetically perfect long-living strains is either not great or absent altogether (Kohn, 1971), and (3) the life-prolonging effect of the antioxidants may be due not to their direct action on the aging processes, but to a decrease in food consumption by the animals whose food has antioxidant (Bender *et al.*, 1970; Kohn, 1971; Sacher, 1977).

Even in the most successful experiments, the life-prolonging effect of the antioxidants is probably due not to a decrease in the aging rate (the maximum life spans of the control and test animals differ less in this respect), but to a decrease in vulnerability (Sacher, 1977).

Influence of the Stabilizers of the Lysosomal Membranes on the Life Span

Many authors working on the ways of prolonging life, the causes of many pathologies and their mechanisms have taken interest in the problem of stabilizing the lysosomal membranes ever since the lysosomes were discovered and deDuve's lysosomal hypothesis of aging was added to the numerous hypotheses of aging. The stability of the lysosomal membranes decreases under the action of many physical (ultraviolet or ionizing radiation, freezing and thawing, etc.), chemical (pyrogens, carcinogens) or biological factors (testosterone, progesterone, an excess or insufficiency of glucose and vitamin A, anoxia, ischemia, shock, starvation, inflammation, virus infections, bacterial endotoxins, the products of antigen-antibody reactions). Consequently, the powerful hydrolytic lysosomal enzymes are released "not according to plan," thus giving rise to consequences which are dramatic for the cell.

Hochschild (1971, 1973a, b) has done a great deal of work on the influence of the lysosomal membrane stabilizers on the life span. He tested the influence of about 40 synthetic and biological preparations of the membrane stabilizers on the life span of the fruit flies and mice. Among the synthetic membrane stabilizers, the following agents produced the greatest life-prolonging effect in the experiments with the fruit flies: aspirin (up to 40 per cent), pantothenic acid (23 per cent), salicylamide (17 per cent), a mixture of salicyl-salicylic acid and aspirin (38 per cent), acetaminophen (20 per cent), chlorpromazine hydrochloride (25 per cent), colchicine (25 per cent), meclofenoxate (39 per cent), triamcinolone (19 per cent), various derivatives of prednisolone (up to 23 per cent), etc. Among the preparations which were tested on mice, meclofenoxate (27 per cent) produced a great life-prolonging effect on the Swiss line (Hochschild, 1973a). However, no positive result was obtained in the experiments with the long-living C57BL/6J mice (Hochschild, 1973b). This was also true of the experiments with the preparations containing dimethylaminoethyl, an active agent of many lysosomal membrane stabilizers that was tried on the Japanese quails (Cherkin, 1975) and nematodes (Zukerman, Berrett, 1978).

Thus, many questions of the influence of the lysosomal membrane stabilizers on the life span must still be solved. As is the case with most of the other chemical factors, experiments with stabilizers are unreproducible to a great extent. According to Sacher (1977), membrane stabilizers do not influence the aging rate, but merely reduce the vulnerability of the test animals.

Influence of Latirogens on the Life Span

The formation of crosslinks between the macromolecules reduces their mobility and functional activity and is one of the most typical features of aging. It is expressed experimentally in an elevation of the melting temperature, a decrease in the extractability of individual fractions of chromatin proteins, callogen solubility, the loss of skin elasticity, etc. Therefore, in order to increase the life span, it is quite natural to use substances (known as *latirogens*) which can prevent the formation of such crosslinks. The main agents which participate in the formation of these chemical links include aldehydes (especially formaldehydes), the oxidation products of lipids (especially the unsaturated ones), sulphide groups, radiomimetic alkylating agents, free radicals, insoluble antigen-antibody complexes, and many ions of polyvalent metals. An incomplete list of the possible participants in the crosslinks suggests that a latirogen capable of neutralizing all the given active groups can hardly exist. Individual compounds, the most effective ones being aminopropionitrile and semicarbazide, were tested instead of the complex preparations of latirogens (especially those combined with antioxidants) in the research works where latirogens were used as a means of increasing the life span (LaBella, Vivian, 1975; Davies, Schofield, 1980).

Thus, just as with antioxidants, the life-prolonging effect of the tested latirogens is not very great, while the experimental results are poorly reproducible (Bender *et al.*, 1970).

Influence of Other Chemical Agents on the Life Span

In literature, mention is made of the possible life-prolonging effect of some other chemical compounds, whose site of action is most probably the autoimmunity processes (azathioprine, cyclophosphamide), the accumulation of lipofuscin (meclofenoxate, Kavazin, magnesium orotate), and various structures of the central nervous system (diiodomethane, Phenoformin, diphenylhydantoin) (Bender *et al.*, 1970; Massie *et al.*, 1978; Dilman, Anisimov, 1980). A great life-prolonging effect has been recorded in one of the latest researches by McCay and his associates (Sperling *et al.*, 1978). It turned out that Sulphomerazin increases the life span of the female rats by 36 per cent when it is added to food in a dose of 250 mg/kg from the very beginning of independent feeding. True, the life-prolonging effect did not surpass 10–15 per cent in the male rats and hamsters of both sexes.

According to Oeriu and Vochitu (1965), aging is connected with an increase in the concentration of cysteine and oxidized glutathione and with a decrease in the activity of the enzymes of thiol metabolism. The authors discovered a small life-prolonging effect when they studied the influence exerted by a combination of thiazolidine carboxylic and folic acids on the life span of the male and female rats and the female guinea pigs. However, it is difficult to definitely state what role the thiol compounds play in both aging and the determination of the mammalian life span owing to both the relatively short life span of the control animals and the life-prolonging effect itself.

Influence of the Biological Factors on the Life Span

The existence of biological subjects whose life span may be hundreds of years is in itself irrefugable evidence of the great possibilities of the biological factors for increasing the life span. Unfortunately, we still do not have enough knowledge to fully use these factors, while the life span of even short-living subjects increased experimentally by means of these factors only by 50–60 per cent.

Influence of the Low-Calorie or Low-Protein Diet on the Life Span

The study of the influence of diets of different composition and caloricity involving different feeding conditions has become one of the most promising models of prolonging the life of warm-blooded organisms (a model which is now being intensively worked out) ever since Osborne and his associates (1915) had shown that limited nutrition can increase substantially the life span of rats. Even in the thirties and the forties, when far less interest was taken in gerontology and the problems of increasing the life span, investigations of the influence of starvation on the life span were being intensively carried out especially by McCay and his associates (1935, 1941). In the subsequent years, the works by Nikitin, Ross, Barrows and their school shed much light on this problem. It was shown that besides increasing the life span of warm-blooded animals, starvation can increase the life span of cold-blooded animals and insects, i. e. fish (Comfort, 1963) and fruit flies (Loeb, Northrop, 1917, and others). Interestingly, limited nutrition increased the mammalian life span in most cases in spite of the different experimental conditions (species and strains of the test animals, the composition and caloricity of the diet, maintenance conditions, etc.) (McCay et al., 1935, 1941; Ross, 1961, 1969; Stuchlikova et al., 1975; Driori, Folman, 1976; Cheney et al., 1980; Everitt et al., 1980). Moreover, there is a direct link between the extent to which nutrition is limited and an increase in the life span. A decrease in daily food consumption by one kilocalorie increased the life span of rats by about 4 days (Ross, 1969). An important fact is that the life span grows when nutrition is limited not because the maintenance conditions of the animals are improved and mortality is reduced at the early stages of life, as is true in most cases, but because mortality is reduced at the later stages of life. Conversely, mortality at the early stages was higher in the starving animals than in the control groups. However, mortality among the starving animals decreased with age. This is probably because various tumours appear less frequently and are manifested only at the later stages of life (Gerbase-DeLima et al., 1975; Cheney et al., 1980; Everitt et al., 1980).

Low-calorie nutrition acts most effectively on the life span if it is started at the early stages of ontogeny. At a mature age, limited nutrition either increases the life span to a smaller extent or even reduces it (Stuchlikova et al., 1975; Everitt et al., 1980). The life span of the animals which began to starve at a mature age can be increased only by gradually reducing the amount of food being consumed (Stuchlikova et al., 1975).

When the diets of different composition were selected freely, the duration of future life inversely depended on the amount of the calories being consumed only during the first 200 days of life. The correlative level dropped with age and the amount of food being consumed did not influence substantially the life span from the age of 400 days (Ross, Bras, 1974). Similar results were obtained by Stuchlikova and her associates (1975), in whose experiments mice, rats and hamsters starved either throughout their life or during the early or late half of their life. The greatest life-prolonging effect was observed in the group of animals which starved only during the early half of their life and which were put on a diet *ad libitum* during the late half of their life. The animals rapidly gained weight (which greatly exceeded the control level) due to excessive obesity, e. g. some rats weighed as much as one kilogram. Nevertheless, the increase in life span of this animal group reached 50–60 per cent of the life span of the animals which were on a diet *ad libitum* all their life.

The wear-and-tear hypothesis is the most generally accepted hypothesis which explains the longer life span of the starving animals. According to it, the rate of metabolic processes decreases when nutrition is limited, as a result of which the level of the damaging influences drops (Ross, 1969; Sacher, 1977; Arshavksy, 1979). According to some authors, however, the life span increases during starvation because RNA polymerases are activated due to slight stress. Obviously, this contradicts the wear-and-tear hypothesis. In their research works, Nikitin (1979) and his associates proved experimentally that such an assumption was wrong. They established that the activity of the RNA polymerases A and B of the liver decreases during starvation. In this respect, there is a sharp decrease in the rate of such well-known age changes as growing polyploidy, the enrichment of chromatin with histone proteins, a decrease in the amount of non-histone proteins, phospholopids, free phosphate groups of DNA, the albumin/globulin ratio in the blood, etc. (Nikitin, 1979). According to Arshavsky (1979), oxygen consumption must be adequately measured. The fact is that the thermoindifferent zone of the starving rats is 3–4 °C lower than that of the control rats. Therefore, at 28 °C, which is an indifferent temperature for control rats but a stress one for starving animals, oxygen consumption and the respiration and heart rates are 30–70 per cent higher in the starving animals, while in the control rats, these indices drop by 15–40 per cent in comparison with the level which exists at ordinary habitation temperatures. Hence, the oxygen consumption of starving animals is 30–60 per cent higher at 28 °C, while at the real temperatures (19–20 °C) of their maintenance, it is 33 per cent lower than in the control animals. According to Arshavsky, the coefficient of the complete thermal insulation of the starving rats is higher (0.38) than that of the intact animals (0.27). A decrease in oxygen consumption is apparently not connected with the reduction of the functional abilities of mitochondria, since there is a certain increase in the third level of respiration, while the values of other levels are virtually unchanged in the preparations of the purified hepatic mitochondria of the starving rats (Weindruch et al., 1980).

According to some authors, the life-prolonging effect of starvation is due to hormonal shifts, such as slight stress, and especially to a decrease in the secretion of the releasing factors of the hypothalamus and the trophic hormones of the hypophysis (Nikitin, 1979; Everitt et al., 1980). In this respect, only the synthesis and secretion of the iodine-containing hormones of the thyroid gland and the thyrotropic hormone of the hypophysis are considerably suppressed, while the secretion of corticosterone and insulin does not decrease, but somewhat increases (Nikitin, 1979). The immunosuppressive effect of limited feeding can also play an important role in increasing the life span of the starving animals; consequently, the immune system matures more slowly and stays "young" longer (Gerbase-DeLima et al., 1975).

In considering the influence of limited nutrition on the life span, it should be taken into account that approximately the same life-prolonging effect is produced by both a low-calorie diet and a high-calorie diet with a low content of proteins. For instance, the life span of the females increases by 28 per cent when the content of the biologically useful proteins is reduced from 12 per cent (ordinary diet) to 4 per cent by adding starch from the age of 120 days. In these experiments, the skeleton dimensions and behaviour of the rats differed hardly from the control ones, while in the experiments involving a low-calorie diet, the weight, dimensions and growth rate of the test rats decreased markedly, the viability of the animals during stress diminished sharply, etc. (Miller, Payne,

1968). Approximately the same life-prolonging effect was observed by several authors when the protein content was reduced in the food of rats (Barrows, 1971; Leato *et al.*, 1976). According to Goodrick (1975), a low-protein diet increases the life span to a greater extent among hybrid animals than among inbred ones.

To increase the life span substantially, it is enough to limit not only the total proteins, but also individual indispensable amino acids, particularly tryptophan (Segall, 1977). A low-protein diet or a diet with a low content of individual indispensable amino acids may possibly reduce the rate of synthesis of the functionally active enzymic proteins. At least, this is indirectly evident from the data on a decrease in the activity of lactate dehydrogenase, malate dehydrogenase, cholinesterase, cathepsins, alkaline phosphatase, succinoxidase, etc. (Ross, 1969; Leato *et al.*, 1976).

Thus, a low-calorie or a low-protein diet or even a diet without one indispensable amino acid may increase substantially the life span. The genetic apparatus and the processes of protein synthesis are obviously one of the most probably "applications" of the given effects. A large amount of experimental material shows that the rate of synthesis of RNA and protein decreases substantially and the existence of these macromolecules increases when there is a deficiency of amino acids and energy in the cells of the most diverse types of differentiation. When these alimentary factors operate, the rate of breakdown and synthesis of macromolecules decreases and the cell passes over to the more economical use of information taken from the genetic apparatus, thus reducing the level of damages to DNA and increasing the life span of the cell and the organism as a whole.

A decrease in the body temperature by 2–3 °C may be of great importance in increasing the life span of the starving animals (Barrows, 1977; Arshavsky, 1979). The energy of activation of the aging processes, being calculated on that basis, is 30–50 kcal/mole. This is more or less in accord with similar values which were obtained from other experimental models. The life-prolonging effect of starvation may possibly be mainly due to a decrease in the body temperature, while starvation should be regarded not as an independent factor of increasing the life span, but as a successful physiological method of reducing the body temperature. This may be more convincing if account is taken of the fact that, unlike the temperature factor, the low-calorie diet and especially the low-protein diet do not increase the life span of many species of cold-blooded animals (Van Harrewega, 1974; Rockstein *et al.*, 1977; Bileva *et al.*, 1978). An analysis of age mortality made on the basis of available experimental material shows that an increase in the life span of the cold-blooded animals during starvation is not connected with a decrease in the real aging rate, and that it is more likely the outcome of the better maintenance conditions and a decrease in mortality at the early stages which are not determined by aging. For instance, the almost 1.5-fold increase in the life span of the starving cold-blooded animals that was discovered by Comfort did not change the slope of the age mortality curve (Sacher, 1977).

Influence of Physical Activity on the Life Span

It is difficult to assess the influence of the physical activity relating to the most diverse biological and metabolic parameters, especially when the life span is involved.

Oxygen consumption increases 40–60 times during the flight of many insects. According to the "rate of living" hypothesis, this should reduce sharply the life span. Indeed, as Sohal and Donato (1979) have shown, the life span of the flies doubles or trebles when their flying ability is almost completely limited by keeping them in a beaker with labyrinth-like barriers. According to Trout and Kaplan (1970), the life span decreased markedly in the mutant flies with extremely high endogenous motoneuron activity and physical activity. But they did not detect any clear-cut inverse relationship between the life span and physical activity of seven different strains of the fruit fly.

Several authors have shown that the activation of the motor system may be a means of preventing many cardiovascular diseases (Muravov, 1976; Arshavsky, 1979). A moderate physical load may influence favourably aging by economizing the metabolic and functional processes and increasing the operating range of the appropriate functional systems. In this respect, it is very important to look for the maximally individualized physical loads, whose optimum is one of the most natural physiological stimuli of the restorative processes. Hypokinesis or maximum physical loads reduce substantially the life span (Muravov, 1976). However, moderate physical activity, such as voluntary or forced walking or slight running for a short time increased the life span of rats (McCay et al., 1941; Retzlaff et al., 1966; Drori, Folman, 1976). In some research works, the life-prolonging effect of heightened physical activity was more pronounced in the females (Sperling et al., 1978), while in others, it was more pronounced in the males (Goodrick, 1980). Interestingly, the female rats, which as a rule have a longer life span, walked almost eight times the distance covered by the male rats daily (Sperling et al., 1978). Edington and his associates (1972) forced rats to run in the treadmill after they were 120, 300, 450 and 600 days old and showed that physical activity increased the life span of animals which were younger than 450 days, while it reduced the life span of animals which were older. Hence, the authors concluded that there was a certain "age threshold" after which physical activity influenced the life span negatively. However, this conclusion was justly criticized by several authors, who maintained that the physical load should be differentiated according to age, while the same compulsory load used by Edington and his associates was too great a test for the untrained mature and old animals. Since obesity is known to reduce the life span, while trained animals have far less weight and fat, some authors concluded that the life-prolonging effect of physical activity is due to the smaller extent of obesity of the test animals. Arshavsky (1977) has worked out an interesting concept. According to him, the positive effect of a physical load is due to the excessive stimulation of the anabolic processes. After comparing several physiological and morphological parameters of the closely related species (the rabbit and the hare, the cow and the horse, the rat and the squirrel) which differed from one another by the extent of physical activity and the life span, the author concluded that hightened physical activity, especially the dynamic component of the muscular load, was a means which increased substantially the life span. Unlike in other researches, it was shown that the optimal physical loads do- not enhance, but reduce basal metabolism by 40–60 per cent and increase the content of ATP, protein, the membrane potential, etc. (Arshavsky, 1977).

Influence of the Hormones on the Life Span

At first, the study of the influence of the hormones on aging and the life span was widely welcomed. Later, however, disappointing results were obtained. When the attempts to rejuvenate the organism by transplanting the sexual glands had failed, the influence of the hormones on the life span was hardly studied for a long time. Attempts to influence the life span by sexual and some other hormones began to be made again only in the fifties and the sixties. In an effort to reveal the reasons why the female mammals have a longer life span, it was shown that testosterone reduced somewhat the life span of castrated males and females, while estradiol increased the life span of only the males (Asdel et al., 1967). The castration of animals and man brought the life span of the males almost up to that of the females, hardly influencing the life span of the latter (Hamilton et al., 1969; Drori, Folman, 1976). Interestingly, the life span increased by almost 25 per cent when the males and the females were kept together than when they were maintained separately (Drori, Folman, 1976). A similar picture was observed among flies, whose life span increased markedly when the number of females and males was in a 3 : 1 ratio (Ragland, Sohal, 1975).

The negative influence of the hormones of the thyroid gland on the life span is quite unequivocal. Mortality increases substantially when thyroxine is administered for a long time, but it returns to the initial level when the hormone is no longer administered (Everitt et al., 1980). In the case of a low-calorie diet, the life span grows while the secretion of the hormones of the thyroid gland is suppressed markedly, and when the rats are maintained at low temperatures (which reduce the life span), the secretion of these hormones increases.

According to several researchers studying the influence of the hormones on the life span, the life span may increase when the trophic influence of the hypophysial hormones is reduced. This has been proved experimentally by comparing the life span of the intact animals and that of the hypophysectomied ones. It turned out that hypophysectomy in itself reduces somewhat the life span, while substitution therapy by only one hormone of the glands regulated by the hypophysis, i. e. hydrocortisone, is enough to raise the life span level of the hypophysectomied animals far above that of the intact ones (Everitt et al., 1980). It has been shown that hypophysectomy by substitution therapy with hydrocortisone acetate can increase the life span almost to the same extent as starvation. In both cases, the life-prolonging effect is produced when the experiments are started at an early age. Hypophysectomy performed at the age of 400 days either with or without substitution therapy had increased mortality and reduced the life span, just as among the animals which were operated at the age of 70 days but which were not given hydrocortisone. It has been shown that corticoids, particularly prednisolone, whose corticotropic action is less pronounced and its growth inhibiting action is more pronounced, influence favourably the life span when they are administered for a long time to mice (Bellamy, 1968; LaBella, Vivian, 1975).

Corticoids played a definite role also when the life span of the rats was increased by many stress effects (Frolkis et al., 1976b). These effects began to be produced at the age of 600 days, and they increased the life span to 1,110 days as compared with 938 days of the control animals, i. e. the life span approximately doubled since the effects began to be produced. When the short-living A/J and the long-living C57BL/6J mice age, the long-living strain is characterized by less affinity for, but a higher content of the glucocorticoid receptors (Bonner, Slavkin, 1975). Hydrocortisone increases substantially (by 30–50 per cent) the life span of the human fibroblast cultures. This is associated with a decrease in the proteolytic rate, the stimulation of rRNA synthesis (and a decrease in the background level of the errors made by the protein biosynthesis apparatus), the stabilization of the lysosomal membranes, a diminution of the age growth of the G_1 and G_2 periods of the cell cycle, an increase in the fraction of the proliferative pool, etc. As we have already seen, the hypothermal action of hydrocortisone and other corticoids should be taken into account when the life-prolonging effects of these hormones are being considered (Putthoff et al., 1977). Unfortunately, most of the authors who studied the influence of various factors on the life span do not given data on a change in this important and rather easily measurable indicator.

Although hypophysectomy increases the life span, it would apparently be wrong to assume that all the hormones which are secreted by this important neurhohormonal centre reduce the life span. A study of the influence of the extracts of the posterior lobe of the hypophysis and vasopressin as well as their combination with corticosteroids has shown (Friedman, Friedman, 1964) that these hormonal preparations with or without steroids can increase the life span. The parallel administration of the extracts of the posterior lobe of the hypophysis and oxytocin to male rats has revealed that the life-prolonging effect of the hypophysial preparations is caused apparently by oxytocin, whose content is much higher in females than in males. This fact is also probably very important when the reasons why females have a longer life span than males are being considered.

Among other mammalian hormones, the influence of the growth hormone on the life span has been studied. This hormone did not influence the aging rate and the life span substantially (Everitt et al., 1980).

In insects, the rate of metamorphosis and moulting is regulated by special juvenile hormones, which can retard and even stop the development of the characteristic features of an adult mate. However, these hormones cannot reverse aging and development. Moreover, all the attempts to increase the insect life span by transplanting the whole brain and a separate round gland, which secretes a juvenile hormone, to young imagoes and the attempts made at the larval stages had failed (Sondhi, 1967, 1970). When the precursors of the steroid hormones were added to the culture medium, it turned out that ergosterol and sterol, unlike cholesterol, increase the insect life span (Norris, Moore, 1980).

Influence of the Inhibitors of Protein Biosynthesis and Energy Metabolism on the Life Span

In gerontology, an indisputable fact is that the life span of a species and the intensity of metabolic processes are inversely related. This has often been confirmed by various cold-blooded and warm-blooded biological subjects. Since the intensity of metabolism is determined largely by enzymic activity, i. e. by the rate of RNA and protein synthesis, the inhibitors of RNA and protein biosynthesis could naturally be an effective means of increasing the life span.

According to our data, the addition of such common inhibitors of transcription as olivomycin and actinomycin D in optimal concentrations to the culture medium of the fruit flies reduced the activity of the protein-synthesizing apparatus and increased the life span by 20–30 per cent. The optimal doses of the inhibitors of translation (cycloheximide, hydroxylamine, tetracycline) and energy (sodium fluoride, dinitrophenol) produced approximately the same life-prolonging effect. Our doses of the inhibitors, while increasing the life span, suppressed strongly RNA and protein biosynthesis in the fruit flies. For instance, the relative specific radioactivity of RNA and protein decreased rapidly by the third hour (by 35 and 33 per cent, respectively) and the 8th hour (by 39 and 44 per cent, respectively) when actinomycin D was added in a dose of $10\,\mu g/ml$ to the culture medium. However, the rate of the synthetic processes gradually increases at the later stages of inhibitor feeding. In all the cases, the inhibitor doses which were smaller than the optimal ones did not influence the life span substantially, while larger doses reduced it sharply (Frolkis et al., 1979b). House flies were used to show that the life span can be increased by the transcription inhibitors (tetracycline, morphocycline, streptomycine) (Yudeleva, 1977).

Such experiments with mammals were carried out for the first time in our laboratory (Frolkis et al., 1976b). When olivomycin was administered from the age of 600 days, the average life span increased to 35.6 months, while that of the control animals was 30.9 months. The maximum life span in this respect was 47.1 and 38.3 months, respectively.

Extremely important is the fact that olivomycin influenced the rate of age changes, since the typical features of the metabolic and structural manifestations of aging had originated 5 or 6 months later in the test animals, while they were far less pronounced than in the intact animals of the same age. This is especially evident when a comparison is made of the structural and ultrastructural changes in various organs of the control and test animals. The structural changes in both the connective tissue and the parenchyma of the organs being examined were less pronounced in rats which received olivomycin than in the control animals. The structural age changes in the test rats 30–32 months old were very similar to those in the intact rats 24–26 months old. For instance, the amount of lipid inclusions in the subcutaneous adipose tissue and the fat reserve as well as those under the epicardium and the liver decreases substantially in comparison with that in the control animals. The hepatic tissue retains its usual architectonics in this respect: the hepatocytes have a fine-grained cytoplasm and very rich glycogen, whose granules are distributed throughout the cytoplasm. Also important is the fact that the dimensions of the hepatocytes and their nuclei are reduced greatly. Pores are clearly seen in the nuclear envelope, and the granular endoplasmic reticulum with many ribosomes is well developed. These ribosomes are also on the outer side of the nuclear membrane.

Olivomycin influences the structure of several endocrine glands substantially. In intact animals, the insular apparatus diminishes with age mainly owing to the disappearance of large stromata and the appearance of small ones, while in animals which were given olivomycin, the number and dimensions of stromata do not diminish and sometimes large and occasionally fused stromata are seen, being characteristic of a younger age. The atrophic changes in the thyroid gland are poorly expressed. The thyroid gland of old intact rats has many large follicles which are lined with a flattened epithelium and are filled with a dense colloid. Animals of the same age that were given olivomycin had no large congested follicles. In them, the colloid in the space between the follicles was light and not dense, while the cells of the thyroid epithelium were not compact and had a cubic shape.

Certain metabolic shifts also indicate that the aging rate slows down in animals which received olivomycin. For instance, gaseous metabolism and oxygen consumption are known to become less intense with age. Olivomycin, however, impedes this process. In the control rats, oxygen consumption diminishes by 29 per cent (from 128 ± 2 to 91 ± 1 ml of oxygen per kilogram of weight per hour) at the age of 20–36 months, while in the test rats, this consumption diminishes only by 9 per cent in that age bracket. Rats which were 36 months old and which were given olivomycin consumed the same amount of oxygen as intact rats 24 months old. Olivomycin has a similar effect on the osmatic resistance of erythrocytes. This indicator in the test rats 28–32 months old was the same as that in the control animals 24 months old.

We have observed that olivomycin exerts considerable influence on lipid metabolism. The prolonged administration of the inhibitors not only reduces the content of lipids in the blood and several tissues, but also changes the ratio of the fractions in them. For instance, olivomycin in therapy reduced the content of total lipids in blood serum by an average of 10 per cent. This reduction was verified statistically ($p < 0.05$) in 73 per cent of the test animals, while the level of total lipids tended to rise (by 13 per cent) in 24 per cent of the rats. Olivomycin reduces the total content of prebeta and beta lipoproteins by an average of 14 per cent. It reduces the total content of lipids by 20 per cent in the myocardium and by 23 per cent in the brain. This reduction is especially great in the skeletal muscle (by 55 per cent). The concentration of total cholesterol also decreases in these organs by 17, 16 and 28 per cent, respectively. The content of triglycerides decreases in the skeletal muscle and the liver by 56 and 44 per cent, respectively. The amount of triglycerides does not change in the myocardium and the brain, but the content of atherogenic beta and prebeta lipoproteins decreases in them by 35 and 22 per cent, respectively. At the same time, the content of the given fractions of lipoproteins increases in the liver and the skeletal muscle by 28 and 62 per cent, respectively. Hence, the therapeutic administration of olivomycin optimalizes lipid metabolism, retards the accumulation of individual lipid fractions and reduces their total content in most of the organs of the test animals, thus showing that the preparation has an inhibiting effect on the development of the age changes in lipid metabolism.

Aging and atherosclerosis are known to be interconnected. The age changes in the metabolism of man creates prerequisites for the development of atherosclerosis, which is connected with the disturbance of protein and lipid metabolism. The given data on the influence of olivomycin on protein and lipid metabolism show that it is necessary to study its effect on the development of experimental atherosclerosis. Anichkov-Khalatov's cholesterol model was used to this end. Cholesterol was administered to rabbits 20 months old in a dose of 100 mg/kg for 3.5 months (control group). Some of the rabbits (experimental group) were given olivomycin besides cholesterol in a dose of 0.15 mg/kg for 10 days. Two more groups of animals were used for control: intact animals and rabbits which were given only olivomycin. An analysis of the data obtained shows that olivomycin retards the accumulation of lipids in the organism when atherosclerosis is simulated experimentally. The content of lipids and their individual fractions increases substantially when the animals are given only cholesterol. However, no differences are observed in animals which are given olivomycin and cholesterol simultaneously in comparison with the intact rabbits and rabbits which were given only olivomycin. In animals with experimental atherosclerosis, for instance, the content of lipids in the blood reached 651 mg per cent, while in rabbits which were given olivomycin and cholesterol simultaneously, the figure did not differ from that of the intact animals (252 and 251 mg per cent, respectively). When olivomycin was administered against the background of cholesterol, it also reduced substantially the content of cholesterol (by 30 per cent), non-esterified fatty acids (by 34 per cent), triglycerides (by 51 per cent) and, what is especially important, atherogenic lipoproteins (by 45 per cent). In the case of experimental atherosclerosis, the administration of olivomycin retarded the accumulation of lipids and their fractions. However, the effect of this inhibitor of protein biosynthesis on lipid exchange is manifested differently in different organs. Among all the organs which were studied, olivomycin exerted the strongest influence on lipid metabolism in the liver, and then in the brain, the heart and the skeletal muscle. Atherogenic prebeta and beta lipoproteins took the longest, while triglycerides took the shortest time to accumulate in all the organs being considered. The lipid content more or less diminished in all the organs of the test animals: it diminished by 46 per cent in myocardium, by 35 per cent in the liver, by 16 per cent in the skeletal muscle, and by 6 per cent in the brain. Just as in the aorta, the atherogenic lipoproteins in the brain took the longest to accumulate (by 65 and 83 per cent, respectively), triglycerides in the liver (by 57 per cent), and non-esterified fatty acids in the skeletal muscle (by 21 per cent). Even at the present stage of the elaboration of the problem, these data show that protein biosynthesis plays a considerable role in the development of atherosclerosis and that the latter can be influenced by acting on transcription and translation.

The data on a decrease in the content of lipids and non-esterified fatty acids in the blood and on the sharp diminution of the content of atherogenic lipoproteins in several organs show that olivomycin prevents both gross changes in protein and lipid metabolism and the development of atherosclerosis.

Just as in the experiments with the fruit flies, the administration of olivomycin to rats considerably reduced the rate of RNA and protein synthesis in the frontal cortex of the brain, the hypothalamus, the liver and especially the muscles. In the hypophysis and the myocardium, however, the rate of biosynthesis increased. An analysis of the mortality curves shows that the life-prolonging effect of olivomycin is connected with both a decrease in the "real aging rate" and a certain improvement of the maintenance conditions as well as a reduction of mortality at the relatively early stages or ontogeny.

Influence of the Genetic Factors on the Life Span

The existence of species which differ from one another in their life span by tens and occasionally hundreds of times even within a single class shows that the genetic factors play the leading role in determining the life span. The development of genetic sciences, especially gene engineering, holds out great prospects for increasing the life span. At present, only one genetic phenomenon which increases the life span is known, i. e. heterosis.

All the attempts to produce long-living strains of animals by genetic modifications have failed. In the course of evolution, the gradual selection of features which are favourable for longevity apparently made it less likely for new favourable features and the modifications of the genetic apparatus to appear. Almost all mutations affecting the most diverse metabolic and regulatory processes at the cellular and higher levels of organization as a rule reduced substantially the life span. The probability of producing a long-living strain is very small. Favourable results were not obtained even by special selection of longevity (Lints et al., 1979).

There is an increasing amount of evidence which shows that the life span of many species gradually increased during their evolution. Cutler (1979) used 59 species of ungulates and 32 species of carnivores to show that their evolution involved a substantial increase in the life span since the Paleogene. For instance, the maximum potential life span of carnivores was 9 years in the Archean era, 14 years in the Paleogene, 17 years in the Neocene, and 21 years in the modern era. The figures are 10, 15, 21 and 30 years, respectively, for ungulates. The life span of the primates grew approximately to the same extent. The only exception was hominids, whose life span grew much more rapidly. For instance, the maximum potential human life span increased by 14 years in the last 100,000 years, being accompanied by the modification of only 0.5 per cent of the genome (Cutler, 1976). The dominant and superdominant inheritance of longevity, being shown by many authors with respect to the most diverse species of insects and mammals, including man, apparently plays in important role in the evolutionary growth of the life span. Studying the general nature of the inheritance of longevity in four inbred and six hybrid strains of mice, Goodrick (1975) showed that the inheritance of longevity was superdominant in 5 out of 6 hybrid strains, while it was dominant in the remaining strain. Genetic analysis shows that the aging factor is represented by one locus, which is the same for all strains, in a genome, and that it acts through the secondary specific factors. Most authors attribute the effect of the superdominant inheritance of longevity to the greater probability of the appearance of heterozygotic genes which can retain the viability of the cell within a wider range of the damaging effects, e. g. temperature, radiation, etc.

Serious discussion of the possibilities of increasing the life span held by scientists in various countries and the attempts to work out scientifically substantiated ways and means of substantially increasing the life span of man and other biological subjects of the animal and vegetable kingdoms are a new important stage in developing not only gerontology, but also biology as a whole. Since this is a difficult problem and there are several differences involving theory and experiments, it is hard to assess all the possible ways of development and the results of the solution of the problem. The matter in question is the frequently unsubstantiated comparison of the experimental results obtained from subjects with different levels of biological organization and the inadequate account taken of the role of the doses, concentrations, the duration of the action of the life-prolonging factors, and so forth. This concerns the nature of the statements made by various authors, including statements which range from senselessly optimistic ones to gloomy and just as senselessly pessimistic ones. There were and will be difficulties in solving such a difficult problem as life prolongation. Some authors will score unexpected successes, while others may be disappointed with their research. This applies to most researchers, too. Even now, the available means make it possible to change the life span of the cold-blooded animals by tens and hundreds of times, regulate the rate of their aging in virtually any set rhythm, model various aging processes, etc. Less successes have been scored in prolonging the life of the warm-blooded animals. It has been prolonged by 25–30 per cent at the most, being within the framework of the life span prolongation reserves inside a species. The subjects of research, their maintenance and the effects of the life-prolonging factors differ from one research to another. Therefore, the results of the researches into life prolongation are poorly reproducible and need to be verified. However, there is no doubt that the average and maximum life spans can be increased by lowering the body temperature and maintaining a certain diet. This has been confirmed in many laboratories in the world.

What is amazing is that old age and death always set in very steadily. Among numerous biological subjects whose life span is known to man, not a single one lived several times longer than the known biological limits. The organism ages as a complex biological self-regulating system. The aging processes are initiated and realized through numerous canals which are connected in a parallel manner and are to a certain extent autonomous, making the system highly reliable. Therefore, attempts to prolong life by reducing the influence of separate damaging factors, which in essence reduce the level of the stimulating signal in one or seven canals, do not increase the life span of species substantially. No wonder that only the factors of total action, such as the type of temperature or diet, produce the most significant and stable results in increasing the life span.

Aging is usually regarded as a process which gradually damages the organism and reduces its viability. However, biological subjects basically differ from such systems, because every cell has, in many respects, a mechanism which heals virtually all the damages by supercompensation. Vitauct, which increases the life span, had originated and has become perfect in the course of evolution. It not only restores the initial state, but also gives rise to a new quality of the basis of the adaptation mechanisms. The life span of the organism is determined apparently by the relationship of at least three parameters: the level of the damaging factors, the effectiveness of eliminating the damages, and the intensity of vitauct as well as the stability of the biological system. Since the nature and structure of the same functional systems as well as the level of the external damaging factors are the same to a certain extent, the different life spans of biological species should be attributed above all to the different level of the vitauct processes, including DNA reparation (Hart, Setlow, 1974). In some cases, e. g. when poikilotherms are being acclimatized to the cold, situations may originate in which the level of the restoring processes of the adaptive mechanisms is higher than the level of the damaging factors, and then the life span grows substantially. In the near future, the life span will be increased mainly by revealing the effects which change the relationship between aging and vitauct as well as the processes which activate restoration at all the levels of biological organization. In this respect, it is not enough to prove the influence which a certain factor exerts on the life span. Moreover, it is necessary to ascertain the "price" which the organism pays for increasing the life span and whether unfavourable changes occur in the activity of individual systems and the organism as a whole in this respect. Therefore, experiments involving life prolongation should be combined with a thorough study of the changes in the organism's metabolism and functions. To this end, it is important to work out effective criteria of biological age, making it possible to assess quickly the action of a geroprotector.

In Lieu of a Conclusion

Creative work in science is a process which involves reason as well as emotion. Every author believes that the subject in which he has recently been taking keen interest is the most interesting subject. Therefore, this section is called "In Lieu of a Conclusion." It not only sums up somewhat the whole monograph, but also contains such new concepts as the "chronobiological" and "ontobiological" manifestations of aging as well as "accelerated" and "retarded" aging and expounds new approaches which interest the author now.

John Bernal wrote that today it is easier to discover a new fact or propose a new theory than to make sure that the given fact has not been discovered or the given theory has not been proposed. The concept of the internal contradictoriness of individual development, i. e. the concept of the life-prolongating mechanisms which originate with age and the existence of the life-prolongating processes, was proposed by us over two decades ago, and it is now the basis of the adaptive regulatory theory. I am glad that we are not the only ones who hold such views today, and that they are being specifically and creatively developed by other researchers.

To propose the concept of the life-prolongating processes and the existence of vitauct, the mechanisms of aging had to be analyzed systematically and the onsetting age changes had to be considered from the standpoint of self-regulation, from the standpoint of two extremely important physiological categories: regulation and adaptation. The age changes in self-regulation determine ultimately the mechanisms of aging and vitauct and the organism's age dynamics.

Vitauct cannot be regarded as simply anti-aging, just as life cannot be regarded as only anti-death. Vitauct cannot be divorced from its biological essence, i. e. from adaptation to the external environment and the inheritance of information. The vitauct mechanism is determined by (a) the original reliability of the biological structures, (b) the extent of the reparative processes, (c) the activity of the defence and preventive systems, and (d) the mechanisms of adaptation and compensation. The vitauct mechanisms can be divided into genotypical ones (genetically programmed ones) and phenotypical ones, which are formed during vital activity due to the self-regulation mechanisms.

The main mechanisms of vitauct are: DNA reparation, the perfection of gene regulation in the course of evolution, gene redundancy, the growth of the potentialities of the protein-synthesizing system, the great mitotic potential of the cells, an increase in their number, the establishment of a relationship between protein biosynthesis and the state of the cell membrane, the origination of the antioxidant systems, microsomal oxidation, the trophic influences of the nervous system and many connective-tissue elements, and the development of many current adaptive regulatory shifts during aging at all the levels of biological organization (polyploidy, compensatory hyperfunction, the activation of several metabolic cycles and local humoral systems, the growth of sensitivity to several mediators, etc.).

The main mechanisms of aging are: the shifts in genome regulation, irreparable DNA alterations, the shifts in the membrane-gene relationships and in the intermolecular links, the disturbances of the active and passive transport of substances through the membrane, the shifts in the reception of cells and their excitability, the changes in the protein-synthesizing system of mitochondria and the limitation of the energy potential of cells on this basis, as well as the disturbances in the intercellular relationships, ending in the destruction of cells. The development of these molecular and cellular disturbances in the neuro-hormonal control structures increasingly limits the organism's adaptation to the environment and to the age changes in other organs and tissues. The attenuation of neural control and the changes in the reactions to the humoral factors at the stages of the direct link and feed-back concerning self-regulation are especially significant in this respect.

The relationship between aging and vitauct determines the rate and extent of the age changes. To understand the life span mechanisms, it is expedient to nominally divide all the age changes into chronobiological and ontobiological ones. Chronobiological changes are connected largely with chronological age (osteoporosis, sclerosis of vessels and some other tissues, arterial pressure, myocardial contractility, blood lipids, etc.). The rate at which ontobiological changes develop correlates with the species life span. The higher the rate of ontobiological changes, the smaller is the species life span (neurohumoral mechanisms of the cessation of growth, the potentialities of the protein-synthe-sizing system, the mitotic potential of the cells, several immune defence factors, the metabolic capacity of the enzymic systems, etc.). The life span grows as the ontobiological changes slow down, and then chronobiological shifts become increasingly important in the mechanisms of aging. Therefore, the relationships between the mechanisms of aging of the short-living and long-living species can differ greatly from one another. The relationship between the chronobiological and ontobiological changes determines the species specificity of age pathology, which is different in the short-living and long-living species. To understand the essence of aging, it is important to divide the age changes into chronobiological and ontobiological ones, since the genetically programmed mechanisms and stochastic influences, which are connected with the inevitable action of the damaging factors and the relative reliability of the biological structures, differ in their significance as the changes develop.

The mechanisms which determine the distinctions of the species' life span cannot be simply transferred in order to explain the intraspecies distinctions of the individual life span. Aging is an individual process. Therefore, its individual course may vary within the limits of the age changes characteristic of a species. In this respect, it is expedient to single out different syndromes of aging (neurogenic, endocrine, hemodynamic and other syndromes) as well as accelerated and retarded aging (taking its average rate for a species). Progeria and early age pathology are the greatest expression of accelerated aging, while great longevity is the extreme expression of retarded aging. The mechanisms of accelerated aging are particular and are not of a single type. They are based on the different relationships of the shifts in the rates of the chronobiological and ontobiological changes. The early origin of atherosclerosis, arterial hypertension, ischemia, diabetes and other diseases is connected largely with accelerated aging.

The existence of a constant link (which is not always mathematically rigid) between the duration of the organism's formation, its progressive development and the life span of a species is an extremely important regularity of ontogenesis. This link is so essential that the life span can be increased to the greatest extent by growth-restraining influences. This confirms the need to develop ontogenology. We believe that the term ontogenology should be applied to the investigation of the age changes at different stages of individual development without artificially separating different age periods and comparing some of them with others. This is the approach that should be taken in order to study the unity of vitauct and aging.

The relationship between individual periods of age development and also the mechanisms that determine the life span can be understood from the standpoint of the genoregulatory hypothesis. The duration of the organism's formation, its progressive development and growth are determined by genome regulation, the rhythm, and the rate at which the genoregulatory mechanisms are switched on. These factors determine the link between the initial periods of ontogenesis and the whole life span.

Thus, the adaptive regulatory theory of aging acknowledges the origin of two opposite processes in ontogenesis, confirms the leading role which the changes in genome regulation play in vitauct and aging, proves the existence of the membranogenetic mechanisms of aging, recognizes that the primary changes in neurohormonal control change decisively the relationship between the organism and the environment and can cause secondary disturbances in the tissues with age, proves that there exists a reduction of reactivity of cells, organs and systems to many physiologically active substances (however changes in responses to small doses, i.e. sensitivity, and large doses of substances, i.e. reactive capacity, are different), and asserts that aging is ultimately due to the diminution of the reliability of self-regulation. This diminution limits the organism's adaptive abilities and promotes age pathology.

In gerontology, only the aging process has been studied in the past. However, due attention should in future be given to the life-prolongating processes. In 1913, Dastre wrote: "To reach the end of the longevity allotted to us, we should not rely on the elixir of life, the alchemists' gold, the stone of immortality, which did not prevent its inventor, Paracelsus, from dying at the age of 58, transfusion, Graham's celestial bed, King David's herocomia, charlatans, and soothsayers . . . The art to prolong life is the art not to curtail it."

That is all quite true. A reasonable mode of life, or Mechnikov's orthobiosis, naturally helps to prolong life. However, gerontological achievements show that not only the struggle against life-reducing factors, but also the search for effective means of retarding aging and activating vitauct will help to prolong human life.

We hope that our concepts will be the focus of lively discussion. As Chenning wrote, nothing helps the triumph of truth so much as resistance to it.

References

Abe, T., Malik, A. B., O'Kane, H. O., Geha, A. S. (1973): Effects of isoproterenol and norepinephrine on function of coronary flow and oxygen consumption of the intact left ventricle. Surgery *74*, 562–569.

Abu-Erreish, G., Wohlrab, H., Sanadi, D. R. (1974): In vitro and in vivo changes of mitochondria from hearts of senescent rats. Fed. Proc. *33*, 1518–1521.

Abu-Erreish, G., Sanadi, D. R. (1978): Age-related changes in cytochrome concentration of myocardial mitochondria. Mech. Ageing Develop. *7*, 425–432.

Adamopoulos, D. A., Loraine, J. A., Dowe, G. A. (1971): Endocrinological studies in women approaching the menopause. J. Obstet. Gynecol. *78*, 62–79.

Adelman, R. C. (1971): Age dependent effects of enzyme induction–a biological expression of ageing. Exp. Gerontol. *6*, 75–87.

Adelman, R. C. (1975): Disruptions in enzyme regulation during aging. In: Enzyme Induction (Parke, P. V., ed.), pp. 304–311. Surrey: Raven Press.

Adelman, R. C., Freeman, C. (1972): Age-dependent regulation of glucokinase, tyrosine amino-transferase activities of rat liver in vivo by adrenal, pancreatic and pituitary hormone. Endocrinology *90*, 26, 1551–1560.

Ahlquist, R. P. (1948): A study of the adrenotropic receptors. Amer. J. Physiol. *153*, 586–592.

Ahn Ho Sam, Makman, M. H. (1977): Neurotransmitter-sensitive adenylate cyclase in hypothalami of guinea-pig, rat and monkey. Brain Res. *138*, 125–138.

Aksyenova, I. Ye. (1971): Age changes in the ultrastructural organization of mitochondria. In: Cellular Aging. Gerontologiya i geriatriya 1970–1971 (yearbook), pp. 131–136. Kiev: Institute of Gerontology.

Aksyenova, I. Ye. (1973): Age changes in the ultrastructure of the neurons of the cortex. Izvest. Akad. Nauk BSSR *4*, 102–105.

Algeri, S., Bonati, M., Brunello, W., Ponzio, F. (1977): Dihydropteridine reductase and tyrosine hydroxylase activities in rat brain during development and senescence: a comparison study. Brain Res. *132*, 569–574.

Almazov, V. A., Tkachenko, B. I., Samoilenko, A. V., Temirov, A. A. (1976): Comparative characterization of the influence of noradrenaline on the hemodynamics in persons and animals. Fiz. cheloveka *6*, 990–996.

Alpatov, W. W., Pearl, R. (1929): Experimental studies in the duration of life. XII. Influence of temperature during the larval period and adult life on the duration of life of the imago of *Drosophila melanogaster*. Am. Nat. *63*, 37–67.

Altman, J. (1968): DNA metabolism and cell proliferation. In: Handbook of Neurochemistry, Vol. 2, pp. 137–182. Oxford: Pergamon Press.

Altshuler, R. A., Granik, V. G. (1976): Pharmacological regulation of the function of the noradrenergic neurons. Zhurn. Vses. khim. ob. im. D. I. Mendeleyeva *21*, 171–179.

Alyeshin, B. V. (1971): Histophysiology of the Hypothalamohypophysial System. Moscow: Meditsina. (In Russian.)

Andrew, W. (1971): The Anatomy of Aging in Man and Animals. New York: Grune and Stratton.

Anisimov, V. N., Pozdeev, V. K., Dmitrievskaya, A. Yu., Gracheva, G. M., Ilin, A. P., Dilman, V. M. (1977): Age changes in the level of biogenic amines in the rat brain. Fiziol. zhurn. SSSR *63*, 3, 353–357.

Anokhin, P. K. (1952): On the two-phase action of adrenaline on the baroreceptors of the carotid nerve. In: Neural Regulation of Blood Circulation and Respiration, pp. 147–158. Moscow: Medgiz. (In Russian.)

Anokhin, P. K. (1968): Biology and Neurophysiology of Conditioned Reflexes. Moscow: Meditsina. (In Russian.)

Aprikyan, G. V., Shaginyan, V. D., Gevorkyan, G. A., Akhverdyan, M. S., Melikyan, A. M. (1978): On the possibility of using the enriched fractions of the glia cells and neurons in studying the transport of neurotransmitter amino acids in old age. In: Age Biology of the Brain, pp. 255–302. Yerevan: Publishing House of the Academy of Sciences of the Armenian Soviet Socialist Republic. (In Russian.)

Arinchin, N. I. (1966): Evolutionary and Clinical Interpretation of Electrocardiograms and Phases of the Cardiac Cycle. Minsk: Belarus. (In Russian.)

Arshavsky, I. A. (1976): Ontogenesis and aging (physiological mechanisms of life prolongation). In: Biological Possibilities of Life Span Prolongation, pp. 29–39. Kiev: Institute of Gerontology. (In Russian.)

Arshavsky, I. A. (1977): Physiological mechanisms of the life span of mammals. Uspekhi sovr. biologii 83, 287–304.

Arshavsky, I. A. (1979): Mechanisms which determine the life span of rats that develop under the conditions of a limited calorie diet from the standpoint of the non-entropy theory of ontogenesis. In: Gerontology and Geriatrics. Life Prolongation: Prognoses, Mechanisms, Control, pp. 135–140. Kiev: Institute of Gerontology. (In Russian.)

Artyukhina, N. I. (1979): Structural and Functional Organization of Neurons and Interneuronal Relationships. Moscow: Nauka. (In Russian.)

Aschheim, P. (1976): Aging in the hypothalamic-hypophyseal-ovarian axis in the rat. In: Hypothalamus, Pituitary and Aging (Everitt, A. V., ed.), pp. 376–418. Springfield, Ill.: Charles C Thomas.

Asdel, S. A. (1946): Patterns of Mammalian Reproduction. New York: Academic Press.

Asdel, S. A., Doornenbel, H., Joshi, S. R., Sperling, G. A. (1967): The effect of sex steroid hormones on the longevity of rats. J. Reprod. Fertil. 14, 113–120.

Astafev, A. K. (1972): Reliability and progressive evolution. In: Laws of Progressive Evolution, pp. 39–48. Leningrad: Institute of the History of Natural Science. (In Russian.)

Atkinson, D. E. (1968): The energy change of the adenylate pool as a regulatory parameter. Interaction with feed-back modifiers. Biochemistry 7, 4030–4034.

Avtandilov, G. G. (1970): Dynamics of the Atherosclerotic Process in Man. Questions of Morphogenesis and Pathogenesis. Moscow: Meditsina. (In Russian.)

Axelrod, I. (1966): Methylation reactions in the formation and metabolism of catecholamines and other biogenic amines. Pharmacol. Rev. 18, 95–102.

Axelrod, I. (1969): Control of catecholamine metabolism. In: Progress in Endocrinology (Gual, C., ed.), pp. 286–293. Amsterdam: Excerpta Med. Found.

Babichev, V. N. (1973): Characterization of the neurons of the hypothalamus that control the gonadotropic function of the hypophysis in old female and male rats. Bull. exp. biol. 75, 3–5.

Baird, M. B., Zimmerman, I. A., Massie, H. R., Pacilio, L. V. (1976): Microsomal, mixed-function oxidase activity and senescence. II. In vivo and in vitro hepatic drug metabolism in rats of different ages following partial hepatectomy. Exp. Gerontol. 11, 161–165.

Balodimas, M. (1967): Abnormal carbohydrate tolerance and elderly persons. Geriatrics 1, 159–166.

Baranov, V. G., Propp, V. M., Savchenko, O. N., Stepanov, G. S. (1972): Some clinical and experimental data on the hypothalamohypophysial-ovary relationships in the genesis of aging. In: Ninth International Congress of Gerontology, p. 71. Kiev: Institute of Gerontology. (In Russian.)

Barondes, S. H. (1968): Further studies of the transport of protein to nerve endings. J. Neurochem. 15, 343–350.

Barrows, C. H. (1960): Age and cellular metabolism of tissues. In: The Biology of Aging, 116–123. Springfield, Ill.: Charles C Thomas.

Barrows, C. H. (1966): Enzymes in the study of biological aging. In: Perspectives in Experimental Gerontology, pp. 650–665. Springfield, Ill.: Charles C Thomas.

Barrows, C. H. (1971): The challenge-mechanisms of biological ageing. The Gerontologist 11, 5–12.

Barrows, C. H. (1977): Nutrition. In: Handbook of the Biology of Aging (Finch, C. E., Hayflick, L., eds.), pp. 561–581. New York: Van Nostrand Reinhold.

Barrows, C. H., Yiengst, M. J., Shock, N. W. (1958): Senescence and the metabolism of various tissues of rats. J. Geront. *13*, 351–368.

Beier, W. (1980): On a mathematical relationship between growth rate and life span. Mech. Ageing Dev. *13*, 401–406.

Bekhtereva, N. P. (1974): Neurophysiological Aspects of Man's Mental Activity, 2nd ed. Leningrad: Meditsina. (In Russian.)

Bellamy, D. (1968): Long-term action of prednisolone phosphate on a strain of short-lived mice. Exp. Gerontol. *3*, 327–333.

Belonog, R. P. (1977): Effect of insulin of brain bioelectric activity in subjects of different age. In: Insulin Provision in Old Age, pp. 73–77. Kiev: Institute of Gerontology. (In Russian.)

Belonog, R. P., Kuznetsova, S. M. (1973): Geneological investigations of the electric activity of the brain in persons with a long life. In: Longevous People, pp. 256–263. Kiev: Institute of Gerontology. (In Russian.)

Bender, A. D., Kormendy, C. G., Powell, R. (1970): Pharmacological control of aging. Exp. Gerontol. *5*, 97–129.

Benedict, F., Talbot, F. (1921): Metabolism and Growth from Birth to Puberty. Washington.

Bergmann, H. (1848): Über die Verhältnisse der Wärmeökonomie der Tiere zu ihrer Größe. Universität Göttingen.

Berkowitz, B. A. (1976): Vascular contraction: effect of age and extracellular calcium. Blood Vessels *13*, 139–154.

Bertolini, A. M., Quardamaqua, C., Massari, N. (1960): L'attivita colesterole-esterasica di alcuni tessuti di ratio nelle varie eta' della vita. Boll. soc. Ital. Biol. *36*, 434–437.

Bezrukov, V. V. (1967): Age specifics of the EEG changes when adrenaline, noradrenaline and acetylcholine are administered intravenously and intraperitoneally. In: Documents of the Eighth Scientific Conference on Age Morphology, Physiology and Biochemistry, part 2, pp. 44–45. Moscow: Institute of Age Physiology. (In Russian.)

Bezrukov, V. V. (1969): On the age specifics of the influence of the stimulation of some structures of the brain on blood circulation. In: Documents of the Ninth Scientific Conference on Age Morphology, Physiology and Biochemistry, Vol. 2, part 1, pp. 74–75. Moscow: Institute of Age Physiology. (In Russian.)

Bezrukov, V. V. (1971): On some specifics of the autonomic shifts when the structures of the brain of animals of different age are stimulated. In: First Byelorussian Conference of Gerontologists and Geriatricians, pp. 102–104. Minsk: Nauka i Tekhnika. (In Russian.)

Bezrukov, V. V. (1972): On a change in the hypothalamic regulation of blood circulation during aging. In: Physiology and Pathology of the Cardiovascular System, pp. 273–275. Moscow: Institute of Pathological Physiology. (In Russian.)

Bezrukov, V. V. (1975): On a change in the hypothalamic regulation of external respiration during aging. In: Respiration, Gas Exchange, and Hypoxic Conditions in Elderly and Old Ages, pp. 63 67. Kiev: Institute of Gerontology. (In Russian.)

Bezrukov, V. V. (1979): On the analysis of the intrahypothalamic relationships during aging. In: Life Prolongation: Prognoses, Mechanisms, Control, pp. 105–111. Kiev: Institute of Gerontology. (In Russian.)

Bezrukov, V. V., Muradian, Kh. K. (1974): Inductive synthesis of some liver enzymes in electrical stimulation of hypothalamic area. In: Pathophysiological Aspects of the Problem of Neural Trophism, pp. 14–17. Kiev: Medical Institute. (In Russian.)

Bezrukov, V. V., Epstein, E. V. (1977): On the peculiarities of the hypothalamic regulation of the insulin level in animals of different age. In: Insulin Provision in Old Age, pp. 66–72. Kiev: Institute of Gerontology. (In Russian.)

Bileva, A. S., Zimina, L. M., Malinovsky, A. A. (1978): Influence of the genotype and environment on the life span of *Drosophila melanogaster*. Genetika *14*, 848–852.

Birnbaum, L., Baird, M. (1978): Induction of hepatic mixed function oxidases in senescent rodents. Exp. Gerontol. *13*, 299–303.

Birren, J., Schaie, W. (1977): Handbook of the Psychology of Aging. New York: Van Nostrand Reinhold.

Biscardi, H. M., Webster, G. C. (1977): Accumulation of fluorescent age pigment in different genetic strains of *Drosophila melanogaster*. Exp. Gerontol. *12*, 201–205.

Blichert-Toft, M. (1975): Secretion of corticotropin and somatotropin by the senescent adenohypophysis in man. Acta Endocrinol. *78*, Suppl. 195, 15–154.

Bobek, S., Krus, P. (1977): In vitro studies of normal human thyroid cells: responses to thyrotropin and dibutyryl cyclic AMP. Biochim. Biophys. Acta *91*, 315–327.

Bogatskaya, L. N. (1968): Age specifics of the relationship between respiration and glycolysis in the cardiac muscle. In: Adaptive Capacities of an Aging Organism, pp. 131–144. Kiev: Institute of Gerontology. (In Russian.)

Bogdanovich, N. K. (1974): Hypothalamohypophysial neurosecretory system during aging. Arkh. pat. *36*, 53–58.

Bogomolets, A. A. (1940): A few introductory words. In: Old Age, pp. 8–11. Kiev: Publishing House of the Academy of Sciences of the Ukrainian SSR. (In Russian.)

Bonner, J., Slavkin, H. (1975): Glucocorticoids and aging in inbred mice. The Gerontologist *15*, part II, p. 30.

Book, J. (1976): Effect of hypoxia and high altitude on thyroidal iodine metabolism in the rat. Endocrinology *85*, 307–315.

Borisov, I. N. (1968): Role of nervous system and especially of the hypothalamus in vertebrates aging. Uspekhi sovr. biol. *62*, 222–236.

Borochov, A., Nalevy, A. H., Shinitzky, M. (1976): Increase in microviscosity with aging in protoplast plasmolemma of rose petals. Nature *263*, 158–159.

Bourlière, F. (1957): Aging and metabolism. In: The Biology of Aging, pp. 27–33. London: Academic Press.

Bourlière, F. (1958): The comparative biology of aging. J. Gerontol. *13*, Suppl. 1, 16–24.

Brizzee, K. R. (1975): Gross morphometric analyses and quantitative histology of the aging brain. In: Neurobiology of Aging, pp. 401–423. New York: Plenum Press.

Brizzee, K. R., Ordy, J. M. (1979): Age pigment, cell loss and hippocampal function. Mech. Ageing Develop. *9*, 143–162.

Brody, H., Vijayashankar, N. (1975): Neuronal loss in the human brain stem and its relation to sleep in the elderly. In: 10th International Congress of Gerontology, Vol. 2, p. 2. Jerusalem.

Brody, S. (1945): Bioenergetics and Growth. New York: Plenum Press.

Bronk, D. W. (1939): Synaptic mechanisms in sympathetic ganglia. J. Neurophysiol. *2*, 380–386.

Brown, H. F., Di Francesco, D., Noble, S. J. (1979): How does adrenaline accelerate the heart? Nature *280*, 2819, 235–236.

Brunelle, P., Bohnon, C. (1972): Baisse de la triiodothyronine serique avec l'age. Clin. Chim. Acta *42*, 201–203.

Brunk, J., Ericsson, L. E., Ponten, J. (1973): Residual bodies and ageing in cultured human glial cells. Exp. Cell Res. *70*, 1–14.

Büffon, G. L. C. (1749): Histoire Naturelle Générale et Particulière. Paris: Impremeré Loyale.

Bulankina, N. I. (1973): Adaptation of Some Enzymes of Nitrogen Metabolism in Ontogenesis. Author's abstract of the dissertation for a candidate's degree (biology). Kharkov: State University. (In Russian.)

Bulos, B. A., Shukla, S. P., Sacktor, B. (1975): Bioenergetics of mitochondria from flight muscles of fruit-flies: partial reactions of oxidation and phosphorylation. Arch. Biochem. Biophys. *166*, 639–644.

Bürger, M. (1960): Altern und Krankheit als Problem Biomorphose. Leipzig: VEB G. Thieme.

Butenko, G. M., Andrianova, L. F. (1979): Influence of the age of the recepient on the immunological cells of the transplanted cells of the marrow and the spleen in a prolonged experiment. Tsitologiya i genetika *13*, 3–7.

Buttlar-Brentano, K. (1954): Zur Lebensgeschichte des Nucleus basalis, tuberomammillaris, supraopticus und paraventricularis unter normalen und pathologischen Bedingungen. Z. Hirnforsch. *1*, 337–419.

Buznikov, G. A. (1971): Role of mediators of the nervous system in individual development. Ontogenez *2*, 5–13.

Buzunov, V. A. (1969): Changes in muscle efficiency during development, maintenance and derangement of dynamic motor stereotype in persons aged 55–60 (experimental investigation). Gigiena truda i professionalnye zabolevaniya *9*, 32–33.

Bylund, D., Tellez-Inon, M., Hollenberg, M. (1977): Age-related parallel decline in beta adrenergic receptors, adenylate cyclase and phosphodiesterase activities in rat erythrocyte membranes. Life Sci. *21*, 403–410.

Caciagli, F., Amato, G., Bertalli, A. (1974): Substances released by trypsin potentiating bradykinin action on smooth muscle. Pharm. Res. Commun. *6*, 319–328.

Calloway, N. O. (1971): Senescence: Identical rates of water loss in various species. J. Amer. Geriat. Soc. *19*, 12–21.

Cannon, W., Rosenblueth, A. (1951): The Supersensitivity of Denervated Structures. London: Pergamon Press.

Cannon, W. G. (1929): Organization for physiological homeostasis. Physiol. Rev. *9*, 399–431.

Carell, A. (1912): On the permanent life of tissues outside the organism. J. Exp. Med. *15*, 516–524.

Carlson, L. A., Floberg, S. C., Nye, E. R. (1968): Effect of age on blood and tissue lipid levels in the male rat. Gerontologia *14*, 65–79.

Carothers, A. D., Collyer, S., De Mey, R., Frackiewicz, A. (1978): Parental age and birth order in the aetiology of some sex chromosome aneuploides. Ann. Hum. Genet. *41*, 277–287.

Chaconas, G., Finch, C. (1973): The effect of aging on RNA/DNA ratios in brain regions of the C57BL/6J male mouse. J. Neurochem. *21*, 1469–1473.

Chaika, L. D. (1977): Age specifics of the influence of adrenaline and somatotropin on free fatty acids under normal conditions and in a pathological state. In: Adaptive Processes in the Organism during Aging, pp. 57–62. Minsk: Science and Technology Publishing House. (In Russian.)

Chakravarti, S., Collins, W. P., Forecast, J. D., Newton, J. R., Orem, D. H., Studd, J. (1976): Hormonal profiles after the menopause. Brit. Med. J. *21*, 784–786.

Chebotarev, D. F., Korkushko, O. V. (1966): Cardiovascular system in elderly and old age. In: Problems of Age Physiology and Pathophysiology of the Cardiovascular System, pp. 147–149. Moscow: Institute of Gerontology. (In Russian.)

Chebotareva, L. L. (1978): Influence of the Midbrain Operculum on the Function of the Supra-opticohypophysial Neurosecretory System. Author's abstract of the dissertation for a candidate's degree (medicine). Kiev: Institute of Physiology. (In Russian.)

Chen, J. C., Warshaw, I. B., Sanadi, D. R. (1972): J. Cell Physiol. *80*, 141–148.

Cheney, K. E., Lui, R. K., Smith, G. S., Leung, R. E., Mickey, M. R., Walford, R. L. (1980): Survival and disease patterns in C57BL/6J mice subjected to undernutrition. Exp. Gerontol. *15*, 237–258.

Cherkin, A. (1975): Dimethylaminoethanol did not extent survival of aged Japanese quail. The Gerontologist *15*, part II, 25.

Chernigovsky, V. N. (1960): Interoreceptors. Moscow: Medgiz. (In Russian.)

Chernukh, A. M., Alexandrov, G. I., Alexeev, O. V. (1975): Microcirculation. Moscow: Meditsina. (In Russian.)

Chernyshev, V. B., Afonina, V. M. (1975): Disturbances of the biological rhythm and the life span of some insects. Zhurn., obshchei biol. *25*, 859–862.

Chihara, E. (1979): Axoplasmic and non-axoplasmic transport along the optic pathway of albino rats. Invest. Ophthalmol. and Visceral Sci. *18*, 339.

Chipens, G. I., Papsuevich, O. S. (1971): Analysis of the signatures of the neurohypophysial hormones. In: Chemistry and Biology of Peptides, pp. 66–112. Riga: Publishing House of the Academy of Sciences of Latvian SSR. (In Russian.)

Chotkowska, E., Rywik, S., Szostak, W. B., Napierala, M. (1977): The distribution of serum cholesterol level in the male population aged 40–59 covered by the Polish trial on multifactorial prevention of IHD (first pair of the Warsaw factories). Przegl. lek. *34*, 627–630.

Chouknyiska, R., Vassileva-Popova, J. G. (1977): Effect of age on the binding of H^3-testosterone with receptor protein from rat brain and testes. C. R. Acad. Bulg. Sci. *30*, 133–135.

Ciaponi, A., Ferrero, E., Casule, G., Pizzamiglio, D. (1978): Insulin secretion in the aged: studies on the double intravenous tolerance test. In: Proceedings of 11th Congress of Gerontology, pp. 107–108. Tokyo: Scimed Publications, Inc.

Cicinotta, D., Carapezzio, P., Mouica, C., Ceccaco, S. (1974): Compartamento della curva della captazione tiroidea del radioiodio, della tiroxinemia L8 della capacità tiroxino fissante del plasma in soggetti presenili, e senili in confronto a giovane eucrini. G. Clin. Med. *55*, 40–54.

Clark, A. J. (1926): The antagonism of acetylcholine by atropine. J. Physiol. *61*, 547–566.

Clark, A. M., Cole, K. W. (1967): The effect of ionizing radiation on the longevity of ploidy types in the wasp *Morminella vitripennis*. Exp. Gerontol. *2*, 89–95.

Clark, A. M., Kidwell, R. N. (1967): Effects of development temperature on the adult life span of *Morminiella vitripennis* female. Exp. Gerontol. *2*, 79–84.

Clarke, P. V., Kisselbak, A. H., Hope-Gill, H., Vydelingum, H., Pulloch, B., Fraser, T. R. (1975): The role of calcium in insulin action. IV. Mechanism of insulin resistance in adipose tissue of mice and old Wistar rats. Eur. J. Clin. Invest. *5*, 351–358.

Clemens, J. A., Meites, J. (1971): Neuroendocrine status of old constant estrous rats. Neuroendocrinology *7*, 249–256.

Coddling, J. A., Kallnins, A., Haist, R. E. (1975): Effects of age and of fasting on the responsiveness of the insulin-secreting mechanism of the islets of Langerhans to glucose. J. Physiol. Pharmacol. *53*, 716–725.

Cohet, Y. (1975): Epigenetic influence on the life span of the *Drosophila:* Existence of an optimal growth temperature for adult longevity. Exp. Gerontol. *10*, 181–184.

Comfort, A. (1963): Effect of delayed and resumed growth on the longevity of a fish (*Labistes recticulatus,* Peters) in captivity. Gerontologia *8*, 150–155.

Comfort, A. (1964): Ageing–the Biology of Senescence. London: Routledge and Kegan Paul.

Comfort, A., Youhotsky-Gore, I., Pathmanathan, K. (1971): Effect of ethoxyquin on the longevity of C3H mice. Nature *220*, 254–255.

Cote, I. J., Kremzner, L. T. (1975): Age-dependent changes in the activities of enzymes related to the formation and degradation of neurotransmitters in human brain, correlating with the level of polyamines. In: 7th International Congress of Neuropathologists, pp. 433–441. Budapest: University Press.

Cowdry, E. (1939): Problems of Aging. Biological and Medical Aspects. Baltimore: Williams and Wilkins.

Cowley, A. W., Switzer, S. J., Guinn, M. M. (1980): Evidence and quantification of vasopressin arterial pressure control system in the dog. Circ. Res. *46*, 58–67.

Crepaldi, G.: Contrainsular hormones and insulin secretion in aging. In: 11th International Congress of Gerontology, Vol. 3, p. 132. Tokyo: Scimed Publications, Inc.

Cristofalo, V. J. (1975): The effect of hydrocortisone on DNA synthesis and cell division during aging in vitro. In: Explorations in Aging, pp. 57–69. New York: Plenum Press.

Curtis, H., Tilley, J. (1970): The role of calcium in chromosomal stability and aging in mammals. J. Gerontol. *25*, 1–3.

Curtis, H. J., Miller, K. (1971): Chromosome abberations in liver cells of guinea pigs. J. Gerontol. *26*, 292–293.

Cutler, R. G. (1973): Redundancy of information content as a protective mechanism determining aging rate. Mech. Ageing Develop. *2*, 381–408.

Cutler, R. G. (1975): Age-dependent accumulation of DNA adducts in chromatin. The Gerontologist *15*, 33–39.

Cutler, R. G. (1976): Evolution of longevity in primates. J. Human. Evol. *6*, 159–204.

Cutler, R. G. (1978): Alteration with age in the informational storage and flow system of the mammalian cell. Birth Defects: Original Articles Series *14*, 463–498.

Cutler, R. G. (1979): Evolution of human longevity: a critical overview. Mech. Ageing Develop. *2*, 337–354.

Czech, M. P. (1976): Cellular basis of insulin insensitivity in large rat adipocytes. J. Clin. Invest. *57*, 694–701.

Dalakishvili, S. M. (1967): Problems of State of Some Cerebral Cortical Area Structure in Aging, Tbilisi, Metsniereba.

Dale, H. H. (1936): On some physiological action of ergot. J. Physiol. *34*, 163–169.

Daniel, C. W. (1972): Aging of cells during serial propagation in vivo. Adv. Gerontol. *4*, 167–199.

Danielson, A. K. (1952): Specifics of the secondary regeneration of the peripheral nerve at various ages of the rabbit. In: Questions of Visceral Biology and Medicine, pp. 38–44. Moscow: Medgiz. (In Russian.)

Darenskaya, N. G. (1978): Influence of the parameters of external radiation on the life span. In: Present Problems of Radiobiology, pp. 7–27. Moscow: Atomizdat. (In Russian.)

David, C., Hartia, L., Stanescu, S. (1963): Modificarile hemodinamice in raport cu virsta. Fisiol. Norm. Pat. *9*, 353–360.

Davidenko, I. P. (1972): Age Morphological and Histoenzymochemical Specifics of the Nerve Ganglia of the Rat Heart. Author's abstract of the dissertation for a candidate's degree (medicine). Kiev: Medical Institute. (In Russian.)

Davies, I., Fotheringham, A. P. (1980): The influence of age on the hypothalamo-neurohypophyseal system of the mouse: a quantitative ultrastructural analysis of the supraoptic nucleus. Mech. Ageing Develop. *12*, 93–105.

Davies, I., Schofield, J. D. (1980): Connective tissue ageing: the influence of a lathyrogen (α-aminopropionitrile) on the life span of female C57BL/Jcrfat mice. Exp. Gerontol. *15*, 487–494.

Deéb, S. S. (1972): Inhibition of cleavage and hatching of sea urchin embryos by serotonin. J. Exp. Zool. *181*, 79–86.

Deerberg, F., Rapp, K., Pittermann, W. (1980): Genetic and environmental influences on life span and diseases in Han:Wistar rats. Mech. Ageing Develop. *4*, 333–343.

Dejmék, J., Preiss, J. (1974): Vek rodicu v etiologii genetickijch poruch. Cas. lek. cesk. *113*, 666–672.

Denckla, W. D. (1974): Role of the pituitary and thyroid glands in the decline of minimal O_2 consumption with age. J. Clin. Invest. *53*, 572–581.

Deyl, Z., Juricova, M., Rosmus, J., Adam, M. (1971): Aging of the connective tissue: collagen crosslinking in animals of different species and equal age. Exp. Gerontol. *6*, 227–233.

Dietrich, L. S., Vero, I. L. (1965): Mitochondrial electron transport: effect of age on sensitivity to inhibitors. Gerontology *11*, 67–73.

Dilman, V. M. (1976a): Ways of increasing the life span of man in the light of the elevation mechanism of aging. In: Biological Possibilities of Life Span Prolongation, pp.129–137. Kiev: Institute of Gerontology. (In Russian.)

Dilman, V. M. (1976b): The hypothalamic control of aging and age-associated pathology: the elevation mechanism of aging. In: Hypothalamus, Pituitary and Aging (Everitt, A. V., ed.), pp. 634–667. Springfield, Ill.: Charles C Thomas.

Dilman, V. M. (1978): Transformation of the development programme in the mechanism of age pathology. Elevation model of age pathology and the natural death of man. Fiziologiya cheloveka *4*, 579–596.

Dilman, V. M., Ostroumova, M. N. (1973): Disturbance of the hormonal regulation of carbohydrate metabolism in the age pathology of man. In: Problems of Medical Chemistry, pp. 147–183. Moscow: Meditsina. (In Russian.)

Dilman, V. M., Anisimov, V. N. (1980): Effect of treatment with phenformin, diphenylhydantoin or L-Dopa on life span and tumour incidence in C3H/Sn mice. Gerontology *26*, 241–246.

Dogiel, A. S. (1922): Old Age and Death. Petrograd: Mysl. (In Russian.)

Dolgo-Saburov, B. A. (1960): Plasticity of the Blood Vessels. Leningrad: USSR Academy of Sciences. (In Russian.)

D'Onfrio (1970): Alcuni aspetti della functionalità del pancreas as endocrino nell'età senile. Giorn. Geront. *18*, 475–482.

Driver, Ch. J., Cosopodiotis, G. (1979): The effect of dietary fat on longevity of *Drosophila melanogaster*. Exp. Gerontol. *14*, 95–100.

Drori, D., Folman, Y. (1976): Environmental effects on longevity in the male rats: exercise, mating, castration and restricted feeding. Exp. Gerontol. *11*, 25–32.

Drozdova, I. L. (1969): Specifics of the gas composition of the blood of elderly and old persons and persons who live to very old age. In: Aging and the Physiological Systems of the Organism, pp. 305–309. Kiev: Institute of Physiology. (In Russian.)

Dubina, T. L., Berlov, G. A. (1974): Life span and the causes of death of white rats when they are regularly fed ethylene diamine tetraacetate for a long time. Byull. exper. biol. *9*, 36–38.

Dubina, T. L., Razumovich, A. N. (1975): Introduction to Experimental Gerontology. Minsk: Nauka i Tekhnika. (In Russian.)

Duckworth, W., Kitabachi, A. (1976): The effect of age on plasma proinsulin-like material after oral glucose. J. Lab. Clin. Med. *88*, 359–369.

Ducoff, H. S. (1975): Form of increased longevity of Tribolium after X-irradiation. Exp. Gerontol. *10*, 189–193.

Dudl, R. J., Ensinck, J. W., Palmer, H. E., Williams, R. H. (1973): Effects of age on growth hormone secretion in man. J. Clin. Endocrinol. Metab. *37*, 11–16.

Dukhovichny, S. M. (1968): Pharmacological analysis of the age changes in the parasympathetic regulation of the heart when a physical load is applied and the pose is changed. In: Muscular Activity and the Functions of the Organism During Aging, pp. 51–53. Kiev: Institute of Gerontology. (In Russian.)

Dukhovichny, S. M. (1974): Influence of some neurotropic agents on arterial pressure in persons of various age. In: Gerontology and Geriatrics, pp. 78–81. Kiev: Institute of Gerontology. (In Russian.)

Duncan, T. G. (1976): Diabetes: diagnosis and management in the older patient. Geriatrics *10*, 161–172.

Dunn, I., Critchlow, V. (1971): Vasopressin-evoked ACTH release in rats following forebrain removal. Proc. Soc. Exp. Biol. Med. *136*, 1284–1288.

Duplenko, Yu. K. (1965): Age Specifics of the Functional State of the Ganglia of the Autonomic Nervous System. Author's abstract of the dissertation for a candidate's degree (medicine). Kiev: Medical Institute. (In Russian.)

Dussault, J., Walker, P. (1979): Effect of age and testicular function on the pituitary-thyroid system in male rats. J. Endocrinol. *82*, 53–59.

Economos, A. C. (1980a): Brain-life span conjecture: a reevolution of the evidence. Gerontology *26*, 82–89.

Economos, A. C. (1980b): Taxonomic differences in the mammalian life span, body weight relationship and the problem of brain weight. Gerontology *26*, 90–98.

Edington, D. W., Cosmas, A. C., McCafferty, W. B. (1972): Exercise and longevity evidence for a threshold age. J. Gerontol. *27*, 341–343.

Emanuel, N. M. (1976): Free radicals and aging. In: Biological Possibilities of Life Span Prolongation, pp. 103–110. Kiev: Institute of Gerontology. (In Russian.)

Emanuel, N. M. (1979): Inhibitors of radical processes (antioxidants) and the possibilities of prolonging life. In: Life Prolongation: Prognoses, Mechanisms, Control, pp. 118–127. Kiev: Institute of Gerontology. (In Russian.)

Emanuel, N. M., Obukhova, L. K. (1978a): Characteristic types of retardation of aging in experiments. In: Artificially Increasing the Life Span of a Species. First Symposium. Theses of Reports, p. 34. Moscow: Institute of General Genetics. (In Russian.)

Emanuel, N. M., Obukhova, L. K. (1978b): Type of experimental delay in aging patterns. Exp. Gerontol. *13*, 25–29.

Engels, F. (1961): Dialectics of Nature. In: K. Marx and F. Engels, Works, 2nd ed., Vol. 20, pp. 339–625. Moscow: Gospolitizdat. (In Russian.)

Enesco, H. B., Holzman, F. (1980): Effect of calcium, magnesium and chelating agents on the life span of the rotifer *Asplanchna brightwelli*. Exp. Gerontol. *15*, 389–392.

Enesco, H. B., Verdone-Smith, C. (1980): Tocopherol increases life span in the rotifer *Philodina*. Exp. Gerontol. *15*, 335–338.

Erisson, E. (1973): Beta-adrenoreceptor activity and cyclic AMP metabolism of rat aorta, variation with age. Acta physiol. Scand. *89*, Suppl. 396, 10–18.

Ermini, M., Verzar, F. (1968): Decreased restitution of creatine phosphate in white and red skeletal muscles during aging. Experientia *24*, 902–904.

Euler, U. S., Lishajko, F. (1961): Improved technique for the fluometric estimation of catecholamines. Acta physiol. Scand. *51*, 348–352.

Evans, C. H. (1979): On the aging of organisms and their cells. Medical Hypotheses *5*, 53–66.

Everitt, A. V. (1970): Food intake, endocrines and aging. Proc. Austr. Ass. Geront. *1*, 65–78.

Everitt, A. V. (1976): Conclusion: aging and its hypothalamic-pituitary control. In: Hypothalamus, Pituitary and Aging (Everitt, A. V., ed.), pp. 676–701. Springfield, Ill.: Charles C Thomas.

Everitt, A. V., Seedsman, N. J., Jones, F. (1980): The effects of hypophysectomy and continuous food restriction, begun at age 70 and 400 days, on collagen aging, proteinuria, incidence of pathology and longevity in the male rat. Mech. Ageing Develop. *12*, 161–172.

Ewer, D. W., Ewer, R. F. (1942): The biology and behaviour of *Pinus tectus Boie*, a pest of stored products. III. The effect of temperature and humidity on ovioposition, feeding and duration of life cycle. J. Exp. Zool. *18*, 290–305.

Fabricant, I. D., Schneider, E. L. (1978): Studies of the genetic and immunologic components of the maternal age effect. Develop. Biol. *66*, 337–343.

Faizulin, V. V. (1978): Age specifics of the adrenergic and cholinergic influences on the level of the electric polarization of the acinar cells of the parotid gland of a rat. In: Laws of the Development of the Organic World and the Scientific Principles of Its Use, pp. 169–170. Minsk: Nauka i Tekhnika. (In Russian.)

Faizulin, V. V. (1979): Age specifics of the influence of acetylcholine, noradrenaline and isadrine on the membrane potential of the acinar cells of the parotid gland of a rat in vitro. Fiziol. zhurn. 25, 566–571.

Falck, B. (1972): Observation on the possibility of the cellular localization of monoamines by a fluorescent method. Acta physiol. Scand. 56, 197–207.

Feldman, L., Plank, M. (1976): Effect of age on intravenous glucose tolerance and insulin secretion. J. Amer. Geriatr. Soc. 24, 1–3.

Felsl, I., Gottsmann, M., Eversmann, T., Jehle, W., Uhlich, E. (1978): Influence of various stress situations on vasopressin secretion in man. Acta endocrinol. 87, Suppl. 215, 122–123.

Ferrendelli, J. A., Segwick, W. G., Suntzeff, W. (1971): Regional energy metabolism and lipofuscin accumulation in mouse brain during aging. J. Neuropath. Exp. Neurol. 30, 638–649.

Finch, C. E. (1973): Catecholamine metabolism in the brains of aging male mice. Brain Res. 52, 261–276.

Finch, C. E. (1976): The regulation of physiological changes during mammalian aging. Quart. Rev. Biol. 51, 49–83.

Finch, C. E., Foster, J. R., Mirsky, A. E. (1969): Aging and regulation of cell activities during exposure to cold. J. gen. Physiol. 54, 690–712.

Finch, C. E., Jonec, V., Wisner, J. R., jr., Sinha, Y. N., de Vellis, J. S., Swerdloff, R. S. (1977): Hormone production by the pituitary and testes of male C57BL/6J mice during aging. Endocrinology 101, 1310–1317.

Fleisch, I. H. (1971): Further study on the effect of ageing on beta-adrenoceptor activity of rat aorta. Brit. J. Pharmacol. 42, 311–313.

Flourens, M. S. P. (1855): De la longevité humaine et de la quantité, de vie sur le globe. Paris.

Flower, R. T. (1978): Biochemistry of prostaglandins. Biochem. Soc. Frans. 6, 713–714.

Folbort, G. V. (1968): Selected Works. Kiev: Publishing House of the Academy of Sciences of the Ukrainian SSR. (In Russian.)

Folbort, G. V. (1969): Selected Works. Kiev: Publishing House of the Academy of Sciences of the Ukrainian SSR. (In Russian.)

Folbort, G. V., Semernina, A. D. (1940): Change in the working ability of the central elements which ensure higher nervous activity in dogs in old age. In: Old Age, pp. 199–205. Kiev: Publishing House of the Academy of Sciences of the Ukrainian SSR. (In Russian.)

Folkow, B. (1960): Role of the nervous system in the control of vascular tone. Circulation 21, 760–772.

Fox, J. H., Parmacek, M. S., Patel-Mandlik, K. (1975): Effect of aging on brain respiration and carbohydrate metabolism of Syrian hamsters. J. Gerontol. 21, 224–230.

Franks, L. M. (1970): Cellular aspects of ageing. Exp. Gerontol. 5, 281–286.

Freddari, C. B., Giuli, C. (1980): A quantitative morphometric study of synapses of rat cerebellar glomeruli during aging. Mech. Ageing Develop. 12, 127–136.

Freeman, C., Karoly, K., Adelman, R. (1973): Impairments in availability of insulin to liver in vivo and in binding of insulin to purified hepatic plasma membrane during aging. Biochem. Biophys. Res. Commun. 54, 1573–1576.

Freji, H. (1966): Changes in mechanical properties of rabbit blood vessels with growth. Fukuoka acta med. 57, 287–291.

Friedenthal (1910): Über die Gültigkeit der Massenwirkung für den Energieumsatz der lebendigen Substanzen. Zbl. f. Physiol. 24, 321–323.

Friedman, S. M., Friedman, C. L. (1964): Prolonged treatment with pituitary powder in aged rats. Exp. Gerontol. 1, 37–48.

Frolkis, I. V. (1973): Influence of RNAase on a change in the membrane potential of muscle fibres caused by the stimulation of the sympathetic nerve. Fiziol. zhurn. 2, 256–257.

Frolkis, I. V. (1978): Functional and Ultrastructural Specifics of the Smooth-Muscle Cells of the Portal Vein of Animals of Different Age. Author's abstract of the dissertation for a candidate's degree (medicine). Kiev: Institute of Physiology. (In Russian.)

Frolkis, V. V. (1959): Reflex Regulation of the Activity of the Cardiovascular System. Kiev: Gosmedizdat. (In Russian.)

Frolkis, V. V. (1963): Self-regulation of the function when the organism ages. Fiziol. zhurn. SSSR *49*, 1221–1229.

Frolkis, V. V. (1966): Neuro-humoral regulations in the aging organism. J. Gerontol. *21*, 161–167.

Frolkis, V. V. (1969): A hypothesis on regulatory mechanism of molecular-genetic changes with aging. In: Aging and Organism's Physiological Systems, pp. 36–44. Kiev: Institute of Gerontology. (In Russian.)

Frolkis, V. V. (1969): Nature of Aging. Moscow: Nauka. (In Russian.)

Frolkis, V. V. (1970): Regulation, Adaptation and Aging. Leningrad: Nauka. (In Russian.)

Frolkis, V. V. (1970): On the regulatory mechanism of molecular-genetic alterations during aging. Exp. Geront. *5*, 37–47.

Frolkis, V. V. (1971): Mechanisms of cell aging. In: Aging of a Cell, pp. 5–23. Kiev: Institute of Gerontology. (In Russian.)

Frolkis, V. V. (1975): Aging and the Biological Abilities of the Organism. Moscow: Nauka. (In Russian.)

Frolkis, V. V. (1978): Neurohumoral mechanisms of the development of pathology in old age. In: Aging and Diseases, pp. 7–8. Kiev: Institute of Gerontology. (In Russian.)

Frolkis, V. V. (1979): Once more on the adaptive regulatory mechanisms of aging. In: Life Prolongation: Prognoses, Mechanisms, Control, pp. 55–69. Kiev: Institute of Gerontology. (In Russian.)

Frolkis, V. V. (1980): On the formation of the hyperpolarizing factor in protein biosynthesis. Fiziol. zhurn. *4*, 38–42.

Frolkis, V. V., Shchegoleva, I. V. (1963): On the mechanism of the changes in the sensitivity of vascular chemoreceptors when the organism ages. Doklady Akad. Nauk SSSR *48*, 481–493.

Frolkis, V. V., Bogatskaya, L. N. (1965): Age specifics of the regulation of the energy processes in the heart. In: Blood Circulation and Old Age, pp. 104–117. Kiev: Zdorovye. (In Russian.)

Frolkis, V. V., Epstein, Ye. V. (1966): Age specifics of the metabolism of some macroergic phosphorus compounds in the skeletal muscles at rest and during work. Voprosy meditsinskoi khimii *12*, 248–253.

Frolkis, V. V., Verkhratsky, N. S., Zamostian, V. P. (1967): Age specifics of the regulation of regional blood circulation. Fiziol. zhurn. SSSR *58*, 330–336.

Frolkis, V. V., Mandelblat, L. S. (1970): Age specifics of the regulation of the inductive synthesis of the tyrosine-amino-transferase of the liver. Doklady Akad. Nauk SSSR *193* (biology series), 1426–1428.

Frolkis, V. V., Bogatskaya, L. N., Bogush, S. V., Shevchuk, V. G. (1971): Content and activity of insulin in the blood and the sensitivity of tissues to it during aging. Geriatrics *8*, 118–129.

Frolkis, V. V., Bezrukov, V. V., Genis, Ye. D., Duplenko, Yu. K., Tanin, S. A. (1972a): Central nervous regulation of the cardiovascular and endocrine systems and the motor apparatus as the organism ages. In: Main Factors of Untogenesis, pp. 93–122. Kiev: Naukova Dumka. (In Russian.)

Frolkis, V. V., Martynenko, O. A., Korotonozhkin, V. G. (1972b): Influence of the inhibitors of protein biosynthesis on the development of the hyperpolarization of individual muscle fibres. Biofizika *5*, 839–843.

Frolkis, V. V., Verzhikovskaya, N. V., Valueva, G. V. (1973): The thyroid and age. Exp. Gerontol. *8*, 255–296.

Frolkis, V. V., Bogatskaya, L. N. (1974): The energy metabolism of myocardium and its regulation in animals of various age. In: Structure and Chemistry of Aging Heart, pp. 23–32. New York: Academic Press.

Frolkis, V. V., Muradian, Kh. K. (1976): Influence of the prolonged administration of hydrocortisone on the activity of glucose-6-phosphatase and fructose-1,6-diphosphatase and the synthesis of the RNA fractions of the liver of rats of different age. Problemy endocrinologii *22*, 83–87.

Frolkis, V. V., Bezrukov, V. V., Muradian, Kh. K. (1976a): Hypothalamic regulation of RNA and protein synthesis during aging. Fiziol. zhurn. *24*, 627–633.

Frolkis, V. V., Bogatskaya, L. N., Stupina, A. S., Verzhikovskaya, N. V., et al. (1976b): Comparative characterization of some influences on life prolongation. In: Biological Abilities of Increasing the Animal's Life Span, pp. 138–150. Kiev: Institute of Gerontology. (In Russian.)

Frolkis, V. V., Martynenko, O. A., Zamostyan, V. P. (1976c): Aging of the neuromuscular apparatus. Gerontologia 22, 244–279.

Frolkis, V. V., Bogatskaya, L. N., Perfilov, V. P., Shevchuk, V. G., Karpova, S. M. (1976d): Mechanisms of the development of cardiac insufficiency in old age. Kardiologiya 3, 44–52.

Frolkis, V. V., Verkhratsky, N. S., Shevchuk, V. G., Pugach, B. V., Timchenko, A. N. (1977a): Role of activation of protein biosynthesis in the mechanism of the negative chronotropic action of the vagus nerve and acetylcholine on the heart. Fiziol. zhurn. SSSR 63, 1662–1667.

Frolkis, V. V., Verkhratsky, N. S., Shevchuk, V. G. (1977b): Neural regulation of the cardiac function during aging. Fiziol. zhurn. SSSR 63, 1134–1143.

Frolkis, V. V., Bogatskaya, L. N., Korkushko, O. V. (1977c): Insulin provision in old age. In: Insulin Provision in Old Age, pp. 5–34. Kiev: Institute of Gerontology. (In Russian.)

Frolkis, V. V., Valueva, G. V., Verzhikovskaya, N. V. (1978): Relationship between the hypothalamohypophysial system and the thyroid gland during various age periods. Byull. exper. biol. i med. 8, 133–137.

Frolkis, V. V., Bezrukov, V. V. (1979): Aging of the Central Nervous System. Basel: Karger.

Frolkis, V. V., Bezrukov, V. V., Muradian, Kh. K. (1979a): Hypothalamic-pituitary-adrenocortical regulation of induction of some enzymes of carbohydrate and amino acid metabolism in aging. Exp. Gerontol. 14, 65–76.

Frolkis, V. V., Bogatskaya, L. N., Stupina, A. S., Muradian, Kh. K., Timchenko, A. N., Kovtun, A. I. (1979b): Inhibitors of protein biosynthesis as a means of increasing of the life span in experiments. In: Life Prolongation: Prognoses, Mechanisms, Control, pp. 148–164. Kiev: Institute of Gerontology. (In Russian.)

Frolkis, V. V., Paramonova, G. I. (1980): Age specifics of the inductive synthesis of the microsomal monooxygenases of the rat liver and the influence of the hyperpolarization of the plasma membrane on them. Doklady Akad. Nauk Ukr. SSR 3, 816–821.

Frota-Pessoa, O. (1978): Riscos geneticos dependentes da idade. Rev. brasil. pezquisas med. e biol. 11, 77–80.

Fudel-Osipova, S. I. (1968): Aging of the Neuromuscular System. Kiev: Zdorovya. (In Russian.)

Fujishima, M., Omae, T. (1980): Brain blood flow and mean transit time as related to aging. Gerontology 26, 104–107.

Galambos, R. (1965): Introductory discussion of glial function. Progr. Brain Res. 15, 267–277.

Gatsko, G. G. (1975): Aging and Insulin. Minsk: Nauka i Tekhnika. (In Russian.)

Gatsko, G. G. (1977): Hormonal regulation of the metabolism of free fatty acids and glucose during aging. In: Adaptive Processes in the Organism During Aging, pp. 21–32. Minsk: Nauka i Tekhnika. (In Russian.)

Gatsko, G. G., Markovsky, Yu. K., Surikov, P. M., Zhukova, A. S. (1977): Age specifics of the metabolism of cyclic adenosine monophosphate in adipose tissue under normal conditions and during starvation. In: Adaptive Processes in the Organism During Aging, pp. 52–57. Minsk: Nauka i Tekhnika. (In Russian.)

Gaubatz, I. W., Cutler, R. (1978): Age-related differences in the number of ribosomal RNA genes of mouse tissues. Gerontology 24, 179–207.

Gavrilov, L. A. (1980): Investigation of the Kinetics of the Life Span by Kinetic Analysis. Author's abstract of the dissertation for a candidate's degree. Moscow: State University. (In Russian.)

Gavrilov, L. A., Gavrilova, N. S., Yaguzhinsky, L. S. (1978): Basic regularities of the aging and death of animals from the standpoint of the theory of reliability. Zhurn. obshchei biologii 39, 734–742.

Gavrilov, L. A., Gavrilova, N. S. (1979): Investigation of the kinetic regularities of human mortality in the historical aspect. Doklady Akad. Nauk SSSR 245, 1017–1020.

Geinisman, Y., Bondareff, Y., Telser, A. (1977): Diminished axonal transport of glycoproteins in the senescent rat brain. Mech. Ageing Develop. 6, 363–378.

Gerasimova, V. V., Levitsky, Ye. L., Obolenskaya, M. Yu. (1980): Age specifics of the macromolecular structure and biosynthesis of DNA. In: Gerontology and Geriatrics, pp. 74–78. Kiev: Institute of Gerontology. (In Russian.)

Gerbase-DeLima, M., Lui, R. K., Cheney, K. E., Mickey, R., Walford, R. L. (1975): Immune function and survival in a long-lived mouse strain subjected to undernutrition. Gerontologia 21, 184–202.

Gey, K. F., Burkard, W. P., Pletscher, A. (1965): Variation of the norepinephrine metabolism of the rat heart with age. Gerontologia 11, 1–11.

Gharib, H. (1974): Triiodothyronine. Physiological and clinical significance. JAMA 227, 302–304.

Gilbert, J. C. (1973): Thirty-five-year follow-up study of intellectual functioning. J. Gerontol. 28, 68–72.

Giudiulli, I., Pecquery, R. (1978): Beta-adrenergic receptors and catecholamine-sensitive adenylate cyclase in rat fat-cell membranes: influence of growth, cell size and aging. Eur. J. Biochem. 98, 413–419.

Glebov, R. N., Kryzhanovsky, G. N. (1978): Relationship between the axonal flow of macromolecules and organelles with a synaptic function. In: Functional Biochemistry of Synapses, pp. 29–46. Moscow: Meditsina. (In Russian.)

Gley, E. (1922): Principal Problems of Endocrinology. Moscow-Leningrad: Nauchnaya Mysl. (In Russian.)

Globus, A., Lux, U. B., Schubert, P. (1973): Transfer of amino acids between neuroglia cells and neurons in the leech ganglion. Exp. Neurol. 40, 104–113.

Gold, P. H., Gee, M. V., Strehler, B. L. (1968): Effect of age on oxidative phosphorylation in the rat. J. Geront. 23, 509–512.

Goldshtein, B. I., Khilko, O. K. (1969): Change in the reaction properties of the sulfhydryl groups of proteins when the organism grows old. Vestn. Akad. Med. Nauk SSSR 12, 610–620.

Goldstein, N. B., Khilobok, I. Yu., Khilko, O. K. (1977): Age-related peculiarities of insulin action on liver chromatin in rats. In: Insulin Provision in Old Age, pp. 93–97. Kiev: Institute of Gerontology. (In Russian.)

Golovchenko, S. F. (1973): Age specifics of the influence of vasopressin on hemodynamics. In: Central Regulation of Hemodynamics, pp. 78–82. Kiev: Institute of Physiology. (In Russian.)

Golovchenko, S. F. (1976): Age specifics of the development of coronary insufficiency simulated by the administration of vasopressin. Bull. exper. biol. 86, 647–651.

Golovchenko, S. F. (1979): Concentration of vasopressin in the blood of persons of different age in the case of hypertension. Problemy endocrin. 4, 31–35.

Golovchenko, S. F., Potapenko, R. I. (1978): Age specifics of the influence of vasopressin on energy metabolism in the myocardium and the brain. Fiziol. zhurn. 14, 45–51.

Gommers, A., Dehez-Delhay, M., Jeanjean, M. (1977): Effet de l'âge sur la réponse à l'insuline in vitro chez le rat. I. Métabolisme glucidique du tissu diaphragmatique. Gerontology 23, 127–133.

Gomozkov, O. A. (1979): Kinine system and the regulation of vascular tonicity. Itogi nauki i tekhniki 23, 107–135. (In Russian.)

Gomozkov, O. A., Shishkovich, T. V., Chernykh, A. M. (1977): The relationship between the kininase activity and the angiotensin-converting activity under normal conditions and during the experimental infarction of the myocardium. Kardiologiya 17, 103–108.

Goodrick, C. L. (1975): Life span and the inheritance of longevity of inbred mice. J. Gerontol. 30, 257–263.

Goodrick, C. L. (1980): Effects of long-term voluntary wheel exercise on male and female Wistar rats. I. Longevity, body weight and metabolism rate. Gerontology 26, 22–33.

Gorban, Ye. N. (1979): Age specifics of the influence of the tyrotropic hormone on the value of the membrane potential of the cells of the thyroid gland. Fiziol. zhurn. 25, 395–401.

Gordienko, E. A. (1975): Age changes in dicarboxylic amino acids and GABA in the brain and the hypothalamic region of rats in the case of endocrine influences. In: Molecular and Physiological Mechanisms of Aging, pp. 231–239. Kiev: Naukova Dumka. (In Russian.)

Gordon, S. M., Finch, C. E. (1974): An electrophoretic study of protein synthesis in brain regions of senescent male mice. Exp. Gerontol. 9, 269–273.

Govoni, S., Loddo, P., Spano, P., Trabucchi, M. (1977): Dopamine receptor sensitivity in brain and retina of rats during aging. Brain Res. 138, 565–570.

Govoni, S., Memo, M., Saiani, L., Spano, P. F., Trabucchi, M. (1980): Impairment of brain neuro-transmitter receptors in aged rats. Mech. Ageing Develop. 12, 39–46.

Govyrin, V. A. (1967): Trophic Function of the Sympathetic Nerves of the Heart and the Skeletal Muscles. Leningrad: Nauka. (In Russian.)

Grabina, L. L. (1971): Age specifics of the changes in the adenosine triphosphatase and cholinesterase activity of myosin under the conditions of a cholinesterase blockade. In: Gerontology and Geriatrics. Aging of a Cell. Yearbook (1970–1971), pp. 195–198. Kiev: Institute of Gerontology. (In Russian.)

Grabina, L. L. (1972): Adenosine triphosphatase and cholinesterase activities of myosin of skeletal muscles in old age. In: Ninth International Congress of Gerontology, p. 322. Kiev: Institute of Gerontology.

Green, M. (1974): Endocrinology in the elderly. In: Geriatric Medicine (Ferguson Anderson, W., ed.), pp. 153–170. London-New York: Academic Press.

Gregerman, R. J. (1959): Adaptive enzyme response in the senescent rat: tryptophan peroxidase and tyrosine transaminase. Amer. J. Physiol. *197*, 63–69.

Grinna, L. S. (1977): Changes in cell membranes during aging. Gerontology *23*, 452–464.

Grinna, L. S., Barber, A. A. (1976): Lipid changes in the microsomal and mitochondrial membranes. Fed. Proc. *35*, 1425–1432.

Groen, J. J. (1959): General physiology of aging. Geriatrics *14*, 318–331.

Gromov, L. A. (1966): On the influence of papaverin on the reactions of the cardiovascular system in animals of different age. In: Regulation of the Functions During Various Age Periods, pp. 97–101. Kiev: Naukova Dumka. (In Russian.)

Gurevich, M. I., Kondratovich, M. A. (1969): Regional vascular reactions when catecholamines are administered. In: Questions of the Regulation of Regional Blood Circulation, pp. 118–124. Leningrad: Nauka. (In Russian.)

Guseinov, D. Yu. (1972): Adaptability of peripheral nervous system (kidneys, liver, heart) of ageing organism at cellular and subcellular levels. In: Ninth International Congress of Gerontology, p. 325. Kiev: Institute of Gerontology.

Guskova, R. A., Vilenchik, M. M., Koltover, V. K. (1979): On the question of the role of free radicals in the aging process. Studia biophysica *77*, 43–50.

Gutmann, E. (1976): Neurotrophic relations. Ann. Rev. Physiol. *38*, 117–126.

Gutmann, E., Hanzlikova, V. (1973): Basic mechanisms of aging in the neuromuscular system. Mech. Ageing Develop. *1*, 327–349.

Habal, F. M., Movat, H. Z. (1976): Rapid purification of human molecular weight kininogen. Agents and actions *6*, 565–568.

Haber, A. H. (1971): Chloroplast senescence in nongrowing tissue in darkness: effect of temperature and age. Exp. Gerontol. *6*, 179–185.

von Hahn, H. P. (1970): Structural and functional changes in nucleoprotein during the ageing of the cell. Gerontologia *16*, 116–128.

Halbach, U. (1973): Life table data and population dynamics of the rotifer Brachionus calycyflorus Pallas as influenced by periodically oscillating temperature. In: Effects of Temperature on Ectothermic Organisms (Wieser, W., ed.), pp. 217–228. New York: Springer.

Hamilton, J. B., Hamilton, R. S., Mastler, G. E. (1969): Duration of life and causes of death in domestic cats: Influence of sex, gonadectomy and inbreeding. J. Gerontol. *24*, 427–437.

Hansche, W. J. (1975): Role of the nervous system in aging–correlations among life span, brain-body weight and metabolism. In: Neurology of Aging, pp. 23–35. New York: Plenum Publ.

Hansford, R. G. (1978): Lipid oxidation by heart mitochondria from young, adult and senescent rats. Biochem. J. *170*, 2, 285–295.

Harman, D. (1962): Free radical theory of aging: prolongation of the normal life span by free radical inhibitors. In: Biological Aspects of Aging, pp. 279–285. New York-London: Academic Press.

Harman, D. (1968): Free radical theory of aging: effect of free radical reaction inhibitors on the mortality rate of male LAF mice. J. Gerontol. *23*, 476–482.

Harrison, D. E. (1975): Normal function of transplanted marrow cell linses from aged mice. J. Gerontol. *30*, 279–285.

Harrison, D. E., Astle, C. M., Doubleday, J. W. (1977): Stem cell lines from old immunodeficient donors give normal responses in young recipients. J. Immunol. *118*, 1223–1227.

Hart, R. W., Setlow, R. B. (1974): Correlation between deoxyribonucleic acid excision repair and life span in a number of mammalian species. Proc. Nat. Acad. Sci. U.S.A. *71*, 2169–2173.

Hart, R. W., Setlow, R. B. (1976): DNA repair in late passage human cells. Mech. Ageing Develop. 5, 67–77.

Hart, R. W., Ambrosio, S. M., Ng, K. J., Modak, S. P. (1979): Longevity, stability and DNA repair. Mech. Ageing Develop. 9, 203–224.

Hartmann, M. (1931): General Biology. Moscow-Leningrad: Medgiz. (In Russian.)

Hayflick, L. (1965): The limited in vitro lifetime of human diploid cell strains. Exp. Cell Res. 37, 614–636.

Hayflick, L. (1972): Cellular aging in the organism and tissue culture. In: Ninth International Congress of Gerontology, pp. 78–80. Kiev: Institute of Gerontology.

Hayflick, L. (1979): Progress in cytogerontology. Mech. Ageing Develop. 9, 393–409.

Hedqvist, P. (1974): Role of alpha-receptor in the control of noradrenaline release from sympathetic nerves. Acta physiol. Scand. 90, 158–165.

Hegel, G. W. (1959): Works, Vol. 1. Moscow-Leningrad: Publishing House of the USSR Academy of Sciences. (In Russian.)

Heldmann, K., et al. (1970): Diabetes mellitus. Die Diagnostik des Diabetes mellitus. Z. ärztl. Fortbild. 64, 25–31.

Hellthaler, G., Reifegerste, D., Kühler, R., Rotsch, W. (1976): Zur Molekularbiologie des Alterns. Z. Altersforsch. 31, 457–460.

Herbener, G. H. (1976): A morphometric study of age-dependent changes in mitochondrial populations of mouse liver and heart. J. Gerontol. 31, 8–12.

Herreid, G. F. (1964): Rat longevity and metabolic rate. Exp. Gerontol. 1, 4–17.

Van Herrewege, J. (1974): Nutritional requirements of adult Drosophila melanogaster: the influence of the casein concentration on the duration of life. Exp. Gerontol. 9, 191–198.

Herrmann, J., Rusche, H., Kröll, H., Hilger, P., Krüskemper, G. (1974): Free triiodothyronine (T_3) and thyroxine (T_4) serum levels in old age. Horm. Metab. Res. 6, 239–240.

Herrmann, R. L. (1975): Age-related changes in nucleic acids and protein synthesis. In: Neurobiology of Aging, pp. 307–327. New York: Plenum Publ.

Hochschild, R. (1971): Effect of membrane stabilizing drugs on mortality in Drosophila melanogaster. Exp. Gerontol. 6, 139–151.

Hochschild, R. (1973a): Effect of dimethylaminoethyl p-chlorophenoxacetate on the life span of male Swiss webster albino mice. Exp. Gerontol. 8, 177–183.

Hochschild, R. (1973b): Effects of various drugs on longevity in female C57BL/6J mice. Gerontologia 19, 271–280.

Hoffmann, H., Kiesewetter, R., Krohs, G., Schmitz, Ch. (1975): Zur Altersabhängigkeit von Katecholaminwirkungen beim Menschen. I. Einfluß von Noradrenalin, Adrenalin und Isoprenalin auf den Blutdruck und die Herzfrequenz. Z. ges. Inn. Med. 30, 89–95.

Hollingsworth, M. J. (1969): Temperature and length of life in Drosophila. Exp. Gerontol. 4, 49–55.

Horsley, V. (1884): Thyroid glands and aging. Proc. Roy. Soc. 38, 158–164.

Horton, E. W. (1972): Prostaglandins. New York: Raven Press.

Hruza, Z. (1973): Catabolism of epinephrine and histamine during aging in rat. Exp. Gerontol. 8, 333–336.

Hruza, Z., Zweifach, B. (1967): Effect of age on vascular reactivity to catecholamines in rats. J. Gerontol. 22, 1469.

Hsu, H. K., Peng, M. T. (1978): Hypothalamic neuron number of old female rats. Gerontology 24, 434–440.

Iversen, L. L. (1967): The catecholamines. Nature 214, 5083, 8.

Jakubczak, L. F. (1976): Behavioral aspects of nutrition and longevity in animals. In: Nutrition, Longevity and Aging (Rockstein, M., Sussman, S., eds.), pp. 103–122. New York: Academic Press.

James, T. C., Kanungo, M. S. (1976): Alterations in atropine sites of the brain of rats as a function of age. Biochem. Biophys. Res. Commun. 72, 170–175.

Jeffrey, P. L., Austin, L. (1973): Axoplasmic transport. Progr. Neurobiol. 2, 205–238.

Johnson, H. A., Erner, S. (1972): Neuron survival in the aging mouse. Exp. Gerontol. 7, 111–117.

Johnson, H. A., Pavelec, M. (1972): Thermal injury due to normal body temperature. Amer. J. Pathol. 66, 557–564.

Johnson, L. D., Hadden, J. (1977): Modification of human DNA-dependent RNA polymerase activity by cyclic GMP. Nucleic Acid Res. *4*, 1007–1009.

Jonec, V., Finch, C. E. (1975): Ageing and dopamine uptake subcellular fractions in the C57BL/6J male mouse brain. Brain Res. *91*, 197–215.

Junghahn, J., Bielka, H. (1974): Regulation der Translation in eukaryotischen Zellen. Acta biol. med. germ. *32*, 267–269.

Kaack, B., Ordy, J. M., Trapp, B. (1975): Changes in limbic, neuroendocrine and autonomic systems, adaptation, homeostasis during aging. In: Neurobiology of Aging (Ordy, J. M., Brizzee, K. R., eds.), pp. 209–231. New York: Plenum Publ.

Kalendo, G. S. (1972): On the abilities of the adaptive stress syndrome at the cellular level and its role in the reaction of the cell to radiation. Usp. sovrem. biol. *73*, 59–80.

Kaliman, P. A., Amiri, A. (1977): Influence of thyroxine on the distribution of the isoenzymes of lactate dehydrogenase and the content of pyroacemic acid in some tissues of white rats of different age. Ukr. biokhim. zhurn. *49*, 78–83.

Kalinovskaya, Ye. G. (1978): Functional and structural changes in the organs and systems during aging: urinary system. In: Guide to Gerontology, pp. 254–261. Moscow: Meditsina. (In Russian.)

Kalish, M. J., Pineyro, M. A., Gregerman, R. I. (1975): Relation of age to hormone sensitive adenylyl cyclases in rat liver. In: 10th International Congress of Gerontologists, Vol. 1, 19. Jerusalem.

Kalk, W. J., Vinik, K. I., Pimstone, B. M., Jackson, W. P. U. (1973): Growth hormone response to insulin hypoglycemia in the elderly. J. Gerontol. *28*, 431–434.

Kallos, J. (1977): Photochemical attachment of cyclic AMP binding protein to the nuclear genome. Nature *265*, 705–710.

Kanmann, A. J. (1977): Relaxation of heart muscle by catecholamines and by dibutyryl cyclic 3,5-monophosphate. Nanyn-Schmiedeberg's Arch. Pharm. *296*, 205–215.

Kanungo, M. S. (1975): Regulation and induction of enzymes as a function of age of the rat. In: 10th International Congress of Gerontology, p. 35. Jerusalem.

Kanungo, M. S., Koul, O., Reddy, K. R. (1970): Concomitant studies on RNA and protein synthesis in tissues of rats of various ages. Exp. Gerontol. *5*, 261–269.

Kaplan, R., Fideleff, H., Banchik, R. (1975): Thyroid function in the elderly. In: 10th International Congress of Gerontology, Vol. 2, p. 77. Jerusalem.

Kapustina, T. M. (1965): Histological data on the innervation of some tubular bones. In: Important Questions of the Clinical Picture and Treatment of Orthopedotraumatological Patients, pp. 212–214. Kiev: Institute of Gerontology. (In Russian.)

Karnaukhov, V. N. (1973): The Function of Carotenoids in the Animal Cells. Moscow: Nauka. (In Russian.)

Karpova, S. M. (1974): Age-related peculiarities of catecholamine effect on acetylcholine metabolism in myocardium. In: Pharmacotherapy of Diseases of the Cardiovascular System in Elderly and Old Age, pp. 22–28. Kiev: Institute of Gerontology. (In Russian.)

Kato, H. (1978): Does the potential of unscheduled DNA synthesis of mammals correlate with their life span? Ann. Report Nat. Inst. Genet. Jap. *28*, 56–58.

Kato, H., Stitch, H. F. (1976): Sister chromatid exchanges in ageing and repair-deficient human fibroblasts. Nature *260*, 227.

Kazue, O., Osamu, K., Tomoo, M., Yoshio, Y., Takakazu, K., Hiroshi, T., Hidenari, T., Ichio, H. (1972): Human liver mitochondria. Clin. Chim. Acta *38*, 385–393.

Keely, S., Lincoln, T. (1978): On the question of cyclic GMP as the mediator of the effects of acetylcholine on the heart. Biochim. Biophys. Acta *543*, 251–257.

Kelley, R. O., Vogel, K. G., Skipper, B. E., Krissman, H. A., Lujan, C. (1979): Development of the aging cell surface. Exp. Cell Res. *119*, 127–143.

Kellogg, E. W., Fridovich, I. (1976): Superoxide dismutase in the rat and mouse as a function of age and longevity. J. Gerontol. *31*, 405–408.

Khayutin, V. M., Sonina, R. S., Lukoshkova, Ye. V. (1977): Central Organization of Vasomotor Control. Moscow: Meditsina. (In Russian.)

Khesin, R. V. (1975): Present problems of molecular genetics. Genetika *11*, 154–163.

Khilko, O. K. (1965): Age changes in the content of the sulfhydryl groups and the ATPase activity of myosin. Ukr. biokhim. zhurn. *37*, 8–13.

Khilko, O. K., Rogova, A. N. (1971): Change in the amount of the disulphide groups of myogen A, depending on an animal's age. In: Aging of a Cell. Gerontologiya i geriatriya 1970–1971 (yearbook), pp. 319–326. Kiev: Institute of Gerontology.

Khilobok, I. Yu., Khilko, O. K., Goldstein, N. B., Frantseva, T. G. (1977): Chromatin of rat liver in aging. In: Genetic Mechanisms of Aging and Longevity, pp. 78–81. Kiev: Institute of Gerontology. (In Russian.)

Kibler, H. H., Johnson, H. D. (1961): Metabolic rate and aging in rats during exposure to cold. J. Gerontol. 6, 13–16.

Kibler, H. H., Johnson, H. D. (1966): Temperature and longevity in male rats. J. Gerontol. 21, 52–56.

King, M. C., Wilson, A. C. (1975): Evolution at two levels in humans and chimpanzees. Science 188, 107–116.

Kirk, J. E. (1959): Enzyme activities of human arterial tissue. Ann. N. Y. Acad. Sci. 72, 1006–1010.

Kirkham, K., Hunter, U., Jeffery, Z., Bennie, J. (1970): Measurement of thyroid stimulating hormone in vitro. In: In Vitro Procedure Radioisotopes Med., pp. 597–610. Basel: Karger.

Klimenko, A. I., Malyshev, O. B., Shevtsova, M. Ya. (1978): Protein composition of the fragmented chromatin of the rat liver in postnatal ontogenesis. Biokhimiya 43, 1757–1762.

Kogan, A. B. (1972): Biological Cybernetics. Moscow: Vysshaya Shkola. (In Russian.)

Kohn, R. R. (1971): Effect of antioxidants on the life span of C57BL/6J mice. J. Gerontol. 26, 378–380.

Kohn, R. R. (1978): Principles of mammalian aging. Englewood Cliffs, N. J.: Prentice-Hall.

Kolchinskaya, A. Z. (1964): Oxygen Deficiency and Age. Kiev: Naukova Dumka. (In Russian.)

Komarov, L. V. (1978): Studies on the problem of artificially increasing the life span of the organisms of a species that were made in 1977–1978 (some results). In: Artificially Increasing the Life Span of a Species. First Symposium, Theses of Reports, pp. 8–9. Moscow: Institute of General Genetics. (In Russian.)

Konigsmark, B. W., Murphy, E. A. (1973): Neuronal populations in the human brain. Nature 228, 1335–1336.

Kononenko, T. K. (1969): Morphofunctional changes in glia and the neuron-glia relationships in the rat brain in old age. Arkhiv anat., histol., embriol. 6, 35–41.

Konovalova, L. K. (1974): Influence of the electric stimulation of various regions of the hypothalamus of rats on the functional activity of hypophysial adrenocortical system. Probl. endokr. 20, 58–62.

Kopieva, S. A. (1978): Specifics of the influence of estrogens on the hypophysial adrenal system of white rats with respect to age and sex. Fiziol. zhurn. 24, 446–450.

Kopin, I. G. (1965): Biochemical aspects of storage and release of biogenic amines from sympathetic nerves. In: Symposium on Mechanisms of Release of Biogenic Amines. New York: Plenum Press.

Kopin, I. G., Axelrod, Z., Gordon, E. (1961): The metabolic fate of H^3-epinephrine and C^{14}-metanephrine in the rat. J. Biol. Chem. 236, 2109–2113.

Korchagin, N. V., Malinovsky, A. A., Anfalova, T. V., Dementev, B. S., Korchagin, M. V. (1973): Correlation between mammalian species. In: Some Problems of the Theory of Evolution, Vol. 7, pp. 128–135. Moscow: Second Moscow Medical Institute. (In Russian.)

Korkushko, O. V. (1969): Clinical and Physiological Specifics of the Cardiovascular System of Elderly, Old and Long-Living Persons. Author's abstract of the dissertation for a doctor's degree (medicine). Kiev: Medical Institute. (In Russian.)

Korkushko, O. V. (1976): Hemodynamics and age. Fiziologiya cheloveka 2, 633–638.

Korkushko, O. V., Orlov, P. A. (1974): Caloric action of glucose in persons of different age. Voprosy pitaniya 1, 54–57.

Korkushko, O. V., Ivanov, L. A. (1980): Hypoxia and Aging. Kiev: Naukova Dumka. (In Russian.)

Korner, P. I. (1971): Integrative neural cardiovascular control. Physiol. Rev. 51, 312–367.

Korotonozhkin, V. G. (1973): Age Specifics of the Regulation of the Level of the Membrane Potential of Cells (as Exemplified by the Muscle Fibre and Hepatic Cells). Author's abstract of the dissertation for a candidate's degree (medicine). Kiev: Medical Institute. (In Russian.)

Koshtoyants, Kh. S. (1938): Trophic influence of the nervous system in animal onthogenesis. Fiziol. zhurn. 29, 221–227.

Koshtoyants, Kh. S. (1951): Protein Bodies, Metabolism and Neural Regulation. Moscow: Publishing House of the USSR Academy of Sciences. (In Russian.)

Kositsky, G. I. (1975): Afferent Systems of the Heart. Moscow: Meditsina. (In Russian.)

Kostikova, S. N., Nikitin, V. N., Pashkova, A. A. (1974): Age specifics of the action of cyclic 3',5'-AMP on the lipolytic activity of the tissues. Doklady Akad. Nauk SSSR *218*, 1236–1238.

Kranz, D., Wollenberger, A., Poppel, M., Hecht, K. (1976): Hormonelle Stimulierung der Bildung von zyklischen Adenosin-3',5'-monophosphate in zellfreien Partikelpräparaten und intakten Zellen der glatten Muskulatur der Aorta und A. femoralis. Acta Biol. Med. Ges. *35*, 819–828.

Kratin, Yu. G., Propp, M. V. (1963): Changes in the bioelectric activity of the cerebral cortex and the hypothalamus of rabbits during aging and the influence of estrogens on this activity. In: Mechanisms of Aging, pp. 216–220. Kiev: Institute of Gerontology. (In Russian.)

Kreteanu, Ch., Hurjui, J. (1972): Clinical and laboratory aspects of the adaptation of glycoregulation in old persons. In: Ninth International Congress of Gerontology, p. 3. Kiev: Institute of Gerontology.

Krohn, P. L. (ed.) (1966): Topics in the Biology of Aging. New York: Wiley.

Kulchitsky, O. K. (1977): Analysis of the mechanism of the action of adrenaline on the metabolism of adenine nucleotides of the myocardium in rats of different age. Fiziol. zhurn. *23*, 307–310.

Kulchitsky, O. K. (1981): Influence of adrenaline on the content of cyclic nucleotides in the tissues of rats of different age. Vopr. med. khimii *27*, 40–43.

Kulchitsky, K. I., Badaeva, L. N. (1972): Synapses of the human heart and their peculiarities in aging. In: Ninth International Congress of Gerontology, Vol. 3, p. 348. Kiev: Institute of Gerontology.

Kulchitsky, O. K., Orlov, P. A. (1977): Tolerance to carbohydrates and functional activity of insulin apparatus in aging. In: Insulin Provision in Old Age, pp. 34–45. Kiev: Institute of Gerontology. (In Russian.)

Kunstyr, I., Leuenberger, H. W. (1975): Gerontological data of C57BL/6J mice. J. Gerontology *30*, 157–162.

Kuprash, L. P. (1974): Age Specifics of the Water-Electrolyte Metabolism. Author's abstract of the dissertation for a doctor's degree (medicine). Kiev: Medical Institute. (In Russian.)

Kuznetsova, S. M. (1970): Age Changes in the Metabolism of Serotonin and Its Influence on the Functional State of the Central Nervous and Cardiovascular Systems. Author's abstract of the dissertation for a candidate's degree (medicine). Kiev: Medical Institute. (In Russian.)

LaBella, F. S., Vivian, S. (1975): Effect of beta-aminopropionitrile of prednisolone on survival of LAF/J mice. Exp. Gerontol. *10*, 185–188.

Lakatta, E. C., Gersteinblith, C., Angell, Ch. S. (1975): Diminished inotropic response of aged myocardium to catecholamines. Circ. Res. *36*, 262–269.

Lakiza, T. Yu. (1979): Analysis of the age specifics of the adrenergic regulation of the cardiovascular system. In: Biochemical and Physiological Mechanisms of Aging, pp. 121–128. Minsk: Nauka i Tekhnika. (In Russian.)

Lamperti, A., Blaha, G. (1980): The numbers of neurons in the hypothalamic nuclei of young and reproductively senescent female golden hamsters. J. Gerontol. *35*, 335–338.

Lansing, A. (1942): Some effects of the hydrogen concentration, total salt concentration, calcium and citrate on longevity and fecundity of the rotifer. J. Exp. Zool. *91*, 195–211.

Lasada, K., Roberts, P. (1975): Variation in the morphometry of the normal human thyroid in growth and ageing. J. Path. *112*, 161–168.

Lasser, R. P., Master, A. M. (1959): Observation of frequency distribution curves of blood pressure in persons aged 20 to 106 years. Geriatrics *14*, 345–360.

Laurenz, A. (1597): Discours de la conservation de la vie, des maladies mélancoliques, des catarrhes et de la vieillesse. Paris.

Leato, S., Kokkonen, G., Barrows, C. (1976): Dietary protein, lifespan and biochemical variables in female mice. J. Gerontol. *31*, 144–148.

Lebedeva, Ye. A. (1965): Free amino acids of blood serum in elderly and old persons. In: Questions of Gerontology and Geriatrics, pp. 50–53. Leningrad: Nauka. (In Russian.)

Lefkowitz, R. J. (1976): [³H](–)-alprenolol: a new tool for the study of beta-adrenergic receptors. In: Methods in Receptor Research, part 1, pp. 53–72. New York: Dekker.

Lehman, H. C. (1943): The longevity of the eminent. Science *98*, 270–276.

Lenin, V. I. (1963): On Dialectics. Complete Works, Vol. 29, pp. 316–322. Moscow: Gospolitizdat. (In Russian.)

Lerman, M. J. (1978): The biological essence of resting cells in cell population. J. Theor. Biol. *73*, 615–625.

Lewis, B. K., Wexler, B. C. (1974): Serum insulin changes in male rats associated with age and reproductive activity. J. Gerontol. *29*, 139–144.

Limas, C. L. (1975): Comparison of the handling of the norepinephrine in myocardium of adult and old rats. Cardiovasc. Res. *9*, 664–668.

Lindblad, L. E. (1977): Influence of age on sensitivity and effector mechanisms of the carotid baroreflex. Acta physiol. Scand. *101*, 43–49.

Lints, F. A., Stoll, J. Grawez, G., Lints, C. V. (1979): An attempt to select for increased longevity in *Drosophila melanogaster*. Gerontology *25*, 192–204.

Lipton, J. M., Whisenunt, J. D., Gean, J. T. (1979): Hypothermia produced by peripheral and central injections of chlorpromazine in aged rabbits. Brain Res. Bull. *4*, 631–634.

Litoshenko, A. Ya. (1977): Hexokinase activity in rat tissues of different age. In: Insulin Provision in Old Age, pp. 88–93. Kiev: Institute of Gerontology. (In Russian.)

Litoshenko, A. Ya. (1981): Age specifics of the content of adenosine phosphate in the regenerating rat liver. Ukr. biokhim. zhurn. *53*, 63–66.

Litoshenko, A. Ya., Levitsky E. L. (1981): Replication of total and mitochondrial DNA in rat liver with aging. Exp. Gerontol. *16*, 213–218.

Litovchenko, S. V. (1973): Experimental investigation of psychic activity in long-living persons. In: Longevous People, pp. 61–66. Kiev: Institute of Gerontology. (In Russian.)

Liu, R., Walford, R. L. (1972): The effect of lowered body temperature on life span and immune and non-immune processes. Gerontologia *180*, 363–388.

Liu, R., Walford, R. L. (1975): Mid-life temperature-transfer effects on life span of annual fish. J. Gerontol. *30*, 129–131.

Livergant, Yu. E., Dutsenko, N. V., Krupchitskaya, K. I., Motova, L. P., Poltorak, V. V. (1974): Content of immunoreactive insulin in the plasma of persons of different age (without any disturbances of carbohydrate metabolism) and the influence of a glucose load on this index. Probl. endokrin. *4*, 3–7.

Lockshin, R. A., Beaulaton, J. (1975): Programmed cell death. Life Sci. *15*, 1549–1565.

Loeb, J. (1908): Über den Temperaturkoeffizienten für die Lebensdauer kaltblütiger Tiere und über die Ursache des natürlichen Todes. Pflügers Arch. *124*, 411–426.

Loeb, J., Northrop, J. H. (1917): On the influence of food and temperature on the duration of life. J. Biol. Chem. *32*, 103–121.

Lowrie, R. A. (1953): The activity of the cytochrome system in muscle and its relation to myoglobin. Biochem. J. *55*, 298–305.

Ludwig, F. C., Elashoff, R. F. (1972): Effect on longevity of parabiosis between syngeneic white rats of different chronological age. In: 9th International Congress of Gerontology, Abstracts, Vol. 3, p. 356. Kiev: Institute of Gerontology.

Lukjan, H., Bielawiec, M., Furman, M. (1975): Experimental studies on activation of the kininogenic system after exclusion of the hepatic circulation. Arch. immunol. et ther. exps. *23*, 831–835.

Luste, L. A. (1973): Morphological characterization of the adaptive abilities of the thyroid gland during various age periods. In: Morphology of the Endocrine System in Some Pathological States. Collection of Scientific Works, 126th ed., pp. 40–47. Leningrad: Nauka. (In Russian.)

Machado-Salas, J., Scheibel, M. E., Scheibel, A. B. (1977): Neuronal changes in the aging mouse spinal cord and lower brain stem. Expl. Neurol. *54*, 504–512.

Machado-Salas, J. P., Scheibel, A. B. (1979): Limbic system of the aged mouse. Exp. Neurol. *63*, 347–355.

Macill, J., Bertilson, L., Cheney, L., Zsilla, C., Corfa, C. (1979): Aging-induced changes in acetylcholine and serotonin content of discrete brain nuclei. J. Gerontol. *32*, 130–134.

Maggi, A., Schmidt, M. J., Ghetti, B., Enna, S. J. (1979): Effect of aging on neurotransmitter receptor binding in rat and human brain. Life Sci. *24*, 367–374.

Makman, M. H., Ahn, U. S., Thal, L. J., Sharpless, N. S., Dvorkin, B., Horowitz, G., Rosenfeld, M. (1979): Aging and monoamine receptors in brain. Fed. Proc. *38*, 1922–1976.

Mako, M., Starr, J. I., Rubenstein, A. H. (1977): Circulating proinsulin in patients with maturity onset diabetes. Amer. J. Med. *6*, 865–869.

Malenkov, A. G. (1976): Ionic Homeostasis and the Autonomous Behaviour of a Tumour. Moscow: Nauka. (In Russian.)

Malinovsky, A. A. (1962): Some biological prerequisites of a long life of mammals and man. In: Problems of a Long Life, pp. 46–51. Moscow: Publishing House of the USSR Academy of Sciences. (In Russian.)

Mankovsky, N. B. (1973): Neurogerontological aspect of the late stage of human ontogenesis. In: Longevous People, pp. 10–26. Kiev: Institute of Gerontology. (In Russian.)

Mankovsky, N. B., Mints, A. Ya. (1972): Aging and the Nervous System. Kiev: Zdorovya. (In Russian.)

Mankovsky, N. B., Belonog, R. P. (1974): Electroencephalography of persons of different age suffering from hypoxia. In: Respiration, Gas Exchange, and Hypoxic Conditions in Elderly and Old Ages, pp. 130–136. Kiev: Institute of Gerontology. (In Russian.)

Mankovsky, N. B., Belonog, R. P., Kuznetsova, S. M. (1975): Genetic specifics of EEG and a long life. In: Biological Possibilities of Life Span Prolongation, pp. 63–74. Kiev: Institute of Gerontology. (In Russian.)

Mankovsky, N. B., Lizogub, V. G. (1976): Age changes in the regional cerebral blood flow. Vrach. delo *10*, 89–93.

Mankovsky, N. B., Belonog, R. P., Gorbach, N. P. (1978): Light-evoked potentials during aging. Fiziologiya cheloveka *4*, 620–629.

Manukhin, B. N. (1968): Physiology of Adrenoreceptors. Moscow: Nauka. (In Russian.)

Marshall, J. F., Berrios, N. (1979): Movement disorders of aged rats: reversal by dopamine receptor stimulation. Science *206*, 4417, 477–479.

Martinez, T. T., McNeill, J. H. (1977): Cyclic AMP and the positive inotropic effect of norepinephrine and phenylephrine. Can. J. Physiol. Pharmacol. *55*, 279–287.

Martynenko, O. A. (1967): Membrane Potential of the Skeletal Muscle Fibres of Warm-Blooded Animals in Ontogenesis. Author's abstract of the dissertation for a candidate's degree (biology). Kiev: Institute of Physiology. (In Russian.)

Martynenko, O. A. (1971): Age specifics of the change in the main electric parameters of the muscle fibres. In: Tenth Conference on Age Morphology, Biochemistry and Physiology, pp. 20–21. Moscow: Institute of Age Physiology. (In Russian.)

Martynenko, O. A. (1974): Age specifics of the electric properties of the membrane of individual muscle fibres of animals of different age. Biofizika *19*, 391–394.

Martynenko, O. A. (1977): Effect of insulin on electrophysiological properties of single muscle fibres in animals of different age. In: Insulin Provision in Old Age, pp. 77–84. Kiev: Institute of Gerontology. (In Russian.)

Martynenko, O. A. (1980): Influence of estradiol dipropionate on the electric properties of the membrane of the cells and their electrolytic composition in animals of different age. Probl. endocrin. *26*, 55–58.

Massie, H. R., Baird, M. B., Williams, T. R. (1978): Increased longevity of *Drosophila melanogaster* with diiodomethane. Gerontology *24*, 104–111.

Massie, H. R., Williams, T. R. (1980): Singlet oxygen and aging in *Drosophila*. Gerontology *26*, 16–21.

Mathews, R. W., Haschemeyer, A. E. (1978): Temperature dependency of protein synthesis in toadfish liver in vivo. Compar. Biochem. Physiol. *61*, 479–484.

Maximov, A. A. (1916): Cellular division. Russkii arkhiv anatomii, histologii i embriologii *1*, 105–110.

McCay, C. M., Crowell, M. F., Maynard, L. A. (1935): The effect of retarded growth upon the length of life span and upon the ultimate body size. J. Nutr. *10*, 63–79.

McCay, C. M., Maynard, L. A., Sperling, G., Barnes, L. (1939): Retarded growth, life span, ultimate body size and age changes in the albino rat after feeding diets restricted in calories. J. Nutrit. *18*, 16–26.

McCay, C. M., Maynard, L. A., Sperling, G., Osgood, H. S. (1941): Nutritional requirements during the latter half of life. J. Nutrit. *21*, 45–60.

McCay, C. M., Pope, F., Lunsford, W. (1956): Experimental prolongation of the life span. Bull. N. Y. Acad. Med. *32*, 91–101.

McGeer, E. G., Fibiger, H. C., McGeer, P. L., Wickson, W. (1971): Aging and brain enzymes. Exp. Gerontol. 6, 391–396.

McGeer, E. G., McGeer, P. L. (1975): Age changes in the human for some enzymes associated with metabolism of catecholamines, GABA and acetylcholine. In: Neurobiology of Aging, pp. 287–305. New York: Plenum Press.

McMartin, D., O'Connor, J. (1979): Effect of age on axoplasmic transport of cholinesterase in rat asciatic nerves. Mech. Ageing Develop. 10, 241–249.

Meadow, N. D., Barrows, C. H. (1971): Studies on aging in a boelloid rotifer. J. Gerontol. 26, 302–309.

Mechnikov, I. I. (1907): Essays on Optimism. Moscow: Nauchnoie Slovo. (In Russian.)

Mechnikov, I. I. (1908): Essays on Human Nature. Moscow: Nauchnoie Slovo. (In Russian.)

Medavar, P. B. (1972): An Unsolved Problem of Biology. London: Levis.

Medved, V. I. (1980): Influence of vasopressin on the content of cyclic AMP and prostaglandins in the myocardium of animals of different age. Doklady Akad. Nauk Uk. SSR 2, 217–219.

Meerson, F. Z. (1978): Adaptation, Deadaptation and Insufficiency of the Heart. Moscow: Meditsina. (In Russian.)

Meites, J., Huang, M., Simpkins, J. (1978): Recent studies of neuroendocrine control of reproductive senescence in rats. In: Aging of Reproductive System, pp. 213–236. New York: Raven Press.

Menninger, J. (1977): Ribosome editing and the error catastrophe, hypothesis of cellular aging. Mech. Ageing Develop. 6, 131–142.

Metalnikov, S. I. (1917): Problems of Immortality in Modern Biology. Petrograd: Nauchnoie Slovo. (In Russian.)

Mezentsev, A. N., Messinova, O. V. (1971): Transport of the axoplasm and biosynthetic processes in the axon. Usp. sovr. biol. 72, 62–76.

Mezhiborskaya, N. A. (1980): Ultrastructural manifestations of the aging of the neurons of the mammilary nuclei. Doklady Akad. Nauk Ukr. SSR, B, 76–80.

Mezin, D. (1977): Life cycle of the cell. In: Molecules and Cells, pp. 216–234. Moscow: Mir. (In Russian.)

Michaelis, L., Menten, M. L. (1913): Die Kinetik der Investinwirkung. Biochem. Z. 49, 333–351.

Mikhelson, M. Ya., Zeimal, E. V. (1970): Acetylcholine. Leningrad: Nauka. (In Russian.)

Miller, D. S., Payne, R. R. (1968): Longevity and protein intake. Exp. Gerontol. 3, 231–234.

Miller, P., Klinger, W. (1978): The influence of age and of the inducer phenobarbital on the cytochrome P-450 dependent monooxygenation of drugs in rat liver. Pharmazie 33, 397–400.

Minot, C. S. (1908): The Problem of Age, Growth and Death. London: Academic Press.

Mints, A. Ya. (1973): Clinical characterization of the functional state of the nervous system in long-living persons. In: Longevous People, pp. 53–61. Kiev: Institute of Gerontology. (In Russian.)

Miquel, J., Johnson, J. E. (1975): Effect of various antioxidants and radiation protectants on the life span and lipofuscin of Drosophila and C5/BL/6J mice. The Gerontologist 15, part II, 25.

Modestov, V. K., Sokolnikov, O. I., Kaperko, F. F., Dolina, O. A., Shtengold, Ye. Sh., Meshine, Ye. M. (1966): Radiometric investigation of hemodynamics in elderly persons. Ter. arkh. 38, 89–93.

Möhring, J., Arbogast, R., Dusing, R., Glanzer, R., Kintz, J., Liard, J. F., Machial, J. A., Montani, J. P., Schoun, J. (1980): Vasopressor role of vasopressin in hypertension. In: Brain and Pituitary Peptides (Wuttke, W., Weindl, A., Voigt, K. H., Dries, R. R., eds.), pp. 157–167. Basel: Karger.

Moibenko, A. A. (1979): Cardiogenic Reflexes and Their Role in Regulating Blood Circulation. Kiev: Naukova Dumka. (In Russian.)

Mollerach, F., Degrossi, O., Scornavachi, J., Carmico et al. (1978): El eje hipotalamo-hipofiso-tiroideo en el geronte. Medicina (Buenos Aires) 38, 276–280.

Molnar, K. (1973): Subbiological aspects of aging and the concept of biological cathode protection. Mech. Ageing Develop. 2, 319–326.

Monastyrskaya, B. I. (1974): Adenohypophysis: Morphology and Function during Adaptation. Leningrad: Nauka. (In Russian.)

Morozova, V. V. (1971): Catecholamine content in healthy persons of different age groups. Zdravookhraneniye Kazakhstana 4, 46–51.

Morrison, W. W., Milkman, R. (1978): Modification of heat resistance in *Drosophila* by selection. Nature *273*, 5657, 49–50.

Muggeo, M., Tienge, A., Valerio, A., Botti, C., Burinaro, V., Fedell, D., Crepaldi, G. (1979): Recettori insulinici e sensibilità insulinica nelle varie età della vita. Giornale di Gerontologia *27*, 727–750.

Muradian, Kh. K. (1977a): Hypothalamohypophysial Adrenal Regulation of the Activity of Glucose-6-Phosphatase and Fructose-1,6-Diphosphatase and the Synthesis of RNA Fractions in Rats of Different Age. Author's abstract of the dissertation for a candidate's degree (biology). Kiev: Institute of Physiology. (In Russian.)

Muradian, Kh. K. (1977b): Synthesis of RNA fractions in liver of rats of different age. In: Genetic Mechanisms of Aging and Longevity, pp. 66–70. Kiev: Institute of Gerontology. (In Russian.)

Muravov, I. V. (1976): Motor activity, biological age and the life span. In: Biological Opportunities of Increasing the Life Span, pp. 88–96. Kiev: Institute of Gerontology. (In Russian.)

Muravov, I. V., Shchegoleva, I. V., Derkach, N. V. (1965): Blood pressure in persons who are 80 years old and more. In: Blood Circulation and Old Age. Kiev: Zdorovye. (In Russian.)

Nachmansonn, D. (1959): Choline acetylase. In: Cholinesterases and Anticholinesterase Agents. London: Academic Press.

Nagorny, A. V., Golubitskaya, R. N. (1947): Influence of thyroidectomy on nitrous metabolism in animals of different age. In: Problems of Aging, Vol. 25, pp. 149–152. Kharkov: Scientific Transactions of Kharkov State University. (In Russian.)

Napier, J., Napier, P. (1967): A Handbook of Living Primates. London-New York: Academic Press.

Naritomi, H., Meyer, J. S., Sakai, F., Yamaguchi, F., Shaw, T. (1979): Effects of advancing age on regional blood flow. Arch. Neurol. *36*, 410–416.

Natsunaga, E. (1972): Effect of changing parental age patterns on chromosomal aberrations and mutations. Ann. Rept. Nat. Inst. Genet. Jap. *6*, 104–110.

Navakatikyan, A. O. (1967): Respiratory Function in the Case of Pneumoconiosis and Dust Bronchitis. Moscow: Meditsina. (In Russian.)

Nedelkina, S. V., Argutinskaya, S. V., Salganik, R. I. (1972): Some regularities of the induction of arylhydroxylase of the rat liver when phenobarbital is administered once and for a long time. Voprosy meditsinskoi khimii *1*, 65–69.

Nikitin, V. N. (1952): On factors of protein synthesis in the ontogenesis of the animal organism. In: Second Conference on Age Morphology, Biochemistry and Physiology, pp. 162–163. Moscow: Institute of Age Physiology, USSR Academy of Pedagogical Sciences.

Nikitin, V. N. (1970): Age and the endocrine situation of the organism. Uspekhi sovremennoi biologii *68*, 288–305.

Nikitin, V. N. (1972): Age changes in the macromolecular composition and the functional abilities of the cell genome. Zhurn. evol. biokhim. *8*, 233–239.

Nikitin, V. N. (1978): Genetic apparatus during aging. In: Manual of Gerontology, pp. 51–60. Moscow: Meditsina. (In Russian.)

Nikitin, V. N. (1979): Biochemism and the endocrine situation of the organism of laboratory animals when life is experimentally prolonged by nutrition which restrains growth. In: Life Prolongation: Prognoses, Mechanisms, Control, pp. 27–34. Kiev: Institute of Gerontology. (In Russian.)

Nikitin, V. N., Golubitskaya, R. I., Silin, N. P., Likushina, N. G., Blok, L. N. (1956): Age changes in the biochemism of the denervated organs. In: Works of the Kharkov State University, Vol. 24, pp. 79–99. Kharkov: State University. (In Russian.)

Nikitin, V. N., Martynenko, A. A. (1963): Concentration of coenzyme A in the tissues of white rats of different age. In: Mechanisms of Aging, pp. 66–68. Kiev: Institute of Gerontology. (In Russian.)

Nikitin, V. N., Persky, Ye. E., Utevskaya, L. A. (1977): Biochemistry of the Collagen Structures with Respect to Age and Evolution. Kiev: Naukova Dumka. (In Russian.)

Nistratova, S. N. (1965): Possible mechanism by means of which the heart of an edentate slips away from under the action of acetylcholine. Fiziol. zhurn. SSSR *51*, 1012–1016.

Novikova, A. I. (1964): Age changes in the ion composition of the muscle fibres and their correlation with the membrane potential. Fiziol. zhurn. SSSR *36*, 626–630.

Novikova, A. I., Malysheva, Zh. B. (1975): Age changes in the mechanisms of active ion transport through the membrane of the muscle fibre. In: Molecular and Physiological Mechanisms of Aging, pp. 342–345. Kiev: Naukova Dumka. (In Russian.)

Novikova, S. N. (1978): Age Specifics of Energy Metabolism and the Protein-Synthesizing Function of the Rat Liver after Acute Bleeding. Author's abstract of the dissertation for a candidate's degree (medicine). Kiev: Institute of Physiology. (In Russian.)

Nomaguchi, T. A. (1974): Seasonal variation of life span of the ascidian *Ciona intestinalis*. Exp. Gerontol. *9*, 231–234.

Nonaka, K., Kono, N. (1978): Glucose intolerance in the elderly subjects–is it diabetes? In: Proceedings of 11th International Congress of Gerontology, pp. 72–73. Tokyo: Scimed Publications, Inc.

Norris, D. M., Moore, C. L. (1980): Lack of dietary delta-7-sterol markedly shortens the periods of locomotor vigor, reproduction and longevity of adult female *Xyleborus ferrugineus (Coleoptera, scolytidae)*. Exp. Gerontol. *15*, 359–364.

Nouel, J., Brunello, P., Chomant, J., Segond, G., Bohuon, C. (1973): Serum triiodothyronine radioimmunoassay in thyroid disease. Preliminary results in 207 subjects. Nouv. Presse Med. *2*, 219–222.

Nuzhny, V. P., Khitrov, N. K., Alaveryan, A. M. (1977): Dissociation of chronotropic and inotropic reactions of an isolated rat heart to noradrenaline in the case of both oxygen deficiency and the action of cyanide and 2,4-dinitrophenol. Fiziol. zhurn. Akad. Nauk SSSR *4*, 539–544.

Ochs, S. (1973): Effect of maturation and aging on the rate of fast axoplasmic transport in mammalian nerve. Prog. Brain Res. *40*, 349–369.

Odell, W. D., Swerdloff, R. S. (1968): Progesterone-induced luteinizing and follicle-stimulating hormone surge in post-menopause women: a stimulated ovulatory peak. Proc. Nat. Acad. Sci. U.S.A. *61*, 529–536.

Oeriu, S. (1972): Some molecular lever changes: an essential factor in the ageing processes. In: Ninth International Congress of Gerontology, Vol. 3, p. 41. Kiev: Institute of Gerontology.

Oeriu, S., Vochitu, E. (1965): The effect of the administration of compounds which contain sulfhydryl groups on the survival rates of mice, rats and guinea pigs. J. Gerontol. *20*, 417–419.

Oganesyan, S. S. (1967): Contractile Proteins in Muscle Pathology. Author's abstract of the dissertation for a doctor's degree (medicine). Moscow: Medical Institute. (In Russian.)

Ohara, H., Kobayashi, T., Shiraishi, M., Wada, T. (1974): Thyroid function of the aged as viewed from the pituitary-thyroid system. Endocr. Jap. *21*, 337–386.

Olefsky, J. M., Reaven, G. M. (1975): Effects of age and obesity on insulin binding to isolated adipocytes. Endocrinology *96*, 1486–1498.

Ono, T., Okada, S., Suguhara, T. (1976): Comparative studies of DNA size in various tissues of mice during the aging process. Exp. Gerontol. *11*, 127–132.

Osadchy, L. I. (1975): Cardiac Activity and Vascular Tonicity. Leningrad: Nauka. (In Russian.)

Osanai, M. (1978): Longevity and body weight loss of silkworm moth, *Bombyx mori*, varied by different temperature treatments. Exp. Gerontol. *13*, 375–388.

Osborne, T. B., Mendel, L. B. (1915): The resumption of growth after long continued failure to grow. J. Biol. Chem. *23*, 439–454.

Orbeli, L. A. (1935): Lectures on the Physiology of the Nervous System. Moscow: Biomedgiz. (In Russian.)

Orgel, L. E. (1970): The maintenance of the accuracy of protein synthesis and its relevance to ageing: a correction. Proc. Nat. Acad. Sci. U.S.A. *67*, 1476–1481.

Orlova, Ye. V. (1973): Clinical and x-ray characterization of the spine of long-living persons. In: Gerontology and Geriatrics (yearbook), pp. 172–175. Kiev: Institute of Gerontology. (In Russian.)

Orlova, Ye. V., Khromyak, Ye. T. (1972): Experimental osteoporosis in animals of different age. In: Ninth International Congress of Gerontology, p. 411. Kiev: Institute of Gerontology.

Overturf, M., Wyatt, S., Bocez, D., Tetz, A. (1975): Angiotension hydrolase and bradykininase from human lung. Life Sci. *16*, 1669–1681.

Pandya, K. H. (1977): Postnatal developmental changes in adrenergic receptor responses of the dog tracheal muscle. Arch. int. pharmacodyn. et ther. *230*, 53–64.

Paramonova, G. I. (1977): Induceable synthesis of some enzymes in rat liver at different ages caused by anode polarization. In: Genetic Mechanisms of Aging and Longevity, pp. 93–98. Kiev: Institute of Gerontology. (In Russian.)

Paramonova, G. I. (1981): Age specifics of the changes in the enzymes of the microsomal oxidation of the rat liver under the influence of barbiturates. Farmakol. i toxikol. *1*, 98–101.

Parchon, K. I. (1959): Age Biology. Bucharest: Publishing House of the Academy of Sciences of Roumania.

Parin, V. V., Meerson, F. Z. (1960): Outlines of the Clinical Physiology of Blood Circulation. Moscow: Medgiz. (In Russian.)

Parina, Ye. V., Solodinskaya, Ye. B. (1965): Age specifics of ATP metabolism. In: Works of the Institute of Biology of the Kharkov State University, pp. 22–28. Kharkov: State University. (In Russian.)

Parina, Ye. V., Drinyaev, V. A., Khotkevich, T. V. (1974): Adaptive changes in the activity of phosphoenolpyruvate carboxykinase of the liver and their mechanisms in rats of different age. In: Problems of Age Physiology, Biochemistry and Biophysics, pp. 97–106. Kiev: Institute of Biochemistry. (In Russian.)

Parina, Ye. V., Shabanova, I. A., Osetinskaya, A. I. (1976a): Role of insulin and the thyroid hormones in regulating the activity of hexokinase in the liver of young and old animals. In: Mechanisms of Hormone Action, p. 98. Tashkent. (In Russian.)

Parina, Ye. V., Shabanova, N. A., Bulankina, N. I. (1976b): Specifics of the age changes in the induction of enzymes with different functions. In: Third All-Union Congress of Gerontologists and Geriatricians, p. 27. Kiev: Institute of Gerontology. (In Russian.)

Parina, Ye. V., Kaliman, P. A. (1979): Mechanisms of Regulating Enzymes in Ontogenesis. Kharkov: Vishcha Shkola. (In Russian.)

Parkhotik, I. I. (1964): Some indices of the age specifics of the denervation processes in the muscle. Fiziol. zhurn. SSSR *10*, 803–805.

Parmacek, M. S., Fox, J. H., Harrison, W. H., Garron, D. C., Swenie, D. (1979): Effect of aging on brain respiration and carbohydrate metabolism of CBF mice. Gerontology *25*, 185–191.

Parsons, P. A. (1977): Genotype-temperature interaction for longevity in natural populations of *Drosophila simulans*. Exp. Gerontol. *12*, 241–244.

Pashkova, A. A. (1965): On the question of the age specifics of the bioenergetics of the cardiac muscle. In: Blood Circulation and Old Age, pp. 125–131. Kiev: Naukova Dumka. (In Russian.)

Pashkova, A. A. (1975): Age specifics of the hormonal regulation of tissue lipolysis. In: Molecular and Physiological Mechanisms of Aging. Kiev: Institute of Gerontology. (In Russian.)

Pashkova, A. A., Popova, L. Ya. (1970): Lipids and lipid metabolism in ontogenesis. In: Molecular and Functional Foundations of Ontogenesis, pp. 158–190. Moscow: Nauka. (In Russian.)

Patel, M. S. (1977): Age-dependent changes in oxidative metabolism in rat brain. J. Gerontol. *32*, 643–646.

Pavlov, I. P. (1938): Twenty-Year Experience Gained in the Objective Study of Higher Nervous Activity (Animal Behaviour). Moscow: Publishing House of the USSR Academy of Sciences. (In Russian.)

Pavlov, I. P. (1951a): Nitrogen Balance in the Submaxillary Gland during Work. Complete Works, 2nd revised ed., Vol. 2, pp. 142–175. Moscow-Leningrad: Publishing House of the USSR Academy of Sciences. (In Russian.)

Pavlov, I. P. (1951b): Laboratory Observations of the Pathological Reflexes of the Abdominal Cavity. Complete Works, 2nd revised ed., Vol. 1, pp. 550–564. Moscow-Leningrad: Publishing House of the USSR Academy of Sciences. (In Russian.)

Pavlov, I. P. (1951c): Centrifugal Nerves of the Heart. Collected Works, Vol. 1, pp. 87–251. Moscow-Leningrad: Publishing House of the USSR Academy of Sciences. (In Russian.)

Pearl, R. (1928): The Rate of Living; Being an Account of Some Experimental Studies on the Biology of Life Duration. New York.

Pedersen, K. (1974): A systematic study of variables affecting protein binding of thyroxine and tri-iodothyronine in serum. Scand. J. Clin. and Lab. Invest. *34*, 247–255.

Peleg, S., Raz, E. (1977): Changing capacity for DNA excision-repair in mouse embryonic cells in vitro. Exp. Cell Res. *104*, 301–307.

Pelz, B., Andrew, H. (1973): Scientists in Organizations. Moscow: Mir. (In Russian.)

Peng, M. T., Peng, J. M. (1973): Changes in the uptake of tritiated estradiol in the hypothalamus and adenohypophysis of old female rats. Fertility, Sterility *24*, 534–539.

Peng, M. T., Peng, Y.-I., Chen, F.-N. (1977): Age-dependent changes in the oxygen consumption of the cerebral cortex, hypothalamus, hippocampus, and amygdaloid in rats. J. Gerontol. *32*, 517–522.

Peng, T. T., Lee, L. K. (1975): Regional differences of neuron loss of rat brain in old age. Gerontology *25*, 205–211.

Perez, V. J., Moore, B. W. (1970): Biochemistry of the nervous system in aging. In: Interdisciplinary Topics in Gerontology, Vol. 7, pp. 22–45. Basel-München-New York: Karger.

Perry, E. K. (1980): The cholinergic system in old age and Alzheimer's disease. Age and ageing *9*, 1–8.

Petrova, M. K. (1946): On the Role of the Functionally Weakened Cerebral Cortex in the Origin of Pathological Processes in the Organism. Moscow: Nauka. (In Russian.)

Planel, M. H., Giess, M. C. (1973): Diminution de la longévité de drosophila melanogaster sous l'effet de la protection vis-à-vis des radiations ionisantes naturelles. C. R. Acad. Sci. (Paris) *276*, 809–812.

Pollack, G. H. (1977): Cardiac pacemaking: an obligatory role of catecholamines. Science *196*, 4291, 731–738.

Ponzio, F., Brunello, N., Algeri, S. (1978): Catecholamine synthesis in brain of aging rat. J. Neurochem. *26*, 215–222.

Popova, E. N., Lapin, S. K., Krivitskaya, L. N. (1976): The Morphology of Adaptive Changes of the Nervous Structures. Moscow: Meditsina.

Potapenko, R. I. (1974): Age Specifics of Energy Metabolism of Various Parts of the Brain. Author's abstract of the dissertation for a candidate's degree (medicine). Kiev: Medical Institute. (In Russian.)

Potapenko, R. I., Paramonova, G. I. (1977): Insulin-inhibiting properties of animal serum at different ages. In: Insulin Provision in Old Age, pp. 52–60. Kiev: Institute of Gerontology. (In Russian.)

Prasanna, H. R., Lane, R. S. (1979): Protein degradation in aged nematodes *(Turbatrix aceti)*. Biochem. Biophys. Res. Commun. *86*, 553–559.

Price, G. B., Modak, S. P., Makinodan, T. (1971): Age-associated changes in the DNA of mouse tissues. Science *171*, 917–920.

Price, G. B., Makinodan, T. (1972): Immunologic deficiencies in senescence. I. Characterization of intrinsic deficiencies. J. Immunol. *108*, 403–412.

Priduba, L. A. (1978a): Influence of manganes on the fruit flies' aging rate. In: Questions of Natural Sciences, pp. 79–82. Minsk: Nauka i Tekhnika. (In Russian.)

Priduba, L. A. (1978b): Life span of the fruit flies which received the disodium salt of EDTA with food. In: Questions of Natural Science, pp. 82–84. Minsk: Nauka i Tekhnika. (In Russian.)

Prinz, P. N., Halter, J., Benedetti, C., Raskind, M. (1979): Circadian variation of plasma catecholamines in young and old men: relation to rapid eye movement and slow wave sleep. J. clin. Endocrin. *49*, 300–304.

Prosser, L. (1977): Oxygen, respiration and metabolism. In: Comparative Physiology of Animals, Vol. 1, pp. 349–429. Moscow: Nauka. (In Russian.)

Protasova, T. N. (1975): Hormonal Regulation of Enzymic Activity. Moscow: Meditsina. (In Russian.)

Pugach, B. V. (1970): On the development of reflexogenous and pituitary experimental hypertension in animals of different age. Fiziol. zhurn. *16*, 832–834.

Puri, S. K., Volicer, L. (1977): Effect of aging on cAMP levels and adenylate cyclase and phosphodiesterase activities in the rat corpus striatum. Mech. Ageing Develop. *6*, 53–58.

Putthoff, D. L., Justesen, D. R., Ward, L. B., Levinson, D. M. (1977): Drug-induced ectothermia in small mammals: The quest for a biological microwave dosimeter. Radio Sci. *12*, Suppl. 72–80.

Quiring, D. R. (1950): Functional Anatomy of the Vertebrates. New York: Plenum Press.

Rafalowska, J. (1980): Some problems of the development and aging of nervous system. III. The motor cell of the anterior horn of spinal cord in various periods of life. Neuropat. Pol. *18*, 83–96.

Rafsky, H. A., Newman, B., Horonick, A. (1952): Age differences in respiration of guinea pig tissues. J. Gerontol. *7*, 38–40.

Ragland, S. S., Sohal, R. S. (1975): Ambient temperature, physical activity and aging in the housefly *Musca domestica*. Exp. Gerontol. *10*, 279–289.

Rahman, Y. E. (1976): Cited by: Sacher, G. A., Life table modification and life prolongation. In: Handbook of the Biology of Aging (1977) (Finch, C. E., Hayflick, L., eds.), pp. 582–638. New York: Van Nostrand Reinhold.

Ramires, S. G., Corrier, O., Turlapaty, P. D., Heaty, M. D. (1976): The influence of reserpine on responsiveness to norepinephrine and electrolyte contents of rabbit atria. Arch. inter. pharmacodyn. et ther. *223*, 324–332.

Rand, A., Ansari, K. A. (1980): Biochemical studies on brains of young and old inbred (B3F1) mice. Gerontology *26*, 76–81.

Randall, W. C. (1965): Past and present hypotheses of cardiac control. In: Nervous Control of the Heart, pp. 1–15. Baltimore: Univ. Park Press.

Ranish, N., Dettbarn, W. (1976): Effects of paraoxon on axoplasmic transport of cholinesterase in rat sciatic nerve. Exp. Neurol. *53*, 620–632.

Razumovich, A. N. (1972): Bioenergetic Processes and the Aging of the Organism. Minsk: Nauka i Tekhnika. (In Russian.)

Reaven, E. P., Gold, G., Reaven, G. M. (1979): Effect of age on glucose-stimulated insulin release by the beta-cell of the rat. J. Clin. Invest. *64*, 591–593.

Reaven, E. P., Gold, G., Reaven, G. M. (1980): Effect of age on leucine-induced insulin secretion by the beta-cell. J. Gerontol. *35*, 324–328.

Reggi, M. L. (1975): Environmental temperature, X-irradiation and ageing in insects. Exp. Gerontol. *10*, 333–340.

Reshef, L., Hanson, R. W. (1972): The interaction of catecholamines and adrenal corticosteroids in the induction of phosphopyruvate carboxylase. Biochem. J. *127*, 807–818.

Resseguie, L. J. (1976): Parental age, stillbirths and mutation. Ann. Hum. Genet. *40*, 213–219.

Retzlaff, E., Fontaine, J., Futura, W. (1966): Effect of daily exercise on lifespan of albino rats. Geriatrics *21*, 171–177.

Riegle, G. D. (1976): Aging and adrenocortical function. In: Hypothalamus, Pituitary and Aging (Everitt, A. V., ed.), pp. 547–553. Springfield, Ill.: Charles C Thomas.

Riegle, G. D., Meites, J., Miller, A. E., Wood, S. M. (1977): Effect of aging on hypothalamic LH-releasing and prolactin-inhibiting activities and pituitary responsiveness to LHRH in the male laboratory rats. J. Gerontol. *32*, 13–18.

Rigby, B. L., Mitchel, T. W., Robinson, M. S. (1977): Oxygen participation in the in vivo and in vitro aging of collagen fibres. Biochem. Biophys. Res. Commun. *79*, 400–405.

Rockstein, M. (1974): Genetic bases for longevity. In: Theoretical Aspects of Aging. New York: Raven Press.

Rockstein, M., Chesky, J. A., Sussman, M. L. (1977): Comparative biology and evolution of aging. In: Handbook of the Biology of Aging (Finch, C. E., Hayflick, L., eds.), pp. 3–34. New York: Van Nostrand Reinhold.

Rocta, G., Chappel, C., Balasz, T., Gaudry, R. (1959): An infarctive myocardial lesion and other toxic manifestations produced by isoproterenol. Arch. Pathol. *67*, 443–455.

Rogova, A. N., Khilko, O. K. (1971): Age-induced peculiarities of the reaction of the cholino-receptors of protein in the cerebral cortex and cerebellum to acetylcholine action. In: Aging of a Cell, pp. 199–204. Kiev: Institute of Gerontology. (In Russian.)

Roitbak, A. B. (1969): Hypothesis of the mechanism of the formation of temporary links when the conditioned reflex is being produced. Doklady Akad. Nauk SSSR *187*, 1205–1208.

Rosenberg, R. S., Zepelin, H., Rechtschaffen, A. (1979): Sleep in young and old rats. J. Gerontol. *34*, 525–532.

Ross, M. H. (1961): Length of life and nutrition in the rat. J. Nutr. *75*, 197–210.

Ross, M. H. (1969): Aging, nutrition and hepatic enzymes activity patterns in the rat. J. Nutr. *97*, Suppl. 1, part II, 563–602.

Ross, M. H., Bras, G. (1974): Dietary preference and diseases of age. Nature *250*, 263–265.

Rost, G. (1967): Der orale 50-g-Glukosetoleranztest zur Labordiagnostik des Diabetes mellitus. Bewertung und Altersverlauf. Z. inn. Med. *22*, 709–714.

Roth, G. (1979): Hormone receptor changes during adulthood and senescence: significance for aging research. Federat. Proc. *5*, 1910–1914.

Roth, G. S. (1976): Reduced glucocorticoid binding site concentration in cortical neuronal perikarya from senescent rats. Brain Res. *107*, 345–354.

Roth, G. S., Livingston, J. N. (1976): Reductions in glucocorticoid inhibition of glucose oxidation and presumptive glucocorticoid receptor content in rat adipocytes during aging. Endocrinology *99*, 831–852.

Rowlatt, C. (1972): Cellular aging: problem of interpretation. In: Ninth International Congress of Gerontology, Vol. 1, pp. 30–33. Kiev: Institute of Gerontology.

Rozanova, V. D., Surovtseva, Z. S., Siryk, L. A. (1978): Differences in the inductive effect of small doses of phenobarbital in rats in conformity with age and sex. Farmakol. i toxikol. *61*, 1, 40–44.

Rubachev, P. G. (1978): DNA reparation under the action of modifying factors. In: Results of Science and Technology. General Genetics Series, Vol. 4: Biological Systems of DNA Reparation in Eucaryotes, pp. 184–209. Moscow: Nauka. (In Russian.)

Rubio, R., Berne, R. M., Dobson, I. (1973): Sites of adenosine production in cardiac and skeletal muscle. Amer. J. Physiol. *225*, 938–953.

Rubner, M. (1902): Die Gesetze des Energieverbrauches bei der Ernährung. Leipzig-Wien.

Rubner, M. (1908a): Das Problem der Lebensdauer und seine Beziehungen zu Wachstum und Ernährung. München-Berlin: Akademie-Verlag.

Rubner, M. (1908b): Problem des Wachstums und der Lebensdauer. Mitt. Ges. Inn. Med. *7*, 58–72. Universität Wien.

Rushkevich, Yu. E. (1980): Influence of prolonged hypothalamic stimulation on some parameters of the cardiovascular system in animals of different age. Fiziol. zhurn. *26*, 3–9.

Sacher, G. A. (1959): Relation of life span to brain weight and body weight in mammals. In: Ciba Foundation Colloquia on Ageing, pp. 115–133. London: Churchill.

Sacher, G. A. (1975): Maturation and longevity in relation to cranial capacity in hominid evolution. In: Primate Functional Morphology and Evolution, pp. 417–441. The Hague: Mouton Publ.

Sacher, G. A. (1977): Life table modification and life prolongation. In: Handbook of the Biology of Aging (Finch, C. E., Hayflick, L., eds.), pp. 582–638. New York: Van Nostrand Reinhold.

Sacher, G. A. (1978): Longevity and aging in vertebrate evolution. BioScience *28*, 497–501.

Sachs, E. S., Yahoda, M. G. I., Neirmeiyer, M. F., Galyaard, H. (1977): An unexpected high frequency of trisomic fetuses in 229 pregnancies monitored for advanced maternal age. Hum. Genet. *36*, 43–46.

Sakai, K. (1980): Coronary vasoconstriction by locally administered acetylcholine, carbachol and bethanechol in isolated donor-perfused rat heart. Brit. J. Pharmacol. *68*, 625–632.

Salganik, R. I. (1972): Hormonal regulation of transcription. In: Mechanisms of the Regulation of the Functions of the Cellular Nucleus, pp. 101–102. Tbilisi: Metsniereba. (In Russian.)

Samorajski, T., Ordy, J. M. (1977): Neurochemistry of aging. In: Aging and the Brain, pp. 41–61. New York: Plenum Press.

Sato, F., Tsuchihashi, S., Kawashima, N. (1973): Life-shortening of mice by whole or partial body X-irradiation. Radiation Res. *14*, 115.

Sawin-Clark, T., Deepak, C., Fereidonn, A., Ellen, M., Pamela, B. (1979): The aging thyroid. JAMA *242*, 247–250.

Sazonova, Ye. A. (1959): On the nature of the age changes in the oxidative processes in the tissues. Age changes in the activity of the succinoxidase and succindehydrase of the liver. Ukr. biokhim. zhurn. *31*, 523–532.

Schacthord, G. (1949): The attractions of proteins for small molecules and ions. Ann. N. Y. Acad. Sci. *51*, 660–672.

Scharrer, E., Scharrer, B. (1963): Neurosekretion. In: Bergman-Mollendorffs Handb. der mikroskop. Anat. d. Menschen *5*, 953–1066.

Schmidt, M. J., Thornberry, J. F. (1978): Cyclic AMP and cyclic GMP accumulation in vitro in brain regions of young, old and aged rats. Brain Res. *199*, 169–177.

Schmukler, M., Barrows, C. (1966): Age differences in lactic and malic dehydrogenases in the rat. J. Gerontol. *21*, 109–114.

Schneider, E. L., Kram, D., Nakanishi, Y., Miticone, R. E., Gilman, B. A., Nieder, M. L., Tice, R. R. (1979): The effect of aging on sister chromatid exchange. Mech. Ageing Develop. *9*, 303–312.

Schneider, H. (1971): Untersuchungen über die Bezeichnungen der postprandialen Glukosetoleranzminderung im Alter. Z. inn. Med. *26*, 592–596.

Schonfeldt, L., Owens, W. (1966): Age and intellectual change: a cross-sectional view of longitudinal data. In: 18th International Psychological Congress, Vol. 29, pp. 25–30. Moscow: Nauka. (In Russian.)

Schrader, J., Gerlach, E. (1976): Compartmentation of cardial adenine nucleotides and formation of adenosine. Pflügers Arch. *367*, 129–135.

Schroeder, H. A., Vinton, W. H., Balassa, J. J. (1963): Effect of chromium, cadmium and other trod metals on the growth and survival of mice. J. Nutr. *80*, 39–47.

Schroeder, H. A., Mitchener, M. (1971): Scandium, chromium (VI), gallium, itterium, rhodium, palladium, indium in mice: effect on growth and life span. J. Nutr. *101*, 1431–1438.

Schwartz, A. G., Moore, G. J. (1978): Inverse correlation between species life span and capacity to metabolize polycyclic hydrocarbon carcinogens. In: Gerontological Society, 31th Annual Scientific Meeting, 121.

Schwegler, M., Jacob, R. (1976): Catecholamine antagonism of acetylcholine and dibutyryl guanosine-3'5-monophosphate in mammalian ventricular myocardium. In: Recent Advances in Studies on Cardiac Structure and Metabolism, pp. 391–399. Baltimore: Univ. Park Press.

Segall, P. E., Timiras, P. S. (1975): Age-related changes in thermoregulatory capacity of tryptophan-deficient rats. Fed. Proc. Fed. Amer. Socs. Exp. Biol. *34*, 83–85.

Segall, P. N. (1977): Long-term tryptophan restriction and aging in the rat. Actuel. Gerontol. *7*, 535–538.

Segall, P. N. (1979): Interrelations of dietary and hormonal effects in aging. Mech. Ageing Develop. *9*, 515–527.

Selye, H. (1952): The Story of Adaptation Syndrome. Montreal: University.

Sergeev, P. V., Seifulla, R. D., Maisky, A. M. (1971): Molecular Aspects of the Action of Steroid Hormones. Moscow: Nauka. (In Russian.)

Shabanova, N. A., Amiri, A. (1975): Influence of thyroxine on the activity of fructose biphosphate aldolase in the liver and kidneys of rats in ontogenesis. In: Molecular and Physiological Mechanisms of Aging, pp. 265–270. Kiev: Naukova Dumka. (In Russian.)

Shagzh, Zh. (1971): On the Analysis of Some Factors which Determine the Potential Life Span of Mammals (and Man). Author's abstract of the dissertation for a candidate's degree (biology). Moscow: State University. (In Russian.)

Sharin, N. I., Podoplanova, I. I., Kovaleva, A. M. (1978): Influence of prolonged hypothermia on the viability of the cellular cultures. In: Artificially Increasing the Life Span. First Symposium, p. 20. Moscow: Institute of General Genetics. (In Russian.)

Sharma, S. P., Ratton, S., Sharma, G. (1979): Temperature dependent longevity of *Zabrotes subfasciatus beh (coleoptera, bruchidae).* Comp. Physiol. Ecol. *4*, 229–231.

Shaw, R. F., Bercaw, B. L. (1962): Temperature and life span in poikilothermous animals. Nature *196*, 454–457.

Shchegoleva, I. V. (1962): On a change in the sensitivity of the carotid sinus when the organism ages. Byull. exper. biol. *8*, 37–40.

Shershevsky, N. A. (1940): Old age and the endocrine system. In: Old Age, pp. 31–40. Kiev: Publishing House of the Academy of Sciences of Ukrainian SSR. (In Russian.)

Shevchuk, I. A. (1963): Morphological and histochemical indices of the aging of the human pancreas. In: Mechanisms of Aging, pp. 439–443. Kiev: Institute of Gerontology. (In Russian.)

Shevchuk, V. G. (1966): Age specifics of the reflex regulation of blood sugar. In: Regulation of the Functions During Various Age Periods, pp. 238–240. Kiev: Institute of Gerontology. (In Russian.)

Shevchuk, V. G. (1971): Age-induced peculiarities of the reaction of cholinoreceptors in the heart to acetylcholine and atropine. In: Aging of a Cell, pp. 214–221. Kiev: Institute of Gerontology. (In Russian.)

Shevchuk, V. G. (1973): Influence of acetylcholine and catecholamines on hemodynamics at various stages of ontogenesis. Vestn. Akadem. Med. Nauk SSSR *12*, 52–55.

Shevchuk, V. G. (1977): Age-related peculiarities of the insulin effect on the cardiovascular system. In: Insulin Provision in Old Age, pp. 84–88. Kiev: Institute of Gerontology. (In Russian.)

Shevchuk, V. G. (1979): Age specifics of the reflexes of the heart. Fiziol. zhurn. *1*, 16–22.

Sheveleva, V. S. (1977): Evolution of the Functions of the Sympathetic Ganglia in Ontogenesis. Leningrad: Nauka. (In Russian.)

Shima, A., Nikaido, O., Shinohara, S., Egami, N. (1980): Continued in vitro growth of fibroblast-like cells (RBCF-1) derived from the caudal fin of the fish *Carassius Auratus*. Exp. Gerontol. *15*, 305–314.

Shimizu, Y., Kibata, M., Shoji, K., Miyahara, K., Kimura, I. (1978): Early insulin secretion after small doses of intravenous administration of glucose in aged. In: 11th International Congress of Gerontology, Vol. 3, p. 108. Tokyo: Scimed Publications, Inc.

Shkhvatsabaya, I. K., Nekrasova, A. A. (1977): The biologically active substances called prostaglandins and quinines; their role in the regulation of arterial pressure and the development of arterial hypertension. Kardiologiya *17*, 136–145.

Shmalgauzen, I. I. (1926): The Problem of Death and Immortality. Moscow: Vremya. (In Russian.)

Shmalgauzen, I. I. (1968): Factors of Evolution, p. 452. Moscow: Nauka. (In Russian.)

Shock, N., Andres, R. (1968): Adaptive responses to glucose in elderly males. In: Adaptive Capacities of an Aging Organism, 269–280. Kiev: Institute of Gerontology. (In Russian.)

Shvarts, A. S. (1976): Ecological approaches to the analysis of the processes of aging and a change in the life span. In: Biological Possibilities of Life Span Prolongation, pp. 19–29. Kiev: Institute of Gerontology. (In Russian.)

Sichinava, G. N. (1963): Some data on the state of the cardiovascular system in long-living persons. In: Mechanisms of Aging, pp. 379–385. Kiev: Institute of Gerontology. (In Russian.)

Sichinava, G. N. (1972): Long-term observations on health of longevous people. In: Ninth International Congress of Gerontology, Vol. 3, p. 392. Kiev: Institute of Gerontology.

Silva, J., Kaplan, M., Cheron, R., Dick, T., Larsen, P. (1978): Thyroxine to 3,5,3′-triiodothyronine conversion by rat anterior pituitary and liver. Metabolism *11*, 1601–1607.

Sincock, A. (1974): Calcium and aging in the rotifer *Mytilina brevispina var redunca*. J. Gerontol. *29*, 514–517.

Sincock, A. (1975): Life extension in the rotifer *Mytilina brevispina var redunca* by the application of chelatous agents. J. Gerontol. *30*, 289–293.

Sineok, L. L. (1975): Acid-base equilibrium and its change with age under the influence of various effects. In: Gerontology and Geriatrics (yearbook), pp. 96–99. Kiev: Institute of Gerontology. (In Russian.)

Singh, S. N. (1973): Effect of age on the activity and citrate inhibition of malate dehydrogenase of the brain and heart of rats. Experientia *29*, 42–43.

Sinitsky, V. N. (1976): Convulsive Readiness and the Mechanisms of Epileptic Seizures. Kiev: Naukova Dumka. (In Russian.)

Skok, V. I. (1970): Physiology of Autonomic Ganglia. Leningrad: Nauka. (In Russian.)

Slotkin, T. A. (1974): Reserpine. In: Neuropoisons. Pathophysiological Actions, Vol. 2, pp. 1–60. New York-London: Academic Press.

Smith, M. (1958): The effect of temperature and of egg-laying on the longevity of *Drosophila subobscura*. J. Exp. Biol. *35*, 832–842.

Smith-Sonneborn, J. (1979): DNA repair and longevity assurance in *Paramecium tetraurelia*. Science *203*, 1115–1117.

Smith-Sonneborn, J., Reed, J. (1976): Calendar life span versus fission life span of *Paramecium aurelia*. J. Gerontol. *31*, 2–7.

Smolyansky, B. A. (1965): Specifics of carbohydrate metabolism with respect to the aging processes. In: Questions of Gerontology and Geriatrics, pp. 73–75. Leningrad: Nauka. (In Russian.)

Soerjodibroto, W. S., Heard, C. R. C., Exton-Smith, A. N. (1979): Glucose tolerance, plasma insulin sensitivity in elderly patients. Age and Aging *8*, 65–74.

Sohal, R. S., Donato, H. (1979): Effect of experimental prolongation of life span on lipofuscin content and lysosomal enzyme activity in the brain of the housefly, *Musca domestica*. J. Gerontol. *14*, 489–496.

Solomatin, S. S. (1970): Rest potentials of the hepatic cells and the skeletal muscle fibres of mammals during different age periods. Zhurn. evol. biokhim. i fiziol. *3*, 345–347.

Soloveichik, D. I. (1938): Disturbance of higher nervous activity when old age begins. In: Works of the Pavlov Physiological Laboratory, Vol. 8, pp. 427–444. Leningrad: Academy of Sciences of the USSR. (In Russian.)

Sondhi, K. C. (1967): Studies in ageing. VII. Integration of genotypes, homeostasis and the expression of ageing processes in *Drosophila*. Exp. Gerontol. *2*, 241–248.

Sondhi, K. S. (1970): Studies in ageing. IX. Brain transplantation in *Drosophila*. Exp. Gerontol. *5*, 77–81.

Sousa, B., Baskin, S. (1977): Na$^+$, K$^+$-ATPase in the central nervous system during aging. In: Gerontological Society, 30th Annual Scientific Meeting, p. 54. San Francisco: Columbia University Press.

Sperling, G. A., Loosli, J. K., McCay, C. M. (1978): Effect of sulfamerazine and exercise on lifespan of rats and hamsters. Gerontology *24*, 220–224.

Stanton, H. C., Brenner, G., Mayfield, E. (1969): Studies on isoproterenol-induced cardiomegaly in rats. Amer. Heart J. *77*, 72–80.

Staroseltseva, L. K. (1976): Hormones of the pancreas. In: Biochemistry of the Hormones and Hormonal Regulation, pp. 93–122. Moscow: Meditsina. (In Russian.)

Stepanov, S. A. (1974): Morphological changes in the anterior hypothalamus in old age and in the case of atherosclerosis and hypertension. In: First All-Union Conference on Neuroendocrinology, pp. 167–168. Leningrad: Nauka. (In Russian.)

Storer, J. B. (1967): Relation of lifespan to brain weight, body weight, and metabolic rate among inbred mouse strains. Exp. Gerontol. *2*, 173–182.

Strandell, T. (1964): Circulatory studies on healthy old men with special reference to the limitation of the maximal working capacity. Acta med. Scand. *175*, Suppl. 414, 44–58.

Strazhesko, N. D. (1939): On the specifics of the occurrence and manifestation of diseases in old persons. In: Old Age, pp. 19–29. Kiev: Publishing House of the Academy of Sciences of the Ukrainian SSR. (In Russian.)

Strehler, B. (1977): Genetic and neural aspects of redundancy and aging. In: 5th European Symposium on Basic Research in Gerontology, pp. 36–61. Erlangen: Perimed Verlag.

Strehler, B., Hirsch, G., Yohrkson, R. (1971): Codon restriction theory of aging and development. J. Theror. Biol. *33*, 429–474.

Strehler, B. L. (1961): Studies on the comparative physiology of aging. II. On the mechanism of temperature life-shortening in *Drosophila melanogaster*. J. Gerontol. *16*, 2–12.

Strehler, B. L., Chang, M.-P. (1979): Loss of hybridizable ribosomal DNA from human post-mitotic tissues during aging. II. Age-dependent loss in human cerebral cortex–hippocampal and Somatosen–sory cortex comparison. Mech. Ageing Develop. *11*, 379–384.

Stuchlikova, E., Juricova-Horacova, M., Deyl, Z. (1975): New aspects of the dietary effects of life prolongation in rodents: what is the role of obesity in aging? Exp. Gerontol. *10*, 141–144.

Stulnikov, B. V. (1973): Role of the lateral and ventromedial parts of the hypothalamus in regulating insulin secretion. Byull. exper. biol. *10*, 3–6.

Stupina, A. S. (1978): Functional significance of the structural and ultrastructural changes in myocardial blood capillaries in late ontogenesis. Fiziol. zhurn. *24*, 358–365.

Stupina, A. S., Shaposhnikov, V. M. (1977): Ultrastructural changes in insulocytes in aging. In: Insulin Provision in Old Age, pp. 45–52. Kiev: Institute of Gerontology. (In Russian.)

Sturrock, R. R. (1977): Quantitative and morphological changes in neurons and neuroglia in the indusium griseum of aging mice. J. Gerontol. *32*, 647–658.

Surikov, P. M., Marakhovsky, Yu. K., Balakleevsky, A. I. (1976): Metabolism of cyclic AMP of some tissues in ontogenesis. In: Third All-Union Congress of Gerontologists and Geriatricians. Theses and Abstracts of Reports, p. 193. Kiev: Institute of Gerontology. (In Russian.)

Suyma, J., Iwasaki, T. (1976): Radiation-induced lifespan shortening of artemia under different temperature conditions. Exp. Gerontol. *11*, 133–140.

Suzuki, K., Hyodo, M., Ishii, H., Morila, J. (1978): A strain of nematode for aging research. In: Proceedings of 11th International Congress of Gerontology, Abstracts, p. 15. Tokyo: Scimed Publications, Inc.

Tallarido, G., Semprium, A. (1973): Reflex cardiovasculatory and respiratory responses caused by injection of bradykinin in the femoral and carotid circulatory areas. Boll. Soc. Ital. Biol. Sperim. *49*, 79–84.

Tanaka, R., Matsuyama, T., Sawazaki, N., Ota, T., Oka, N., Tanaka, A., Shima, K., Tarni, S., Kamahara, Y. (1978): Influence of age on pancreatic alpha and beta cell functions in rat. In: 11th International Congress of Gerontology, pp. 54–55. Tokyo: Scimed Publications, Inc.

Tang, F., Phillips, I. G. (1978): Some age-related changes in pituitary-adrenal function in the male laboratory rat. J. Gerontol. *33*, 377–382.

Tanin, S. A. (1971): Age Specifics of the Regulation Levels of Motor Reactions. Author's abstract of the dissertation for a doctor's degree (medicine). Kiev: Medical Institute. (In Russian.)

Tanin, S. A. (1976): On the characterization of the functional properties of the motoneurons of the spinal cord of old rats. Byull. exper. biol. *82*, 911–913.

Tanin, S. A. (1977): Effect of hormones stimulating protein biosynthesis on polarization of neurons of the spinal cord in rats of different age. In: Genetic Mechanisms of Aging and Longevity, pp. 90–93. Kiev: Institute of Gerontology. (In Russian.)

Tauchi, H., Hasegawa, K. (1977): Change of the hepatic cells in parabiosis between old and young rats. Mech. Ageing Develop. *6*, 333–339.

Tereshchenko, O. Ya. (1978): Reparation and aging. In: General Genetics, pp. 210–246. Moscow: All-Union Institute of Scientific and Technical Information. (In Russian.)

Tikhonov, V. Kh., Valeeva, R. M., Mezentsev, A. N. (1973): Influence of Na$^+$ and K$^+$ on the inclusion of amino acids in the proteins of the sections of the cerebral cortex of rats. Ukr. biokhim. zhurn. *45*, 116–121.

Timchenko, A. N. (1972): Age specifics of the miniature potentials of the end plate of the muscle fibres. In: Ninth Congress of the Ukrainian Physiological Society, Zaporozhye, p. 18. Kiev: Naukova Dumka. (In Ukrainian.)

Timko, N. A. (1971): Effect of experimental ischemia on rate excitement propagation in motor axons of the peripheral nerve in elderly and old persons. In: Aging of a Cell, pp. 184–195. Kiev: Institute of Gerontology. (In Russian.)

Tkachenko, B. I., Polenov, S. A., Agnaev, A. K. (1975): Cardiovascular Reflexes. Leningrad: Meditsina. (In Russian.)

Tokar, A. V. (1977): Arterial Hypertension and Age. Kiev: Zdorovya. (In Russian.)

Tokin, B. A. (1972): On the Death of Protozoans. In: Adaptation of the Aging Organism, pp. 79–90. Kiev: Institute of Gerontology. (In Russian.)

Tonkikh, A. V. (1912): On the question of conditioned reflexes in an old dog. In: Works of the Russian Doctor's Society, pp. 1745–1746. St. Petersburg: Znanie. (In Russian.)

Travis, D. F., Travis, A. (1972): Ultrastructural changes in the left ventricular rat mitochondrial cells with age. J. Ultrastruct. Res. *39*, 124–148.

Trendelenburg, U. (1976): Mechanism of action of drugs acting on sympathetic nerve endings. Acta endocrinol. *82*, Suppl. 202, 18–19.

Tretyak, T. M., Vilenchik, M. M., Smirnova, G. S. (1977): Age specifics of the synthesis of the DNA of the rat brain when tritiated thymidine is administered intraperitoneally. In: Physiology and Biochemistry of Ontogenesis, pp. 136–139. Leningrad: Nauka. (In Russian.)

Tribe, M. A., Ashhurst, D. E. (1972): Biochemical and structural variations in the flight muscle mitochondria of aging bowflies, *Calliphora erythrocephala*. J. Cell Sci. *10*, 443–469.

Trout, W. E., Kaplan, W. D. (1970): A relation between longevity, metabolism rate and activity in shaker mutants of *Drosophila melanogaster*. Exp. Gerontol. *5*, 83–92.

Tsipriyan, V. I. (1969): Influence of Fluorine of Drinking Water on the Age Changes in the Regulation Processes. Author's abstract of the dissertation for a candidate's degree. Kiev: Medical Institute. (In Russian.)

Turaeva, N. M. (1978): Specifics of the adrenergic influences on the electric properties of individual muscle cells in animals of different age. Fiziol. zhurn. *2*, 224–228.

Turaeva, N. M. (1979): Adrenergic Influences on the Electric Properties of the Muscle and Hepatic Cells in Animals of Different Age. Author's abstract of the dissertation for a candidate's degree (medicine). Kiev: Medical Institute. (In Russian.)

Turpaev, T. M. (1962): Mediatory Function of Acetylcholine and the Nature of the Cholinoreceptor. Moscow: Publishing House of the USSR Academy of Sciences. (In Russian.)

Tuttle, R. S. (1966): Age-related changes in the sensitivity of rat aortic strips to norepinephrine and associated chemical and structural alteration. J. Gerontol. *21*, 510–516.

Udelnov, M. G. (1975): Cardiac Physiology. Moscow: Publishing House of the Moscow State University. (In Russian.)

Udelnov, M. G., Yasinovskaya, F. P. (1969): On adequate stimulation for the mechanoreceptors of the auricles. Fiziol. zhurn. SSSR *55*, 321–332.

Utevsky, A. M. (1967): Catecholamines as the regulatory and biocatalytic factors in the general system of biogenic amines. In: Biogenic Amines, pp. 286–287. Moscow: Meditsina. (In Russian.)

Uzbekov, G. A. (1967): Stage (phase) changes of respiration and oxidative phosphorylation in brain hemispheres of animals in the postnatal period. Byull. exper. biol. *43*, 52–54.

Valueva, G. V. (1978): The role of extra- and intracellular factors in the age changes of the metabolism of the thyroid hormones. Fiziol. zhurn. *4*, 18–23.

Valueva, G. V., Verzhikovskaya, N. V. (1977): Thyrotropic activity of hypophysis during aging. Exp. Gerontol. *12*, 97–105.

Vanyushin, B. F., Nemirovsky, L. E., Klimenko, V., Vasiliev, V. K., Belozersky, A. N. (1973): The 5-methylcytosine in DNA of rat tissue and age specificity and the change induced by hydrocortisone and other agents. Gerontologia *19*, 138–192.

Vanyushin, B. F., Berdyshev, G. D. (1977): Molecular and Genetic Mechanisms of Aging. Moscow: Meditsina. (In Russian.)

Vasyukova, Ye. A., Zefirova, G. S., Smirnova, O. I. (1979): Age disturbance of glucose tolerance and diabetes mellitus. Fiziologiya cheloveka *2*, 203–207.

Venkstern, T. V. (1976): Biosynthesis of transport ribonucleic acids. In: Successes of Biological Chemistry, Vol. 17, pp. 3–25. Moscow: Nauka. (In Russian.)

Verkhratsky, N. S. (1962): Age specifics of the sensitivity of the vessels to humoral factors. In: Questions of Gerontology and Geriatrics, pp. 50–55. Kiev: Gosmedizdat. (In Russian.)

Verkhratsky, N. S. (1970): Acetylcholine metabolism peculiarities in aging. Exp. Gerontol. *5*, 49–56.

Verkhratsky, N. S. (1971): Mediator metabolism and the reaction of the effectors to cholinergic and adrenergic influences in old age. Author's abstract of the dissertation for a doctor's degree (medicine). Kiev: Institute of Physiology. (In Russian.)

Verkhratsky, N. S. (1972): Noradrenaline metabolism and the reaction of the effectors to adrenergic influences in old age. In: Ninth Congress of the Ukrainian Physiological Society, pp. 69–70. Zaporozhye: Medical Institute. (In Russian.)

Verkhratsky, N. S. (1977): Age specifics of the influence of noradrenaline on protein biosynthesis. In: Genetic Mechsnisms of Aging and Longevity, pp. 81–86. Kiev: Institute of Gerontology. (In Russian.)

Verkhratsky, N. S. (1978): Specifics of the influence of acetylcholine on protein biosynthesis in the parts of the heart of adult and old rats. Voprosy med. khimii *24*, 648–652.

Vernadakis, A. (1975): Neuronal-glial interactions during development and aging. Fed. Proc. Fed. Amer. Socs. Exp. Biol. *34*, 89–95.

Verzar, F. (1963): Lectures on Experimental Gerontology. Springfield, Ill.: Charles C Thomas.

Verzar, F. (1968): Aging of macromolecules. In: Adaptive Capacities of an Aging Organism, pp. 93–105. Kiev: Institute of Gerontology. (In Russian.)

Verzar, F. (1972): Regulation of the adaptive processes in the mechanism of aging. In: Ninth International Congress of Geronotology, Vol. 1, pp. 40–45. Kiev: Institute of Gerontology.

Verzhikovskaya, N. V. (1971): The Thyroid Gland and Age. Dissertation for a doctor's degree (medicine). Kiev: Medical Institute. (In Russian.)

Verzhikovskaya, N. V., Valujeva, G. V. (1977): Thyrotropic activity of hypophysis during aging. Exp. Gerontol. *12*, 97–105.

Verzhikovskaya, N. V., Valueva, G. V., Sabolch, I. V. (1978): Age specifics of the deiodization of thyroxine and the extrathyroidal formation of triiodothyronine and reverse triiodothyronine. In: Questions of Gerontology, pp. 43–49. Kiev: Institute of Gerontology. (In Russian.)

Vichert, A. M. (1977): Some aspects of the etiology and pathogenesis of atherosclerosis. Med. red. zhurn. *1*, 11, 25–31.

Vilenchik, M. M. (1970): Molecular Mechanisms of Aging. Moscow: Nauka. (In Russian.)

Vilenchik, M. M. (1976): Instability of the gene under physiological conditions: biophysical, molecular, genetic and gerontological aspects. Usp. sovrem. biol. *82*, 371–386.

Virkkunen, P., Lybeck, H., Ranta, T., Leppabuoto, Y. (1974): A serum factor influencing the physiological activity of thyrotropin-releasing hormone (TRH). II. Studies with rat serum in vivo and in vitro. Acta physiol. Scand. *92*, 526–529.

Vlk, Y., Tucek, S. (1964): The formation of acetylcholine in isolated heart auricles of white rats and guinea pigs. Physiol. Bohemoslov. *13*, 310–314.

Voitenko, V. P., Bogush, S. V. (1969): Age specifics of the influence of insulin and adrenaline on the content of nicotinamide adenine nucleotides (NAN) in the liver. In: Documents of the

Ninth Scientific Conference on Age Morphology, Physiology and Biochemistry, Vol. 2, part 1, pp. 152–153. Moscow: Institute of Age Physiology. (In Russian.)

Voitkevich, A. A. (1963): Change in the thyrotropic properties of the hypophysis of amphibians in ontogenesis and after the extirpation of the preoptic region of diencephalon. Doklady Akad. Nauk SSSR *150*, 221–224.

Voronkov, G. S. (1975): Age Specifics of the Content of Adrenaline and Noradrenaline in the Blood and Urine and Some Aspects of their Metabolism During Various Functional States of the Organism. Author's abstract of the dissertation for a candidate's degree (medicine). Kiev: Medical Institute. (In Russian.)

Wagner, H., Zierden, E., Wessals, R., Mollmann, H. (1977): Zur Alternsabhängigkeit von Kohlenhydrattoleranz und Insulinsekretion. Aktuelle Gerontologie *7*, 405–411.

Watkins, B. E., Meites, J., Riegle, G. D. (1975): Age-related changes in pituitary responsiveness to LHRH in the female rat. Endocrinology *97*, 543–548.

Wechsler, D. (1961): Intelligence, memory and the aging process. In: Psychopathology of Aging (Hoch, H. P., Lubin, J., eds.), pp. 275–291. New York: Raven Press.

Weeke, Y. (1973): Circadian variation of the serum thyrotropin level in normal subjects. Scand. J. Clin. Lab. Invest. *31*, 337–342.

Weinbach, E. C., Garbus, I. (1956): Age and oxidative phosphorylation in rat liver and brain. Nature *178*, 1225–1226.

Weindruch, R. H., Cheung, M. K., Verity, M. A., Walford, R. L. (1980): Modification of mitochondrial respiration by aging and dietary restriction. Mech. Ageing Develop. *12*, 375–392.

Weismann, A. (1882): Über die Dauer des Lebens. Jena.

Weismann, A. (1889): Über die Dauer des Lebens. Jena.

Weiss, B., Greenberg, L., Cantor, E. (1979): Age-related alterations in the development of adrenergic denervation supersensitivity. Fed. Proc. *5*, 1915–1920.

Weiss, P. A. (1944): Damming of axoplasm in constricted nerve: a sign of perpetual growth in nerve fibers. Anat. Res. *88*, 48–52.

Weniger, P., Warara, E., Dolejs, J. (1979): Die Wirkung von Hyperthermic auf DNA-Reparaturvorgänge. Radiat. and Environm. Biophys. *16*, 135–141.

Wenzel, K., Memhold, M., Herpich, F. (1974): TRH-Stimulationstest mit Älteren und Geschlechtsabhängigen. TSH-Anstieg bei Normalperson. Klin. Wschr. *52*, 722–727.

Wexler, B. S. (1979): Carotid artery ligation-induced cerebral ischemia in old, male, Sprague-Dawley rats. Age *2*, 39–43.

Wilkes, M., Finch, C., Bonner, Z. (1978): Selective changes during aging in the content of pituitary protein species in mouse. In: 11th International Congress of Gerontology, pp. 39–41. Tokyo: Scimed Publications, Inc.

Williams, G. C. (1957): Pleotropy, natural selection and the evolution of senescence. Evolution *11*, 398–411.

Wilson, D. L. (1974): The Programmed Theory of Aging. London: Academic Press,

Wilson, P. D., Franks, L. M. (1975): The effect of age on mitochondrial ultrastructure and enzyme cytochemistry. Biochem. Soc. Trans. *3*, 126–128.

Winokur, A., Utiger, R. (1974): Thyrotropin-releasing hormone: regional distribution in the rat brain. Science *185*, 265–267.

Wise, A. J., Gross, M. A., Schalch, D. S. (1973): Quantitative relationship of the pituitary gonadal axis in post-menopausal women. J. Lab. Clin. Med. *4*, 81–82.

Woodruff, L. L. (1929): Thirteen thousand generations of paramecium. Proc. Soc. Exp. Biol. *26*, 707–708.

Wool, I. G. (1960): Incorporation of C^{14}-amino acids into protein of isolated diaphragms. Amer. J. Physiol. *198*, 54–56.

Wright, W. E., Hayflick, L. (1975): Nuclear control of cellular aging demonstrated by hybridization of anucleate and whole cultured normal human fibroblasts. Exp. Cell Res. *96*, 113–121.

Yankovskaya, A. S., Podrushnyak, Ye. P. (1979): Human Muscle System During Aging. Kiev: Zdorovye. (In Russian.)

Yarkin, G. A. (1977): Influence of the stimulation of the preganglionic trunk of *Ganglion cervicale superius* on the automatic activity of its neurons. In: Physiology and Biochemistry of Ontogenesis, pp. 41–45. Leningrad: Nauka. (In Russian.)

Yarovaya, G. A., Dotsenko, V. L., Krizhevskaya, Yu. V., Morozova, N. A., Orekhovich, V. N. (1979): Activation of the prekallikrein of the human blood serum by various activating agents. Biokhimiya *44*, 7, 1279–1285.

Yefimov, A. S., Povolotskaya, G. M., Slavnov, V. N. (1973): Diabetes mellitus and age. Sov. med. *12*, 21–26.

Yekhneva, T. L. (1976): Age specifics of the immune response of rats when various doses of the ram erythrocytes are administered many times. Byull. exper. biol. i. med. *81*, 572–574.

Yudeleva, I. V. (1977): Experimental investigations of the possibility of using tetracycline for increasing the species lifespan of organisms. In: Questions of Genetics and the Biosphere, pp. 33–34. Moscow: Nauka. (In Russian.)

Yuhas, J. M. (1969): The dose response curve for radiation-induced life shortening. J. Gerontol. *24*, 451–456.

Yuhas, J. M. (1971): Age and susceptibility of reduction in life expectancy: an analysis of proposed mechanisms. Exp. Gerontol. *6*, 335–343.

Zaichenko, A. P. (1977): Autoimmune responses of humoral and cellular types to antigens of the pancreatic gland and insulin in subjects of different Age. In: Insulin Provision in Old Age, pp. 60–66. Kiev: Institute of Gerontology. (In Russian.)

Zamostyan, V. P. (1963): On the age specifics of the influence of adrenaline on the trophism of the skeletal muscles. In: Mechanisms of Aging, pp. 177–183. Kiev: Institute of Gerontology. (In Russian.)

Zamostyan, V. P. (1964): Age Specific of Neurohumoral Regulation of the Trophism of the Skeletal Muscles. Author's abstract of the dissertation for a candidate's degree (medicine). Kiev: Institute of Physiology. (In Russian.)

Zamostyan, V. P. (1971): On the mechanisms of maintaining long muscular working ability in animals of different age. In: First Byelorussian Conference on Gerontology and Geriatrics, pp. 129–130. Minsk: Nauka i Tekhnika. (In Russian.)

Zavadovsky, M. M. (1931): Contradictory Relationship in the Body of a Developing Animal. Moscow: Moscow State University Publishing House. (In Russian.)

Zerkal, V. P., Nikitin, V. N. (1979): Age changes in the content of prostaglandins in the organs of white rats. Doklady Akad. Nauk Ukr. SSR *5* (biology series), 374–377.

Zhinkin, L. N. (1966): Manual of Cytology. Moscow: Nauka. (In Russian.)

Zhubrikova, L. A., Gordienko, E. A. (1980): Ontogenetic specifics of the metabolism of mediatory substances in the brain structures. In: Problems of Ontogenesis, Heterosis and Ecology of Animals, pp. 18–22. Kharkov: State University. (In Russian.)

Zierler, V. L. (1960): Effect of insulin on potassium efflux from rat muscle in the presence and absence of glucose. Amer. J. Physiol. *198*, 1066–1070.

Zotin, A. I. (1974): Thermodynamic Approach to the Problems of Development, Growth and Aging. Moscow: Nauka. (In Russian.)

Zotin, A. I., Zotina, R. S., Prokofyev, Ye. A., Konoplev, V. A. (1978): Use of growth equations for determining the maximum lifespan of mammals and man. Izv. Akad. Nauk SSSR (biological series) *1*, 87–96.

Zs.-Nagy, I. (1979): The role of membrane structure and function in cellular aging. Mech. Ageing Develop. *9*, 237–246.

Zs.-Nagy, I., Zs.-Nagy, V. (1975): Age dependence of heat-induced strand separation of DNA in situ in postmitotic cells of rat brain as revealed by acridine oragne microfluorometry. Mech. Ageing Develop. *4*, 349–360.

Zuckerman, B. M., Barrett, K. A. (1978): Effect of dimethylaminoethanol (DMAE) and para-chlorophenoxyacetic acid (PCA) on the nematode *Caenorhabditis briggsae*. In: Proceedings of 11th International Congress of Gerontology, Abstracts, p. 16. Tokyo: Scimed Publications, Inc.

Zuckermann, K. (1933): Functional Affinities of Man, Monkeys and Apes. London: Pergamon Press.

Subject Index

Actinomycin D 7, 121, 135, 270, 335
Adenosine 196
Adenylate cyclase 58, 77, 122, 132, 270
ADP 47, 196
Age
– biological 15
– chronological 15, 19
Aging, clonal 253
AMP 58, 77, 122, 195
Antioxidants 326
Arterial pressure, age changes in 280
Atherosclerosis 32
ATP 47, 48, 194
Axovasal synapses 108

Barbiturates 66
Baroreceptors 299
Biosynthesis 3
Bradykinin 198
Brain 33
– aging of 33
– functional changes in 52
– metabolic changes in 36
– structural changes in 36

Calorie effect 243
Cardiac output 282
Cardiovascular system
– age changes in 280
– cholinergic effects on 297
– neurohumoral regulation of 280
– reflexes of 298
Carotid sinus, chemoreceptors of 299
Centre, hemodynamic 286
Cephalization 34
Chromatids 208
Chromatin 11
Collagen 262
Coronary vessels 303

Corticotropin-releasing factor 80
Cycloheximide 271, 272

Energy processes, neurohumoral regulation of 230
Enzymes, genetic induction of 214
Estrogens 66, 87, 94

Feedback
– hormonal 88
– hypothalamic 91
– negative 88, 91
– positive 91
Fibroblasts 253
Follicle-stimulating hormone (FSH) 79, 88, 94

Genes
– pleiotropic 7
– suicide 213
Gland
– endocrine 157
– thyroid 157
Gliacytes 38
Glucagon 144, 150
Glucocorticoids 99
Glycogen 237, 244, 246
Glycogenolysis 154
Glycolysis 6, 27, 48, 119
GMP 58, 132, 195
Gonadotropin-releasing factor 79, 80
Growth hormone (GH) 79
Guanylate cyclase 132

Hepatectomy 254, 260, 271
Heteroplasmones 209
Heterosis 338
Histones 210
Homeorhesis 2, 91

Homeostasis 2, 4, 14, 70, 71, 87, 91, 96
Hormones
- steroid 218
- thyroid 157, 245
Hydrocortisone 334
Hyperglycemia 100, 144
Hyperpolarization 56, 271
Hypertension, arterial 282
Hyperthyroidism 173, 245
Hypophysectomy 333
Hypothalamic misinformation 72
Hypothalamus, regulatory effects of 70
Hypothesis
- genoregulatory 22, 49, 205
- wear-and-tear 329
Hypothyroidism 177, 245, 298
Hypoxia, tissue 282

Influences, hypothalamohypophysial 79
Inosine 196
Insulinemia 83, 142, 148, 149, 153
Iodothyronines 158
Iodotyrosines 158
Ionol 59
IRI 142
Isoprenaline 101

Kallikrein 198
Kallikreinogens 198
Karyotype, abnormal 94
Kinin 198
Kininogens 198

Life span
- criteria of 307
- growth of 314
- influence on 314
Lipofuscin 39, 72, 73
Lipogenesis 156
Luteinizing hormone (LH) 79, 88, 94

MAO 118
Mechanoreceptors, vascular 302
Membrane
- cell 40
- lysosomal 326
- nictitating 102, 175
Memory
- long-term 50
- short-term 50
Metabolic changes 36
Metabolism, acetylcholine 124

Neuroglia 10, 262
Neurons 36
- bulbar 287
- loss of 36
- membrane potential of 54
- types of 39
Noradrenaline 290
Nucleosomes 209
Nucleotides
- adenine 196
- cyclic 194, 270

Olivomycin 24, 335
Ontogenology 343
Orbeli-Ginetsinsky phenomenon 188
Osteoporosis 17, 106, 191
Ouabain 55, 277
Oxidation, microsomal 10
Oxygen consumption 45, 47, 230, 282
Oxytocin 334

Phosphorylation
- glycolytic 230
- oxidative 230
Potentials, inhibiting postsynaptic 55
Pressure, arterial calculation of 284
Proinsulin 143, 154
Prostaglandins 202
Proteins
- errors in 211
- genetic induction of 270
- non-histone 210
- receptor 270
- thyroxine-binding 171

Radiation, ionizing 322
Reflexes
- conditioned 54, 61
- spinal cord 68
Reserpine 117
Rule, age synchronization 20

Serotonin 76, 94, 201
Somatotropic hormone 144
Somatotropin-releasing factor 80
Stroke volume 282
Syndrome, normal aging 20

Tachyphylaxia 86
Tetrodotoxin 276

Theory, adaptive regulatory 4, 26, 36,
    40, 307
Thyroid regulation 157
Thyroidectomy 173, 246, 248
Thyrotoxicosis 247
Thyrotropin-releasing factor 80, 167
Thyrotropin-stimulating hormone (TSH)
    80
Tissue, osseus 191

Trophism, tissue 179
Trophogens 185
Tryptophan 201

Vagus nerve, influence of 295
Vasodilation 196
Vasopressin 83
Vitauct 1